CELEBRATING 50 YEARS OF BRAIN RESEARCH

50th

ANNIVERSARY

NINDS AT 50

An Incomplete History Celebrating the
Fiftieth Anniversary of the
National Institute of
Neurological Disorders and Stroke

LEWIS P. ROWLAND, M.D.

Name Changes for the Neurology Institute

1951	NINDB	National Institute of Neurological Diseases and Blindness
1968	NINDB	National Institute of Neurological Diseases and Stroke
1975	NINCDS	National Institute of Neurological and Communicative Disorders and Stroke
1988	NINDS	National Institute of Neurological Disorders and Stroke

CONTENTS

SECTION 5

APPENDICES

PREFACE

The origins of this book can be dated precisely. One fine day in April 1999, I visited the office of Gerald D. Fischbach, who was then the Director of NINDS. I was there as a representative of the Parkinson's Disease Foundation. Our goal was an action that has made some NIH institute directors uncomfortable; we were promoting "targeted research." More specifically, we were advocating increased NINDS funding for research on Parkinson disease.

This book arose from the introductory small talk that day. Dr. Fischbach asked what I had been doing in the year since the end of my term as Chair of Neurology at Columbia University. I replied that I had planned to write a history of the Neurological Institute of New York and its role in the rise of scientific neurology in the years since I started training in neurology in 1950.

His response was immediate. "Why don't you write a history of NINDS? We are about to celebrate its fiftieth anniversary."

It was as simple as that. Well, the agreement was as simple as that, but the details of an arrangement took some time to work out. I was granted permission to take sabbatical leave from Columbia and arrived to work fulltime in Bethesda on March 1, 2000. The original plan for the book was continuously modified. We had several discussions about my capacity – or that of any other single person, historian or neurological professional – to write such a book. On several occasions I suggested that a multi-authored book would better serve the record of scientific advances. Dr. Fischbach, however, wanted the perspective of a single senior person in the field.

So, what are my credentials?

In 1950, I started training at the Neurological Institute of New York with H. Houston Merritt. My professional life therefore coincides with the life of NINDS.

In 1953, I was in the first group of Clinical Associates at NINDB. We were appointed even before Milton Shy had been selected as Intramural Clinical Director. We were rushed to NIH for the scheduled opening of the Clinical Center on March 1, 1953. In fact, the hospital did not open until September 1, so I had to look around for something to do. By blind good fortune, I had the opportunity to work with Seymour Kety, Louis Sokoloff, William Landau, and Water Freygang. That experience had a profound impact on my views about neuroscience, and it generated lasting friendships. Afterwards, I worked with Milton Shy, who allowed me to do my own patient-oriented research.

I left NIH in 1954 and then had an academic career at Columbia that brought even more gratification. In the process I spent four years in the laboratory of David Shemin, a leading biochemist in the days when the biosynthesis of complex molecules was being worked out.

Shemin was largely responsible for delineating the formation of porphyrins and heme. With that background, I was able to set up my own laboratory and work on the biochemical genetics of human neurological diseases. In 1961, I became the co-principal investigator, with Robert A. Fishman, of one of the first NINDB Clinical Center grants (now called program projects). I maintained that grant in one incarnation or another for almost 40 years, thanks to my later partner, Salvatore Demure. I hold no claims to major scientific contributions, but my experience kept me informed of the impending molecular changes in clinical neurology.

In 1967, I became Chair of Neurology at the University of Pennsylvania, followed by my stint at Columbia from 1973 to 1998. Those positions gave me another view of the activities of NINDS and how important the Institute is to academic departments throughout the country. My contacts with NIH were reinforced by interactions with NINDS staff when I was an officer of the Association of University Professors of Neurology (comprising the heads of neurology training programs), the American Neurological Association, and the American Academy of Neurology. I came to know personally every director of NINDS now alive except for Edward MacNichol.

I saw the world of NIH from another side, too. I served on the Training Grant Committee of NINCDS, on site visit teams, on the Board of Scientific Counselors (which provides peer review for the intramural programs), and also on the National Advisory Council – just when the Decade of the Brain was being formulated.

One more possible attribute is that I like to write. I have been on the editorial boards of several journals and was editor-in-chief of *Neurology*, the official journal of the American Academy of Neurology.

Putting that record together, it might seem that, if any single author could write the book, it would be someone like me. However, I cite my credentials less as boasting than as apology. As I started to collect information, carry out interviews, and write the book, I soon became aware that I had never done anything like this before, that the task was enormous, and that I might not be up to it. To some degree, I shifted from institutional history to personal histories and focused more on the people involved than the organizational structure. I started to write mini-biographies. In doing so, I had to learn details of basic neuroscience that had gone by me.

I became so preoccupied with the biographies that my son, Andrew, told me I should have written the entire history of modern neuroscience in the form of Paul de Kruif's *Microbe Hunters*, a book that had enthralled me in adolescence and had also affected many of the investigators described here. By that time, however, we were nearing the absolute deadline for completion of the book. A more comprehensive history-as-biography seems a good idea for neuroscience, but I leave that to another generation.

The biographies of the prizewinners need some explanation. I did not think I could cover all of the neuroscientists who had won Nobel Prizes since 1950, so I started with investigators only from the NINDS intramural program. When I wrote about Carleton Gajdusek, an intramural researcher who won the Nobel Prize in 1976, I realized I also had to write about Stanley Prusiner, an extramural grantee (who won the Lasker Award in 1994 and the Nobel in 1997), because both worked on Creutzfeldt-Jakob disease. Dr. Prusiner's chapter was the first about an extramural investigator, and it was written just as the 2000 winners were announced: Drs. Carlsson, Kandel, and Greengard – they had to be included. The resulting mix of prizewinners seems to be a somewhat inconsistent group, and I must apologize to the several extramural Nobelists who have not been included because there was insufficient time.

As for the text itself, I know that some readers will pick up errors, and I know that I have omitted mentioning many people who deserve applause, both investigators and administrators. I have become especially impressed by the Program Directors in the NINDS extramural program. My office at NINDS was close to theirs; I ate lunch with them, and went to their weekly staff meetings. Part of their job is to arrange workshops to initiate research programs throughout the country, as well as guide university investigators through the process of preparing grant applications. With involved clinical investigators and statisticians, they initiate and carry out therapeutic trials. In every way, the success of university research depends on the knowledge, skills, and devotion of these scientist-administrators.

Early in the year, a friend asked me: "Who is going to read this book?" I was haunted by that question for months, as the answers gradually emerged. First, there will be people who will immediately look in the index to find out if their names are listed.

I hope that general readers will find the biographies illuminating and informative. I hope that others will find out how NINDS works and what it has achieved. In all of this I have tried to write in a way that is comprehensible to non-scientists but not offensive to scientists.

So, here it is, a book for the record, not a novel and perhaps not even a true history.

A caveat is in order. This book is a celebration. I have deliberately omitted rumors of fights and debates between investigators. I have tread lightly on conflicts between institutional chiefs and NIH leaders or between institute leaders themselves. Celebration it is. NINDS has been one of the most powerful motors that pulled and pushed the rise of modern neuroscience. In the pages that follow I applaud the administrators and the scientists involved.

This could be called the Andy Warhol approach. In his autobiography the artist wrote: "When I did my self-portrait, I left all the pimples out because you always should. Pimples are a temporary condition and they don't have anything to do with what you really look like. Always omit the blemishes – they're not part of the picture you want."

A long list of acknowledgements appears near the end of this book, but a few people merit special recognition. The first is Gerald D. Fischbach, who started the project. Then come Audrey S. Penn, now NINDS Acting Director, and Kevin Kirby, NINDS Acting Deputy Director, who kept the project going through times of stress. My Columbia Chairman, Timothy A. Pedley, and Columbia Vice-President Morton Grusky arranged the sabbatical leave.

Four others were closely associated with the project: Robin Latham, a science writer/editor in the NINDS Office of Communications and Public Liaison, used her talents as a perceptive reader and writer to shape and focus the book, and her skills as a project manager to keep it on track. Nancy Berlage, Ph.D., an historian with History Associates, Incorporated, acted as a fact-detective and constructive reader. Among other contributions, she compiled the information to track NINDS officials through the years, which proved to be a formidable task. Brenda Van Hook, remarkable secretary and Internet whiz, served for a year from the start of the project in March 2000; she transcribed most of the interviews and came up with numerous valuable documents, including one that led to the oral histories of Mary Lasker. Larissa Markarian picked up when Ms. Van Hook left and completed more work in a few weeks than most could do in months. Pamela Jones, chief of publications in the NINDS Office of Communications and Public Liaison, took on the responsibility of deftly moving the book through the publication process, coping with missed deadlines and last-minute additions with grace and good cheer. Marian Emr, director of the NINDS Office of Communications and Public Liaison, ably guided and supported the entire effort.

To all of these NIH workers, I owe not only thanks but also apologies for my inability to finish the text until the very last moment. I surely did not make it easy for them.

Victoria Harden, Historian of the National Institutes of Health, gave encouragement, counsel, support, and pertinent documents; her own writing on the history of NIH served as a model. The staff of the NIH history office provided assistance in locating background information. Mary Marshall Clark is Director of the Oral History Project of Columbia University, where we found the transcripts of recorded interviews with several of the people who profoundly affected the history of NINDS. She was also a most helpful advisor.

I thank all 48 people[1] who consented to be interviewed. Several of them became involved again by reading and editing the sections in which they were mentioned. All of them should have had that opportunity, but the deadline precluded completion of the total task.

Guy McKhann came from Johns Hopkins University on a special assignment from the Director; our earlier friendship became stronger and I was grateful for his advice on important matters.

Many staff members at NINDS, and indeed many of the other institutes, served as sources of information. In particular, Andy Baldus, chief of the NINDS Financial Management Branch, provided historical information about the NINDS budget. Constance Atwell, director of the Division of Extramural Research, patiently made sure the details of the extramural program were accurate.

The list of acknowledgements serves to recognize the many who helped in multiple ways: librarians and archivists at remote university and presidential libraries, staff members of foundations and voluntary health agencies, and professional friends. Although we cannot list everyone, others, too, surely deserve appreciation for their contributions.

With special pleasure, I thank members of my family, starting with my partner of 49 years, Esther E. Rowland. She served as psychotherapist and – as an expert professional proofreader – she was the first serious reader and critic of the emerging manuscript. My son, Steven S. Rowland, is a producer of public radio programs; he provided recording equipment and instructed me in the art of the interview. Others in the family were dragooned, including Amy Edelman, a senior editor at Random House; Eileen Rowland, former Chief Librarian at the John Jay College of the City University of New York; my brother Ted, also a writer and critic; my son, Andrew S. Rowland, Ph.D., an epidemiologist at the University of New Mexico; and my daughter, Joy Rosenthal McIntyre, who is a talented writer and clear-eyed reader as well as a public interest lawyer.

A final comment. This preface has been egotistically sprinkled with the word "I." That single-letter word should not appear anywhere in the text from now on.

Lewis P. Rowland, M.D.
New York, New York
August 2001

1 Constance Atwell, Julius Axelrod, Katherine Bick, Roscoe O. Brady, Thomas N. Chase, Maynard Cohen, Francis Collins, Sam Drage, Marian Emr, Stanley Fahn, Gerald D. Fischbach, Kenneth Fischbeck, Joseph Gibbs, Murray Goldstein, Paul Greengard, Zach W. Hall, Mark Hallett, Victoria Harden, Richard Hodes, Steven Hyman, Eric R. Kandel, Seymour S. Kety, Ruth Kirschstein, Irwin Kopin, Leonard Kurland, William M. Landau, Story C. Landis, Carl Leventhal, John Marler, Joseph H. Martin, Richard L. Masland, Henry F. McFarland, Ronald D.G. McKay, Mary Miers, Karin Nelson, Paul Nichols, Edward Oldfield, Eugene Oliver, Audrey S. Penn, Stanley B. Prusiner, Thomas S. Reese, Louis Sokoloff, Mathilde Solowey, Eugene Streicher, Donald B. Tower, Craig Venter, Michael Walker, and Nancy Wexler.

NTRODUCTION

Writing the history of an institution whose influence has been as deep and wide as the NINDS was not an easy assignment. The author of this history of the NINDS not only had to research and write about five decades of institutional change and progress, but also had to encompass within that story the incredible advances that have occurred in neuroscience and neurology over the past 50 years.

Lewis P. "Bud" Rowland, M.D., was willing to tackle the task and his worthy accomplishment follows in the pages of this text. As an esteemed neurologist and teacher whose specialty is neuromuscular diseases, Dr. Rowland's career has spanned both clinical and academic neurology. It has given him an advantageous place from which to view the course of neuroscience over a lifetime devoted to unraveling the mysteries and mechanisms of neurological disorders.

When Dr. Rowland came to the institute as a clinical associate in the early 1950s, he was one of the first in a distinguished group of post-war M.D.-investigators to find their passion and direction in the freewheeling atmosphere of Seymour Kety's intramural laboratory – a place that accommodated researchers from both the NINDS and the NIMH. This is how neuroscience began at NIH, in tandem with the behavioral sciences, as a fluid exchange between the physiological and psychological study of the brain. When the laboratory split in 1960, the two Institutes diverged and established their own interests and "turf." Over time, the National Eye Institute and the National Institute on Deafness and Other Communication Disorders also split off from the NINDS. Now, as the new National Neuroscience Research Center goes from dream to reality on the NIH campus, all of the neurosciences will once again be united in the same building.

The story of the NINDS is also the tale of how post-war political forces were employed and directed by charismatic individuals such as Mary Lasker, Florence Mahoney, and Senator Claude Pepper, who believed not just in the advancement of neuroscience, but in the ways in which these advances could be used to improve public health. During the time they worked together with politicians and policymakers to create the NINDS, little was known about neurodegenerative diseases and there was little, if any, productive research on Parkinson disease, Huntington disease, stroke, spinal cord injury, or traumatic brain injury – just to name a few areas in which the Institute has spurred research during the past five decades.

Even more telling, at the time of NINDS's first steps, the locus of neurological research was in Cambridge, England, in the labs of Hodgkin and Huxley. Only a decade or so later, due to the steady, thoughtful stimulation of the science by NINDS both on and off the campus, the locus had changed. The most interesting and advanced work was now being done in the United States. Future Nobel and Lasker award-winners bore witness to the ascendancy of American and American-trained neuroscientists.

Within this book you will find the stories of some of the extraordinary individuals, who – either as intramural researchers, administrative directors, or extramural grantees – encouraged exploration or made discoveries themselves that permanently changed how we understand the workings of the brain. You will also find evidence for the continuous emphasis of moving basic science to clinical application – from "bench to bedside."

No single history could possibly include the totality of the influence the NINDS has had on neuroscience and neurology in the past five decades. This book is one person's view of the central role the Institute has played in the lives of particular neuroscientists whose discoveries have been shaped in important ways by their relationship to NINDS. The author of the book calls it an "incomplete history," partly because of its use of individuals to illuminate broader concepts and trends in neuroscience, but also because the history of neuroscience is still far from complete.

Clinical and basic neuroscience is evolving in new and exciting ways. The NINDS will continue to nourish and skillfully direct the growth of the field in the coming decades. This volume celebrates 50 years of advances. There are many more years – and countless new discoveries – yet to come.

Audrey S. Penn, M.D.
Acting Director
National Institute of Neurological
Disorders and Stroke
Bethesda, Maryland
August 2001

SECTION 1

IRTH OF AN INSTITUTE

The National Institute of Neurological Diseases and Blindness (NINDB) and the National Institute of Mental Health (NIMH) were not quite twins, but they were born only a year apart and they were tethered by a conjoint intramural research program. How and why they were created is a story that involves several different plot lines – all of them coming together at the right time. The time was just after World War II, in the five years between 1945 and 1950.

The story revolves around several trends that drove the need for biomedical research just after the war: a new recognition of the burden of illness; an increasingly favorable national opinion about the role of the federal government in scientific research and everything else that governments do (as opposed to private industry or philanthropy); competition between federal agencies for control of biomedical research; and, not least, the impact of remarkable individuals, both within and outside the federal government, who pushed for a federal agenda.

But even after the National Institutes of Health had been established, the outcome of proposals to establish a neurological institute within the NIH was uncertain until the last moment because it could not be taken for granted that the President would sign the final bill and make it a law.

The Growth of NIH After World War II

The modern National Institutes of Health arose from inauspicious beginnings soon after the American Revolution. In 1798, the fledgling government created a Marine Hospital Service (MHS) to provide medical care for merchant seamen.[1] By the 1880s, the MHS was charged by Congress to examine immigrants on arriving ships for signs of infectious diseases. This was the time when Robert Koch in Germany and Louis Pasteur in France became famous for proving

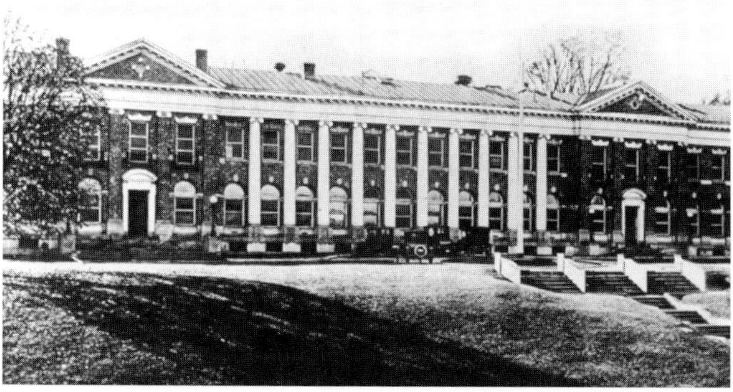

U.S. Hygienic Laboratory, U.S. Public Health Service

that infectious diseases could be caused by bacteria. In 1887, MHS officials authorized Joseph J. Kinyoun, a physician and bacteriologist, to set up a laboratory in the Marine Hospital on Staten Island in New York City. Within a few months he had identified the organism that causes cholera, one of the most deadly and feared diseases of the late nineteenth century. That was medical research of the day – bacteriology and preventive medicine.

In 1891, the laboratory was moved to Washington, D.C., and, for a decade, Kinyoun was the sole fulltime staff member. Rather than research, Kinyoun focused primarily on teaching and applying health science to practical purposes; for example, he taught bacteriology to MHS officers and tested water purity. That changed, however, when the laboratory became the Hygienic Laboratory and acquired research functions.

Two acts, both passed in 1902, set the stage. First, the MHS was reorganized as the Public Health and Marine Hospital Service (PH-MHS), a step toward the modern Public Health Service. The same act launched a formal research program for the Hygienic Laboratory, setting up one division for pathology and bacteriology, one for chemistry, another for pharmacology, and one for zoology.

The second influential act in 1902 charged the Hygienic Laboratory with regulating the production of vaccines and antitoxins, tasks that, according to NIH historian Victoria Harden, "protected the Hygienic Laboratory from political assault because of its value for the U.S. citizenry." In 1912 another reorganization changed the name of the PH-MHS to the Public Health Service and formalized research functions pertaining to non-contagious diseases and water pollution. These changes paid off: during World War I, the PHS traced the origin of an outbreak of anthrax to contaminated shaving brushes, another research achievement of bacteriology and epidemiologic detective work.

After the war, chemists hoped that a philanthropic patron would support their basic research, but none materialized. Proponents within the scientific community turned, for the first time, to the federal government for research support. One chemist thought that research in chemistry would benefit medicine and he persuaded Senator Joseph E. Ransdell of Louisiana to take up the issue. Ransdell worked with officials of the PHS and, with an eye to research, prepared a bill that would change the name of the Laboratory to the National Institute of Health (singular).

At the time, officials of the PHS were of two minds about the proposed name change. They were reluctant to change anything and they also thought the Hygienic Laboratory already had a legislative mandate to carry out research. However, if there was to be a new agency, they wanted it to be located within the PHS where they could retain control over research agendas.

Ransdell collaborated with PHS officials to make the proposals a reality. In 1930, after four years of Congressional hearings and lobbying, the Ransdell bill became law; it extended the scope of research by the Hygienic Laboratory of the PHS from infectious disease to include chronic diseases as well.[2-4] This achievement led Harden to consider Ransdell "the unsung but true father of the modern NIH."[1]

The Great Depression of the 1930s blocked any expansion of medical research, but a new medical institute was nevertheless in the offing. In 1937, the National Cancer Institute (NCI) was created as the first of the individual institutes that make up the modern National Institutes (plural) of Health. Every member of the Senate sponsored the legislation, a show of almost unbelievable unanimity.

NCI became the model for all the other categorical institutes that would be created in subsequent years. There was ample room for expansion because the Luke I. Wilson family (of the local Woodward & Lothrop department stores) had donated – as a gift to the federal government – the land that became the Bethesda campus. President Franklin D. Roosevelt formally dedicated the new campus in 1940.[5]

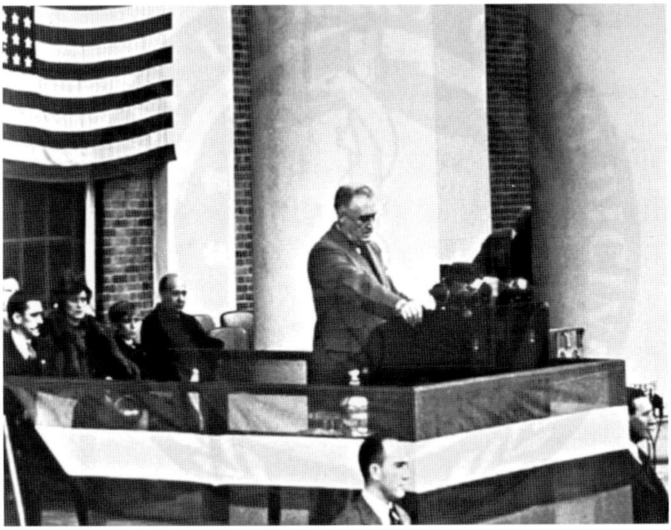

President Franklin D. Roosevelt formally dedicates the NIH campus, October 31, 1940

World War II, however, put further development on hold. The exigencies of the war diverted to other needs money that might have supported biomedical research. Congressional appropriations for the NIH were paltry – just enough to maintain an administration and a smattering of wartime research.

When victory and peace seemed to be in the offing in 1944, the NIH Director, Rolla E. Dyer, and Surgeon General Thomas Parran guided legislation through Congress so that NIH was permitted to award grants and conduct clinical research, the two powers that have been the basis for the continuing expansion of NIH ever since. The stage was set for a new era of biomedical research.

The Burden of Neurologic Illness

The American people had been surprised by the high proportion of young men rejected by the World War II military draft for medical or educational reasons. Fifteen million men had been examined by December 1944. A third of them had been rejected – 4.8 million – including 1.7 million who had neuropsychiatric or learning disorders. Almost one in nine of all American men had a neuropsychiatric disability.[6,7]

Then, during the war, military personnel incurred numerous traumatic injuries to the brain and nerves. Infections of the nervous system followed the injuries, as did epileptic seizures. Psychiatric casualties were widespread. These neurological and psychiatric conditions persisted when the veterans returned to civilian life and the Veterans Administration had to increase neurologic services to care for them. The new medical specialty of rehabilitation medicine developed to deal with the disabling war injuries.

According to one estimate,[8] neurologically disabled veterans in the postwar years accounted for about 25 percent of the patients in general hospitals and 10 percent of those in psychiatric hospitals. Wartime experiences also affected ideas about patient care: during the war, American soldiers had come to appreciate good medical care, and postwar expectations were high that it would continue.

Later calculations set the need for neurologists in peacetime, estimating that one percent of the population would have a disorder appropriate for a physician with training in neurology.[9,10] Yet there were almost no neurologists in the United States. In 1950, only 250 physicians claimed to be neurologists,[11] and only 30 three-year neurology training programs were available; seven were in federal institutions. Combined, these programs provided training for only 139 neurologists annually.[4] Without an adequate number of training programs, neurologists had good reason to fear for the future of their specialty.

In 1950, there was a serious mismatch between the number of patients with neurological disorders (estimated to be 15-25 percent of all hospital admissions) and the number of neurologists. Several states, including Connecticut, as well as such cities as Detroit, had no neurologists at all. James Shannon[13] later acknowledged the shortage when he became Director of NIH.

In striking contrast to the paucity of clinical activity in neurology, there had been a rich tradition of Nobel Prizes for basic research on the biology of the nervous system in the first 50 years of the twentieth century. Among the luminaries were Camillo Golgi and Santiago Ramón y Cajal (1906), E. D. Adrian and Sir Charles S. Sherrington (1932), Sir Henry Dale and Otto Loewi (1936), Joseph Erlanger and Herbert S. Gasser (1944), and Walter R. Hess and Egas Moniz (1949).

Nevertheless, in 1950, the word "neuroscience" was not used. In medical schools, neurophysiologists, neuroanatomists, and neuropathologists were scattered within different departments. Financial support was limited to that provided by universities and foundations. Neuroradiology had barely emerged. Clinical research was mostly restricted to description, electroencephalography, and neuropathology.

Toward Legislation: A National Mood

In the decades between 1925 and 1945, there was a profound shift in the American ethos – from a belief that government should be as small as possible to the view that government should be the agent for improving the lives of all citizens. That belief was embodied in the New Deal policies that Roosevelt implemented during the 1930s.

However, it took the legacies of World War II for political leaders to conceive a new role for the federal government in medical research. During the war, centralized research had been successful in developing the atom bomb, antibiotics, and drugs for malaria. During World War II, the Medical Research Committee of the Office of Scientific Research and Development (OSRD), set up in 1941, directed these efforts.[14,15]

After the war, OSRD was shut down, and the new National Science Foundation was intended by scientific leaders to encompass all scientific research. However, officials of the PHS pressed to keep any new medical research programs within their purview. Although there had been a Division of Mental Hygiene in the PHS since 1930, it had been devoted to psychiatric service, not research.

Thoughtful scientists who had different answers to the central question led the contending factions. Should biomedical research be assigned, with all other scientific research, to the NSF? Or should there be a new biomedical research agency within the PHS? President Truman wanted medical research to be not only part of a unified scientific research program but also part of a national health program. The two needed coordination.

In any case, the national state of mind in 1945 was far different from the current wariness about the role of Washington in the administration of large public programs. Confidence in federal action and involvement was bolstered by a concurrent belief in the power of science and the promise of new drugs – a belief that arose with the wartime discovery and development of antibiotics.

Setting a Legislative Pattern: Mary Lasker, Claude Pepper, and the Heart Institute

On the NIH campus, Building 31 now houses the Directors' offices for NCI, NIMH, NINDS, NEI, and other institutes. In 1988, it was designated the "Claude Denson Pepper Building." A plaque at the entrance notes that he had served in Congress for 41 years and had "sponsored the legislation that established the majority of the NIH Institutes."

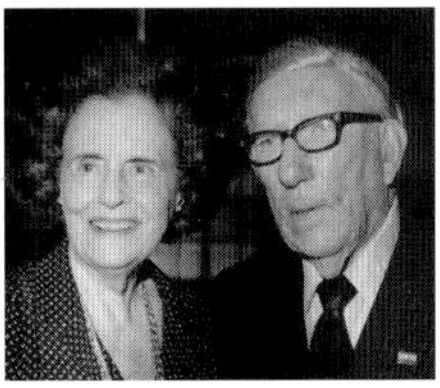

MARY LASKER AND SENATOR CLAUDE PEPPER, 1980

Pepper was born in 1900 and grew up on a farm in rural Alabama. He graduated from the University of Alabama and then from Harvard Law School. Elected to the U.S. Senate from Florida in 1936, he was a staunch supporter of President Franklin D. Roosevelt and the New Deal. Pepper had the typical New Dealer's ethos – using federal agencies to improve social conditions. He was especially dedicated to health issues. Among Pepper's first legislative forays was a bill to establish the NCI in 1937. As he gained influence in Washington, he assumed positions in which he could affect federal health policy. During World War II, for example, he chaired the Senate Select Subcommittee on Wartime Health and Education and vigorously endorsed the view that medical research could improve the health of the nation's citizens. By the time NINDB was established in 1950, Pepper had sponsored bills that created five of the first six disease-oriented institutes.

In 1950, Pepper lost his Senate seat in a bitter campaign. Pepper's national legislative career, however, was far from over. In 1962, Florida voters elected him to the House where he would remain in office until he died in 1989. As a Representative, Pepper continued his efforts to improve health care, and he championed causes of the elderly. As Chairman of the House Select Committee on Aging, he was responsible for the law that abolished mandatory retirement. In addition, he sponsored innovative legislation to establish research centers for Alzheimer disease. For his achievements, Pepper gained an Albert and Mary Lasker Foundation award in 1967.

Pepper's partner in pushing for NIH legislation was Mary W. Lasker, a wealthy New Yorker who had been an entrepreneur before she became the wife of millionaire Albert Lasker, her second husband. Albert had made his fortune as an advertising executive and encouraged his wife's efforts in public affairs. Together, the couple established The Albert and Mary Lasker Foundation, which has given influential awards for contributions to medical research.

The daughter of a banker, Mary grew up in Wisconsin, graduated from Radcliffe, and studied at Oxford. Besides her intellectual pursuits, Mary had diverse interests, such as collecting art. She was active in the Democratic Party and ardently supported urban beautification. City planner Robert Moses[16] described her personal qualities: "Intelligence, vision, generosity, charm, kindness – Mary has them all." He could have added initiative, perseverance, doggedness, gregariousness, leadership, and more.

The papers of Mary Lasker at Columbia University document her unusual ability to influence major figures in Washington. She had direct access to Presidents, congressional leaders, and NIH officials. If she wrote a note to one, there was a prompt response. Moreover, she was not shy about stating her concerns or about claiming credit for the beneficial results of her efforts. During an oral history interview in 1966,[17] she asserted:

> I had been the first one to urge the establishment of the National Heart Institute and to urge the establishment of the Neurology and Blindness Institute.

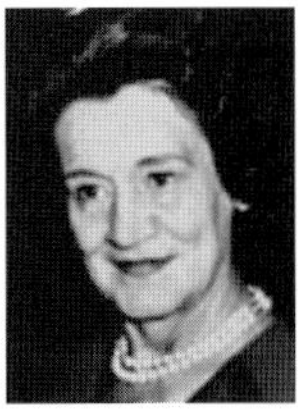

FLORENCE MAHONEY

Mrs. Lasker had a strong ally in Florence Mahoney, another remarkable woman of wealth and personal influence. Mahoney's husband's father-in-law by a previous marriage was James Cox, a newspaper publisher who had been the Democratic candidate for President in 1920; his Vice-Presidential candidate in that unsuccessful campaign had been Franklin D. Roosevelt. Mrs. Mahoney lived in Florida, where her husband Daniel Mahoney was the publisher of the *Miami Daily News* and had an interest in the Cox chain of papers. Like Mary, Florence was active in politics. They backed Pepper's campaign for re-election to the Senate in 1944, and they supported his failed attempt to have Congress pass legislation for national health insurance.

How effectively Mrs. Lasker and Senator Pepper worked together was illustrated by their successful postwar campaign to increase funding for the Cancer Institute. In his memoirs, Pepper described how their collaboration ensured adequate funding for the NCI:

> For many years, only the $500,000 appropriation was available for cancer research. It was totally inadequate. One of the first to sense this was Mary Lasker, a genuine "angel" who has done so much to obtain federal aid for disease research. She urged me to seek $100 million for cancer research, to remain available until it was spent. She asked Representative Matthew Neeley of West Virginia to lead the fight in the House. For months, I held hearings, with Mrs. Lasker producing the nation's leading cancer authorities to serve as witnesses. Finally, Senator Robert A. Taft . . . introduced a bill calling for a $75 million cancer research fund . . . . We joined forces and boosted the annual appropriation for the National Cancer Institute from $500,000 to more than $8 million.[18]

They repeated that pattern with legislation for the Heart Institute; the law included wording that made plural the National Institutes of Health. In that effort, they went two steps further, not merely holding hearings.

First, they obtained the wording of the 1937 NCI law and changed it; wherever "cancer" appeared, they changed it to "heart." The bill contained the same elements as the original law for the Cancer Institute: research, training, construction of research facilities, and efforts for disease control.

Second, Mrs. Lasker collected data to provide a factual background of the need for more research. Then Pepper introduced the legislation and worked with a parallel committee in the House to hold hearings. Once again, Mrs. Lasker selected the research experts who were eloquent and effective witnesses, armed with the facts.

Mary Lasker explained how they devised a bill to establish the Heart Institute:[19]

> In the fall of 1946 I was very much concerned about the fact that there were no funds whatever earmarked in the NIH of the USPHS for diseases of the heart and circulation, the number-one cause of death of people in the United States.
>
> I was tremendously influenced by the illness and death of my father due to a stroke and the illness and death of my mother due to a stroke, which was due to arteriosclerosis, and this certainly influenced me. And when I found that there was no effort whatsoever being made by the federal government in this major cause of death – almost 50 percent of the people were dying of this, and it was just considered the will of God, which God knows it was not and is not – I was furious, as usual.
>
> I considered various means of how to attract attention to this deficit. . .. Between '46 and '47, I spent some time with my husband in Florida and then I went to Washington and spoke to Senator Pepper about the need for a heart research bill similar to the cancer research bill which had been passed in 1936 but which, as I explained, didn't have any money at all, not more than 500,000 dollars until fiscal '46.
>
> Pepper said he would be glad to introduce a bill for heart research and asked me what I had in mind . . . . I stopped in Cincinnati on the way to California . . . . I remember it was the 8th of February 1947. I mailed a draft of the bill very similar to the cancer research bill, providing for a hundred million dollars to be set aside in a fund, to be available until spent; for a group of experts drawn from all over the world to be brought together in one place or a number of places; and provided with funds to make extensive research in the field of heart disease and circulation.

Mrs. Lasker was not daunted by requests for what seemed to be large sums. She explained:

> I was encouraged to think in large sums because of my husband, because of his experience in government, since he was the head of the Shipping Board in the early 20s, which was then the agency that had the largest amount of assets . . . . Also, in his business, he wouldn't speak to anyone who wanted to spend less than a million dollars to advertise his product and he felt 15 million dollars to advertise tobacco in a year wasn't too much at that time. He would be horrified if he knew that smoking had something to do with lung cancer or any other kind of cancer, which was really only made certain only since his death. It was really his scale on which he thought and operated that influenced me. I thought that if a toothpaste, which he owned or had an interest in, deserved advertising at the rate of two or three or four million dollars a year then research against disease maiming and crippling people in the United States and in the rest of the world deserved hundreds of millions of dollars. It seemed perfectly simple and natural to me.[20]

Once the Heart Institute was achieved in 1948, the pattern was set; it worked for the National Institute of Mental Health (NIMH) in 1949 and for the National Institute of Neurological Diseases and Blindness (NINDB) in 1950. Mrs. Lasker also lobbied on behalf of the Arthritis Institute in 1950. Her diverse research interests arose from her personal experiences – one of her house workers had had cancer and, later, Albert Lasker would die of prostate cancer; both her parents had strokes, leading to her interest in diseases of the heart, circulation, and brain; and an acquaintance with a blind relative described the effects of blindness to Mrs. Lasker during the NINDB hearings, leading to her concern with vision – and the "B" in NINDB.

Prelude to NINDB: A National Institute of Mental Health

The Division of Mental Hygiene of the PHS, established in 1930, was largely concerned with drug addiction.[21,22] After the creation of NCI in 1937, Lawrence Kolb headed the Division and formulated legislation to create a national mental health institute but World War II intervened. (Kolb's son, Lawrence J. Kolb was Chair of Psychiatry at Columbia University and, like his father, was a national leader in that field. Kolb, the younger, also played a role in the creation of NINDB.)

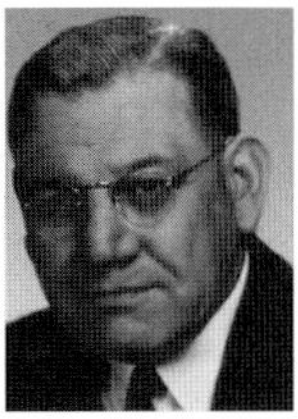

ROBERT H. FELIX, M.D., WAS NAMED DIRECTOR OF NIMH IN 1949

Robert H. Felix succeeded Kolb as Director of the Division of Mental Hygiene and drafted legislation for a National Neuropsychiatric Institute. He enlisted the aid of Mrs. Lasker, Congressman J. Percy Priest, and Senator Pepper. Felix was credited with remarkable political skills and developed close Congressional ties. He also encouraged a citizens' lobby and facilitated a new federal role – as opposed to the previous monopoly of the states – in psychiatric patient care and research.

The hearings included testimony by General Lewis Hershey, who described the high rate of draft rejections. Surgeon General Parran documented the high prevalence of psychiatric disorders, and was supported by the heads of neuropsychiatry in both the army and navy.

Mrs. Lasker's personal experience with mental disorders led to her interest in mental health. Her first husband had had an alcohol problem. Trying to help him, she became interested in psychoanalysis and served on the Board of Franz Alexander's Institute for Psychoanalysis in Chicago before 1940. She later commented on the establishment of the National Institute of Mental Health, the direct predecessor of the one for Neurology and Blindness.[23]

> In connection with the beginning of our efforts to establish the Mental Health Institute, around 1942 or '43, Blanche Ittleson asked me to be a member of the National Committee for Mental Hygiene, which was then the only so-called voluntary agency in the mental illness field. There was a group of psychiatrists and laymen who were very decent and well intentioned but did not have the knowledge or skill for fund raising or propaganda that was needed to make an important voluntary agency out of it. I tried in various ways to improve its situation but was unsuccessful. The only important thing that got accomplished was the National Mental Health Institute Bill and that finally went through the Senate because Florence [Mahoney] and I had influence with Senator Pepper and I had paid for a lobbyist to watch the status of the bill and keep in touch with Dr. [Lewis] Stevenson and me about it. Dr. Stevenson was then the Executive Director of the National Committee for Mental Hygiene.
>
> I had asked Dr. Stevenson to suggest to the PHS in early '45 that a National Mental Health Institute similar to the National Cancer Institute would be a very good idea. The Public Health Service had started to work on such a bill as a result of Stevenson's suggestion.
>
> I then got some figures together showing the small number of psychiatrists trained to take care of the mentally ill and gave them to Dr. [Lawrence] Kubie, who gave them to Tom Stokes for his column in a newspaper, I think the *Post* or the *World-Telegram*. Representative Percy Priest read the Stokes column, which was syndicated, and had been interested in the sad situation in the mental health hospitals he had seen. He, in turn, asked the PHS to give him a bill to introduce. They gave him the Mental Health Institute bill, which was similar to the

National Cancer Institute bill, which Dr. Stevenson had suggested they prepare as a result of my suggestion to him. Percy Priest got the bill through the House, but it probably would have died in the Senate without help.

We urged Pepper on, who got it though the Senate in June 1946.

Q. Why was he interested?
A. He had a son who was a psychiatrist.

Q. You say through "our help" it got through the Senate. Is that you and Mrs. Mahoney?
A. Yes, Florence and I. We were friends with Pepper, who was chairman of the subcommittee that reported on the bill and who was on the full committee and urged the full committee to report the bill, and then the bill got on the consent calendar of the Senate.

Well, the bill contained an appropriation of 17 million dollars for training and research and we thought – Florence and I were so naïve at the time – that if the bill contained a specific amount of money that was tantamount to getting the money. We didn't realize that you had to start . . . entirely with new subcommittees on appropriations . . . and then get it through on the appropriations bills that were going through or get it into a supplemental bill.

So, in this year, in '46, we didn't even know enough to ask for the money, and Pepper was busy with a lot of other things and he didn't, so there was no money for one year. I finally hired a lobbyist to try to work on this, but we finally had to do the bulk of the work ourselves as usual.

As a result, a bill establishing NIMH was passed in 1946 but there was no appropriation for funds. Felix had to apply to a private foundation for the $15,000 needed to support the first meeting of the National Advisory Council.[24] The institute formally opened in 1949, coincident with termination of the Division of Mental Hygiene in the PHS. Its tripartite mission included research, training, and service.

With the establishment of NIMH, the stage was set for the creation of a national neurological institute.

Toward Neurology Legislation: Neurologists and Psychiatrists

In 1948, the American Academy of Neurology was founded and led by the dynamic Abe Baker, Chair of Neurology and Psychiatry at the University of Minnesota. He was a staunch and early advocate of a neurological institute at NIH. So was H. Houston Merritt, Chair of Neurology at the Columbia-Presbyterian Medical Center then. In looking back on those early years, Francis Forster, one of the

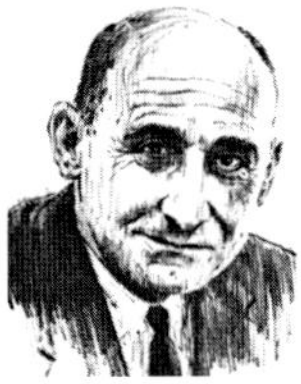

A.B. Baker, M.D., American Academy of Neurology

four founding fathers of the American Academy of Neurology, said that support for NINDB was the only thing Baker and Merritt ever agreed upon.[25]

Their goals differed. Baker wanted to train neurologists and Merritt thought research was the answer to the poverty of neurological therapy. But both addressed unmet needs, and both were driven by the precarious state of clinical neurology. Merritt[26] wrote:

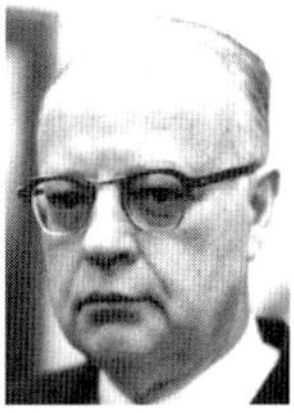

H. Houston Merritt, M.D., Chair of Neurology, Columbia-Presbyterian Medical Center

> Even as late as 1936, there were only 16 hospitals listed in the United States as having approved training for residency in neurology. In addition, most of the physicians who took a residency in neurology went on to practice neuropsychiatry. A few turned to internal medicine or neurosurgery. This was perhaps due to two factors: first, the training they received in neurology was very scant, usually only a year, and as a result they did not know much more about diseases of the nervous system than did the internists who received several years of training in internal medicine. In addition there was great pressure for the care of patients with mental illnesses and most of those who had any training in psychiatry gradually became almost totally concerned with the treatment of psychoneurotic and psychotic patients.

Comments by contemporaries such as Lawrence Kolb, the younger, and Francis Forster, suggest that an early NIMH research grants committee was also influential in establishing NINDB. Interviewed in 2000,[27] he recalled that 52 years earlier he had served on an NIMH grants committee with Houston Merritt (then still at Harvard) and Samuel Wortis of New York University. According to the custom of the time, all three had been trained in both psychiatry and neurology. They were impressed with the number of research grant applications that could have been considered neurological rather than psychiatric, and they conceived a neurological institute by itself. Francis Forster confirmed the story.[6]

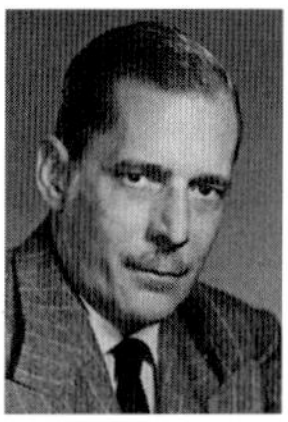

Pearce Bailey, Jr., M.D.

Pearce Bailey was a key player, another son of a well-known neurologist with the same name. Pearce Bailey, Senior, was one of the founders of the New York Neurological Institute and, in 1913, had been elected President of the elite senior organization, the American Neurological Association. Bailey, Junior, had served in the U.S. Navy and, on his discharge in 1946, became Chief of Neurology for the Veterans Administration and rapidly discerned the need for neurological care, training, and research.

During his tenure at the Veterans Administration, Bailey thought he had two major missions: to provide the veterans with high-quality medical service and to establish neurology as a specialty. At that time, university departments of neurology were still either divisions within a department of medicine or were submerged in departments of neuropsychiatry. Seeking to increase the training of neurologists,

Bailey had allies in the American Academy of Neurology because he had been one of its founders and served as its second president in 1949-1950.

Toward Neurology Legislation: Voluntary Health Agencies

According to Bailey,[8] the enabling legislation for NINDB developed mainly in response to the rising power of voluntary health agencies. The 1949 House of Representatives hearings on several related bills tell the story.

Each agency proposed separate institutes: one each for multiple sclerosis, cerebral palsy, and epilepsy. Arthritis and leprosy were also considered. The House committee, led by Representatives Robert Crosser, Percy Priest, and Andrew Biemiller, however, argued that such an approach was wasteful because it duplicated functions. Instead, they presented an Omnibus Bill that was linked to a national health insurance proposal and also to a bill for the training of nurses and other health professionals, as well as other measures. Representative Biemiller introduced the final bill in the House and Senator Pepper introduced a parallel bill in the Senate.

Toward Legislation: Congressional Hearings

The bills that would ultimately establish NINDB led to hearings on the proposals in the House of Representatives.[28] Witnesses met with the committee in May and June 1949. Several separate disease-specific institutes were considered along with one for national health insurance. The research proposal featured training for neuroscientists, provided grants, and established an intramural program.

Supporting witnesses who gave testimony, however, were few in comparison with today's activist advocates. The witnesses emphasized the need to improve research. The Multiple Sclerosis Society, only two years old, was well represented by a team that included Sylvia Lawry, its founder, Cornelius Traeger, its executive director, and two famous neurologists who served on its board, Tracy Putnam and Houston Merritt.

Others, such as Senator Charles W. Tobey, a Republican from Maine, described how their lives had been affected by neurological disease. Tobey presented an emotional depiction of his daughter's struggle with multiple sclerosis. He also told of his chance encounter with the eminent shipbuilder Henry Kaiser, whose son had also been affected, and how the fathers had commiserated over the plight of their children. These personal revelations made Tobey's testimony all the more poignant.

Eleanor Gehrig also testified for the MS Society. Her husband, Lou Gehrig, the famous Columbia University athlete and New York Yankee slugger, had died of amyotrophic lateral sclerosis. The word "sclerosis" served to link two quite different diseases but nevertheless made the point; research was needed.

Representatives for two other voluntary agencies also testified. One persuasive witness was William Lennox, a highly regarded professor of neurology at Harvard and one of the first superspecialists, a pioneer in the clinical investigation of epilepsy. It was up to members of local organizations to support cerebral palsy because no national organization had yet been formed. Leonard Goldenson testified (he was later to head ABC television) and became the leader of the ultimately unified national voluntary group, United Cerebral Palsy. In that capacity he became a driving force for research in birth injuries and perinatal diseases.

Tracy Putnam reappeared; he had first testified for multiple sclerosis, now, he spoke for both epilepsy and cerebral palsy. Several individuals supported victims of leprosy. Proponents of an arthritis institute also appeared. Whatever their particular interests, all the advocates emphasized the paucity of knowledge, the severe limitations of available treatment, and the difficulty of finding physicians expert in the diseases.

But the committee heard nothing of stroke, brain or spinal cord injury, brain tumors, muscular dystrophy, other genetic diseases, or infections of the nervous system – diseases and conditions that also desperately needed research but had no advocates. Neither the American Neurological Association (founded in 1874) nor the American Academy of Neurology (founded a year before the hearings) sent a representative or a statement. By today's standards support for the bill was limited, but it was sufficiently powerful to garner votes for the bill and the time was ripe.

How Blindness was Added

Not a single witness mentioned blindness at the hearings on the bill for the neurological institute. Mrs. Lasker related how vision research became part of the institute's mandate.[29]

> Now, the way the word "blindness" got into the Neurological Diseases Institute is this: during the Spring of 1949, Miss Mildred Wiedenfeld, Dr. Hinsey of Harvard, and Mr. Ulmer of Ohio came to see me about the problem of blindness in the United States. I had not thought much about this problem, as I had not had anybody close to me who was blind, and I had not realized how little was being done for research in this field. I was grateful to them for pointing this problem out to me, so I telephoned Congressman Biemiller of Wisconsin, who was in charge of the legislation in the Interstate and Foreign Commerce Committee, and asked him if he wouldn't like to introduce a blindness institute bill. Biemiller said "Why yes I will." This surprised me, this prompt agreement, and I

said, "Well, you sound very cooperative, Andy; how do you happen to be so interested?" He replied to me quite simply, "My mother was blind."

He did introduce the bill in the House, and as it was too late to have a separate bill introduced in the Senate, I asked Senator Murray, who was holding the hearings, as he was the Chairman of the Committee on Labor and Public Welfare, to include blindness in the omnibus bill. It was included with the neurological diseases in an institute called the National Institute of Neurological Diseases and Blindness, entirely as a result of my suggestion. The whole blindness thing was just done like that, because these men were all in sympathy with the idea.

But it came about after a big debate which Senator Pepper had with Norman Topping [Associate Director, NIH] about the need for additional institutes, which Pepper naturally won.

The Bill Becomes Law

The compromise "Omnibus Medical Research Bill," rather than creating multiple institutes, called for the establishment of two separate institutes, a National Institute of Neurological Diseases and Blindness and one for Arthritis and Metabolic Diseases. It also gave the Surgeon General an important new power, the option of creating new institutes – or discontinuing old ones. All previous NIH laws had stipulated governance by Advisory Council; the bill for NINDB, for the first time, required layperson members of the Council. It included provisions for constructing laboratory facilities throughout the country and for training investigators. Representative Percy Priest[30] introduced the bill in the House and Claude Pepper[31] sponsored the Senate version. Slight differences between the two chambers were resolved in a compromise bill that was passed by voice vote.[32]

President Harry S. Truman ultimately signed the bill into law, but he apparently had concerns about increasing institutional compartmentalization. Roger W. Jones (Assistant Director, Legislative Reference in the Bureau of the Budget, Executive Office of the President) summed up these concerns in a letter dated August 10, 1950,[33] and addressed to William J. Hopkins (Executive Clerk of the Office of Management and Budget):

> For some time there has been concern within the Executive Office of the President over the proliferation of separate institutes within the Public Health Service for each disease category. S. 2591 will bring the total of separate statutory institutes to six. As late as June 15, 1949, the Director of the Bureau of the Budget indicated that the legislative proposals to continue the

authority of the Surgeon General to establish additional institutes and to abolish institutes created by administrative order in the Public Health Service were meritorious because they would "avoid the rigidity and administrative complexity which inevitably results from the creation of a series of statutory research institutes, each for the purpose of doing research in a particular segment of the medical field."

Jones also mentioned that President Truman might veto the bill:

> The addition of these two new statutory institutes makes even more serious the departure from the desired fluidity of organizations stressed in the above-mentioned letter. While a veto does not seem feasible because of the worthiness of the objectives and the popular support and need for medical research, it is our conviction that the defects of this bill should be stressed so as to discourage future attempts to establish by statute other separate institutes. It is therefore recommended that upon signing the enrolled bill, the President issue the enclosed statement, noting the undesirable aspects of the trend toward separate institutes and calling upon the Surgeon General of the Public Health Service to coordinate his research and research grant programs as much as he can.

Truman never publicly made that statement. At the bottom of a copy of this letter, a handwritten note added by William Hopkins remarked that: "After discussion with Mr. Murphy, the President decided not to issue a statement." Hopkins was referring to Charles S. Murphy, Special Counsel to the President. Hopkins, however, did not offer any explanation for the change in plans.

Naturally, Mrs. Lasker commented on the next dramatic scene,[34] including the views of Norman Topping, then Associate Director of NIH:

> When Biemiller let me know of the passage of the bill, I had no apprehension there would be any difficulty getting it signed. I phoned Matt Connolly at the White House to say that I thought the sponsors of the two new institutes bill should be photographed with the President when he signed it. Matt Connolly said he'd let me know when the bill came to the President's desk. Within a week he phoned me and dropped what for me was a bombshell. He said, "I'm afraid the bill won't be signed." I gasped, "Why not?" He said, "The Budget has written a memorandum attached to the bill saying, 'While the purposes of the bill are all right, the methods of establishing more institutes to get these results are bad.'"
>
> I suspect that the Public Health Service, in order to save face, had gotten after the Budget or written the memo and got somebody low down in the Budget to attach this to the bill.

Q. This was Topping's point of view?
A. Yes, I suspect that. I hung up the phone in despair and I called Anna Rosenberg and Florence Mahoney. Anna called David Niles. I called Clark Clifford. Florence called, I'm sure, Clifford, too. Between us all, the memorandum of the Budget was detached from the bill and lost, and within a few days President Truman signed the bill.

Q. He had not seen the memo?
A. Evidently not. These are the chances—

Q. There was no further effort on the part of the Budget people then?
A. Yes. I took a deep breath but next came getting the supplementary appropriations so that the two new institutes just established would mean something. The Public Health Service was willing to put a few funds that had been used for similar purposes in the NIH into these two new institutes to start, but it didn't amount to much. They had amounted to $578,000 for the National Institute of Arthritis and Metabolic Diseases and for Neurological Diseases and Blindness nothing at all in fiscal '51, not one cent.

The bill became law when the President signed it on August 15, 1950,[35] and a new world of neuroscience commenced.

1 Harden VA. National Institutes of Health. In Kurian GT, ed. *A Historical Guide to the U.S. Government.* New York: Oxford University Press, 1998:409-414.

2 Harden VA. *Inventing the NIH. Federal Biomedical Research Policy, 1887-1937.* Baltimore: Johns Hopkins University Press, 1986.

3 Strickland SP. *Politics, Science and Dread Disease: A Short History of United States Medical Research Policy.* Cambridge, Mass.: Harvard University Press, 1972.

4 Spingarn ND. Heartbeat: *The Politics of Health Research.* Washington-New York: Robert B. Luce, Inc., 1976.

5 President Extends Olive Branch to Organized Medicine in Dedicating Health Institute: Reassures Physicians Against Socialization. Transcripts of Radio Recording of Speech by President Franklin D. Roosevelt, October 31, 1940; copy in National Institutes of Health History Office, Bethesda, Md.

6 Miller WB. Written statement. U.S. Congress. House. Committee on Interstate and Foreign Commerce. *National Neuropsychiatric Institute Act: Hearing before a Subcommittee on Public Health.* 79th Cong., 1st sess., September 18, 19, 21, 1945, p. 5.

7 Hershey LB. Statement. U.S. Congress. House. Committee on Interstate and Foreign Commerce. *National Neuropsychiatric Institute Act: Hearing before a Subcommittee on Public Health.* 79th Cong., 1st sess., September 18, 19, 21, 1945, p. 36.

8 Bailey P Jr. Government Organization of Neurological Research and Development in the Veterans Administration and the National Institute of Neurological Diseases and Blindness, 1876-1975. In Denny-Brown D, ed. *Centennial Anniversary Volume of the American Neurological Association.* New York: Springer Publishing Company, 1975:509-531.

9 Kurtzke JF. The current neurologic burden of illness and injury in the United States. *Neurology* 1982;32:1207-1214.

10 Kurtzke JF, Sacco RL, Mayeux R, Hauser WA. Neuroepidemiology. *Continuum* 1998;4:1-137.

11 Severinghaus AE. A medical discipline takes stock. *Arch Neurol* 1967;17:461-470.

12 Cohen MM. Introduction. In Cohen MM. *The Academy of Neurology: The First Fifty Years*, 1948-1998. St. Paul, Minn.: The American Academy of Neurology, 1998:1-8.

13 Shannon JA. The National Institutes of Health: some critical years, 1955-1957. *Science* 1987;237:865-868.

14 Stewart I. *Organizing Scientific Research for War.* Boston: Little Brown, 1948.

15 Richards AN. The impact of the war on medicine. *Science* 1946;193:578.

16 Pace E. Mary W. Lasker, Philanthropist for Medical Research, Dies at 93. Obituary. *The New York Times*, February 23, 1994.

17 *The Reminiscences of Mary Lasker* (April 18, 1966) in the Oral History Collection of Columbia University, New York, pp. 13-14.

18 Pepper CD, with Gorey H. *Pepper – Eyewitness to a Century.* New York: Harcourt Brace Jovanovich, 1987:256.

19 *Reminiscences of Mary Lasker.* Series 1 (1965), vol. 2/7, p. 188.

20 *Reminiscences of Mary Lasker.* Series 1 (1965), vol. 2/7, p. 182.

21 Grob GN. Creation of the National Institute of Mental Health. *Pub Health Rep* 1996;111:378-381.

22 Judd LL, ed. The fiftieth anniversary of the National Institute of Mental Health. *Am J Psychiat* 1998;155 (special supplement):1-40.

23 *Reminiscences of Mary Lasker.* Series 1 (1965), vol. 4/7, pp. 543-545.

24 *Reminiscences of Robert H. Felix* (February 8, 1963) in the Oral History Collection of Columbia University, New York, Health Science Series (1097); p. 45.

25 Forster F. Telephone interview with author, July 14, 2000.

26 Merritt HH. The Development of Neurology in the Past Fifty Years. In Denny-Brown D, ed. *Centennial Anniversary Volume of the American Neurological Association, 1875-1975.* New York: Springer Publishing Company, 1975:3-10.

27 Kolb LC. Telephone interview with author, June 13, 2000.

28 U.S. Congress. House. Committee on Interstate and Foreign Commerce. *National Health Plan: Hearings before a Subcommittee on Public Health, Science, and Commerce.* 81st Cong., 1st sess., 1949.

29 *Reminiscences of Mary Lasker.* Series 1 (1965), vol. 2/7, p. 236.

30 U.S. Congress House *Omnibus Medical Research Bill.* 81st Cong., 2nd sess., June 27, 1950. H. Rep. No. 2352. Committed to the Committee of the Whole House on the State of the Union and ordered to be printed.

31 U.S. Congress. Senate. *Providing for Research and Training in Rheumatism and Arthritis, Multiple Sclerosis, Cerebral Palsy, Epilepsy and Blindness, and Other Diseases.* 81st Cong., 1st sess. September 22, 1949. S. Rep. 1102 (to accompany S. 2591).

32 *Congressional Quarterly Almanac.* 81st Cong., 2nd sess., vol. VI, Washington, D.C.: Congressional Quarterly News Feature, 1950:182-183.

33 August 15-16, 1950, Folder, White House Records Office Files (White House Bill File); Staff Member and Office Files; Harry S. Truman Papers; Harry S. Truman Library, Independence, Mo.

34 *Reminiscences of Mary Lasker.* Series 1 (1965), vol. 2/7, p. 244.

35 *Public Health Act, Amendment: An Act to Amend the Public Health Service Act to Support Research and Training in Matters Relating to Arthritis and Rheumatism, Multiple Sclerosis, Cerebral Palsy, Epilepsy, Poliomyelitis, Blindness, Leprosy, and Other Diseases.* 81 P.L. 692. August 15, 1950. 81st Cong., 2nd sess., chapter 714, 64 Stat. 443.

'IRST STEPS

The Fifties

In 1950, when legislation carved out the Institute of Neurological Diseases and Blindness from the National Institute of Mental Health, the new institute had a mandate but no budget from Congress. Robert H. Felix, the director of NIMH, was given responsibility for establishing the structure and leadership of the fledgling organization.

Trained in psychiatry at the University of Colorado, Felix had joined the Public Health Service in 1933. For a time he was Director of the federal Narcotics Treatment Center in Lexington, Kentucky, and then chief of the Mental Hygiene Division of the Public Health Service from 1944 to 1949. In that position, he helped formulate the law that established NIMH and was then appointed director of the new institute.

Felix had spent his early years working in a state mental hospital system where he recognized several major problems in the delivery of mental health care. The first was that each state controlled its own programs and policies, which led to uneven quality of care and accessibility from place to place. Within a state, local bureaucracies resisted change. There was also little or no antipsychotic drug therapy and virtually no biologic research.

To correct these deficiencies, Felix envisioned a new role for a federal research center in mental health, one that could also confront a fourth challenge – the dominance of psychoanalysis in medical schools and training programs. Felix wanted to take advantage of the unique resources at NIH to create a new brain "science" for psychiatry, one that would rely more on biology than biography to explain and treat mental illness.

At NIMH, Felix soon consulted with the renowned academicians, Houston Merritt in neurology and John Romano in psychiatry.[1] Then, Felix had the foresight and courage to hire Seymour Kety as the first scientific director at NIMH. Kety had had no training in psychiatry and was only 35 years old, but he was already famous because of his studies of cerebral blood flow in humans. Felix[2] told Kety: "I am a psychiatrist, not a scientist. You are the scientist. You will have free range to hire staff, an unrestricted budget, and beds in the new Clinical Center, scheduled to open in 1953."

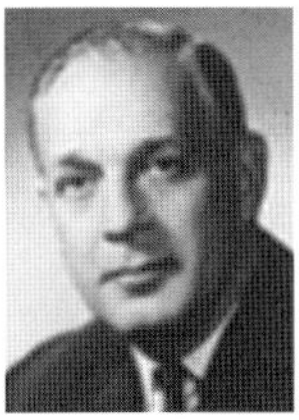

SEYMOUR KETY, M.D., WAS THE FIRST SCIENTIFIC DIRECTOR OF NIMH AND FIRST DIRECTOR OF THE INTRAMURAL PROGRAM AT NINDB

Before he came to NIH, Kety had been quite comfortable in his position as a Professor of Physiology in the Graduate School of the University of Pennsylvania, where he worked in a department headed by pulmonary physiologist Julius H. Comroe, Jr., whom Kety admired as a scientist and teacher. Kety recognized the directorship as a matchless opportunity, and he grasped it, assuming his new responsibilities in 1951.

The same year, Felix hired Pearce Bailey as the first director of NINDB. The NIH itself provided administrative funds, but there was nothing for training or research. Bailey had to depend on NIMH. What otherwise might have been restrictive turned out, in retrospect, to be most fortunate because Kety became director of the intramural programs for both NINDB and NIMH.

Kety had a remarkable ability to spot talent. His stature and personality also made it possible for him to attract talented scientists to what might otherwise have seemed a shaky and risky new venture. Twenty of the investigators he appointed to the intramural programs at NINDB and NIMH were later elected to the National Academy of Sciences and others attained different forms of high public recognition. Later, he was appropriately proud of his hiring record, recalling that he had been grateful to discover that the NIH had the resources to match leading universities in recruiting.

Among the early arrivals were the following research leaders (in alphabetical order to avoid inappropriate comparisons):

Wayne Albers, a biochemist, joined NIH in 1954, served in Sanford Palay's laboratory, and helped organize the Neurochemistry Laboratory under Donald Tower. His career continues at NINDS as Chief of the Enzyme Chemistry Section.

Julius Axelrod, another biochemist, had been working in the Heart Institute with Bernard Brodie. In a desire for more independence he approached Kety; Felix approved a transfer to NIMH in 1954. In the years that followed, Axelrod elucidated the biosynthesis of epinephrine and initiated the modern study of neurotransmitters. He received a Nobel Prize in 1970.

Roscoe O. Brady, lipid chemist and biochemist, worked out the pathogenesis of the sphingolipid storage diseases, including Gaucher disease, Fabry disease, and Tay-Sachs disease. He won a Lasker Award for that achievement in 1982.

Giulio L. Cantoni, a biochemist, discovered and elucidated the role of S-adenosyl-methionine, a key factor in the activity of folic acid, essential for the biosynthesis of nucleic acids, and needed for detoxification of some drugs and chemicals.

Kenneth S. Cole directed the Laboratory of Biophysics in NINDB. He was one of the pioneers in the use of the squid axon to study nerve functions and he was also one of the first to use patch clamping to analyze nerve impulses. He was called "the father of membrane biophysics" when the Biophysical Society named a medal in his honor.

Edward Evarts, trained as a psychiatrist, became a neurophysiologist and was the first to record the intracellular electrical activity in the brain cells that control limb movements. Remarkably, he did this in awake monkeys (with sensitive concern for the animals comfort and safety).

Karl Frank was a premier spinal cord neurophysiologist, one of the first to record intracellularly in spinal motor neurons. He was appointed in 1951 and was an early student of motor control. He served as Associate Director of NINDB from 1965 to 1968.

Seymour Kaufman, a biochemist, elucidated the biochemical abnormality involved in children with phenylketonuria, a reversible cause of mental retardation.

Irwin J. Kopin worked first with Kety, then with Julius Axelrod. For 10 years he headed the Laboratory of Clinical Science in NIMH and then moved to become director of intramural research at NINDS.

Wade H. Marshall was an early Kety appointment. He was one of the first to use microelectrodes to study the sensory functions of the cerebral cortex. He elucidated a phenomenon called *spreading depression*, which became important in understanding normal brain physiology and, also, migraine headache. His laboratory continued to bridge both NIMH and NINDS. He died in 1972.

Sanford Palay headed the section of neurocytology, pioneering the use of the electron microscope to study brain ultrastructure. He became the Bullard Professor of Anatomy at Harvard in 1961, and later served as editor of the *Journal of Comparative Neurology*.

Alexander Rich is a renowned expert in x-ray crystallography and a pioneer in learning the detailed structure of nucleic acids. After leaving NIH he moved to the Massachusetts Institute of Technology. He was given a Presidential Medal of Science in 1995.

Louis Sokoloff, student, colleague, and close friend of Kety's for decades, became a notable investigator himself and won a Lasker Award in 1981 for developing a method to study metabolism of small regions of the nervous system. This "deoxyglucose" method was the basis for functional studies of the human brain by positron emission tomography (PET). After that achievement, Sokoloff solved a mathematical problem that accelerated the development of PET.

Ichiji Tasaki was another outstanding peripheral nerve physiologist who studied the process of transmission of the impulse along a nerve.

William F. Windle, a neuroanatomist, was a pioneer in studies of the developing brain and developed a primate NINDS study center in Puerto Rico.

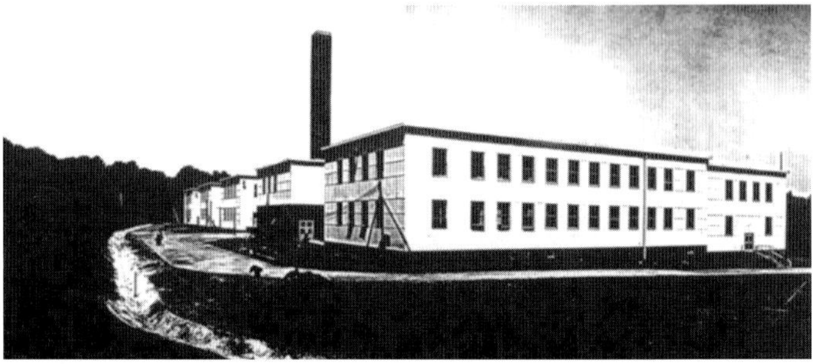

Building T-6, probable site of the joint NIMH/NINDB laboratory

Brady, Cole, Frank, Tasaki, and Windle were assigned to NINDB, the others to NIMH. Both institutes sponsored Marshall's laboratory, but all the laboratories of NINDB and NIMH were contiguous, and the scientists maintained interactive and productive relationships. There were no inhibiting boundaries between the laboratories and it is not clear how the laboratories were assigned to one institute or the other. In terms of work, it seemed not to matter. Interests drove research, not institutional boundaries.

By 1956, Kety had completed the first stages of the organization of the intramural program – recruiting and assigning laboratories – and he resigned as scientific director. He continued his own research in cerebral blood flow. Robert Livingston became the new intramural scientific director but the independent development of NIMH and NINDB in the next few years led to a permanent separation of their laboratories in 1961. After that, there were no formal attempts to integrate laboratories of the two institutes, organizationally or physically.

Starting up the NINDB Intramural Program

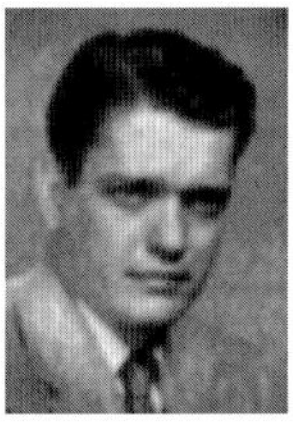

G. Milton Shy, M.D., was named Intramural Clinical Director of NINDB in 1953

The independent development of intramural research for NINDB, distinct from that of NIMH, overlapped with the Kety era. In 1953, G. Milton Shy was appointed Intramural Clinical Director of NINDB, while Kety directed the more basic science laboratories. Shy was only 33 years old and had not yet published much. Director Pearce Bailey picked Shy on grounds of promise.

Shy was born in Colorado, went to college and medical school in Oregon, and interned at the Royal Victoria Hospital in Montreal. During World War II, he served as a physician with the U.S. infantry and was seriously wounded but recovered. He left the army in 1947 and then started training in neurology at the National Hospital, Queen Square, London. He finished his training with Donald McEachern at the Montreal Neurological Institute and became interested in muscle disease. In 1951, he became the first head of neurology at the then new medical school of the University of Colorado. There he established his lifelong friendship and association with Eli Goldensohn, who became a leader in epilepsy research.

While he was still in Colorado, Shy made an important finding, describing two patients with what came to be known as Shy-Drager syndrome. This is now recognized as one form of multiple system atrophy, a neurodegenerative disease that causes – in varying combinations – orthostatic hypotension, cerebellar ataxia, parkinsonism, and motor neuron dysfunction.

Shy also gained a reputation as both a brilliant lecturer and clinician. He became famous, feared, and applauded for his aggressive Socratic style of teaching. He would challenge anyone with seemingly obscure questions in order to make a point, and he would use as a foil even the most distinguished visitor to one of his conferences. Confronted with possible embarrassment, Shy's colleagues, whatever their rank, were likely to prepare well in advance for his conferences. After a conference, the path to the library was well trod. Learning was expedited – defensively.

Shy's main interest was muscle disease. When he started at NINDB, research was largely confined to electromyography and observations of muscle biopsies. Shy extended those techniques and introduced new ones, especially the electron microscope, tissue staining (histochemistry), and intracellular electrical recording from nerve and muscle. At NINDB, he combined these approaches to study familial periodic paralysis. In subsequent investigations, he was the first to recognize and classify diseases according to the site of molecular pathology: muscle membranes, mitochondria, or contractile proteins. Shy was a true innovator in this field.

With his student, W. King Engel, Shy described early cases of mitochondrial diseases of muscle as well as those diseases characterized by structural abnormalities that led to names such as central core disease and nemaline myopathy (*nemaline* from a Greek word meaning "thread" to describe unusual conglomerations in muscle). While he had administrative responsibilities, Shy found the time to teach himself about electrolytes, isotopes, electrophysiology, and histology. His broad range of interests even led him to publish a monograph in a field far from muscle disease, the use of radioisotopes to localize brain tumors.

Shy's clinical associates in the new institute held the lowest staff positions, repeating tasks they had already completed as residents in their earlier training programs, because almost all of them had come to NINDB to fulfill their military obligations during the Korean War and thereafter. While they were medical students, they had been deferred from service, but after postgraduate residencies, they had become subject to a mandatory draft of physicians. Since the United States Public Health Service was considered a "uniformed service," physicians could meet this obligation, either by acting as doctors where the PHS was responsible for medical care (for example, on Native American reservations) or doing research at the NIH.

As a result of these policies, during the first three decades of its existence, the NIH was staffed by a generation of physicians who also learned how to do research. When they returned to medical schools throughout the country, they became academic leaders with skills as both researchers and clinicians. When the doctor draft ended, recruitment of young physicians to NIH became more difficult.

The early NINDB was an example of that pattern. Among those who worked with Milton Shy were several who rose to become recognized investigators or departmental chairs in neurology, including Andrew G. Engel, Daniel B. Drachman and David A. Drachman, Donald H. Silberberg, Leonard Berg, Gunther Haase, and Lewis P. Rowland.

Under Shy, there were two strong intramural research programs, his own in neuromuscular disease and another in epilepsy research. Shy appointed several former colleagues of his at the Montreal Neurological Institute, which was then a prominent center for the study of epilepsy. Among those who came from Montreal was the first NINDB neurosurgeon, Maitland Baldwin, who established the epilepsy surgery program. Baldwin graduated from Harvard College and the medical school at Queens University in Kingston, Ontario, in 1943. He interned at the Massachusetts General Hospital and then served in the Naval Medical Corps with the U.S. Marines during the battles of Iwo Jima and Okinawa. He was one of the best known of Wilder Penfield's trainees and co-authored the landmark 1950 paper on temporal lobectomy for the treatment of seizures originating in that part of the brain. He was instrumental in obtaining congressional approval for the NIH operating rotunda. He had personally directed the design of the neurosurgical operating suites with special recording rooms and electronic equipment.[3] Baldwin died at age 52 in 1970.

Cosimo Ajmone-Marsan came from Montreal to head the EEG Laboratory in the epilepsy program, which he directed for 25 years[4] until he left for the University of Miami.

Donald B. Tower, another Montreal recruit, had been trained in neuronal biochemistry when there were few others in the field. He helped establish a neurochemistry laboratory at NINDB and, among

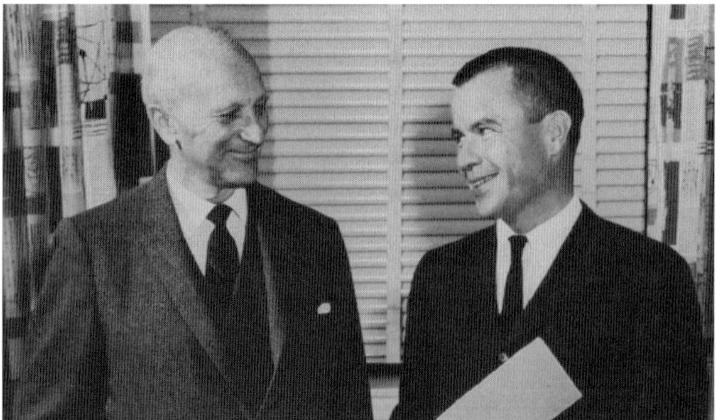

Wilder Penfield, M.D. (left) and Maitland Baldwin, M.D. Baldwin established the epilepsy surgery program at NINDB

other interests, he was one of the first to study the biochemistry of tissue removed in the course of brain surgery for epilepsy. Highly respected by his peers at home and nationally, Tower went on to became Director of the Institute in 1973.

Shy was able to lay the foundations for a strong NINDS epilepsy program by recruiting specialists with research interests in epilepsy. Under his tutelage, the epilepsy program became an important component of the intramural program, and would continue to expand in different directions in later years, as discussed in Chapter 6.

Shy was in a highly productive phase of his career when he was at NINDB, but he missed contact with medical students and other academic attractions.[5] Shy left NINDB in 1961 to become Chair of Neurology at the University of Pennsylvania. He revitalized that department, spurred on by fruitful research collaboration with Nicholas Gonatas, a neuropathologist and cell biologist. In 1967, Shy moved again to head neurology at the Neurological Institute at the Columbia-Presbyterian Medical Center in New York. Three weeks after he arrived he suffered a fatal heart attack at the age of 47. His death was a great loss to the field of neurology.

W. King Engel, a former student of Shy, was branch chief of Clinical Neurology from 1963 to 1978. Engel continued the neuromuscular research emphasized by Shy. He revolutionized the study of muscle disease by introducing histochemical studies as criteria for the classification and understanding of muscle disease. Among his numerous innovative contributions were the use of corticosteroids to treat myasthenia gravis, inflammatory myopathies, and other autoimmune diseases; the use of acetazolamide to prevent attacks of periodic paralysis (remarkably including both hypokalemic and hyperkalemic varieties); and recognition of "ragged red fibers" as a histochemical sign of mitochondrial disease. He was the first neurologist to call for the abolition of boxing, arguing that it was the only sport in which the goal is to injure the brain of an opponent (because brain injury is the result of a knockout blow). His position was later adopted officially by the American Academy of Neurology.

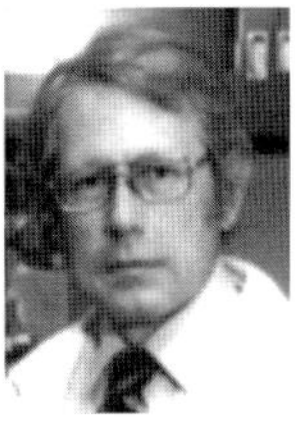

W. King Engel, M.D., was branch chief of Clinical Neurology at NINDB from 1963 to 1978

After 29 years, Engel left NIH in 1990 to join the medical faculty at the University of Southern California in Los Angeles, where he set up a new center for neuromuscular diseases. There, he still collaborates on scientific projects with his wife, Dr. Valerie Askanas, to illuminate the many proteins deposited in muscle in inclusion body myositis.

In 2000, his former students gave an educational course on neuromuscular disease at the annual meeting of the American Academy of Neurology.[6] They toasted their golden days of NIH research with Engel. The list of participants comprised almost all the leaders of current investigation of neuromuscular disease: Steven Ringel, Jerry Mendell, Michel Fardeau, Robert Griggs, John Morgan-Hughes,

Tulio Bertorini, Alberto Dubrovsky, Ferdinando Cornelio, Bruce Adornato, John Whitaker, John Griffin, David Pleasure, George Karpati, and Fernando Tomé. The late Dale McFarlin, who was to lead the NINDS program in neuroimmunology, was another alumnus. Some of the American alumni may have come to NIH for mandatory public service but half of these alumni investigators had come to NIH from abroad – attracted by the intellectual leadership and contributions of Engel.

The NINDS Neuromuscular Diseases Section, now in its 47th year and its third generation of leadership, is currently headed by Marinos Dalakas, himself a student of Engel's. Dalakas, trained also in neurovirology by John Sever, is an authority on inflammatory muscle diseases and post-polio syndrome, among other conditions. His interests extend from molecular pathology to the conduct of therapeutic trials.

The intramural program has encompassed more than the programs in epilepsy and neuromuscular disease. In the early years, when NINDS was still NINDB, intramural researchers also focused on hearing and blindness. One of the early discoveries was the association between blindness in infants called retrolental fibroplasia and the administration of oxygen to low birth-weight babies. Institute researchers found that proper precautions would prevent this pandemic complication. Additionally, some of the earliest work on the cochlear implant was carried out in NINDB laboratories.

A major intramural achievement in the early days was the recognition by virologist John Sever that a horrible brain disease (subacute sclerosis panencephalitis or SSPE) was due to persistent infection by an altered measles virus. That discovery and the development of the measles vaccine led to the virtual elimination of SSPE.

Other than neuromuscular disease, through the years the intramural program has developed along several different lines, as discussed in subsequent chapters.

1 Kety S. Transcript of Oral Interview with Philip S. Holtzman, 1992. Countway Library of Medicine, Rare Books and Special Collections, Harvard University, Cambridge, Mass.

2 Kety S. Recorded interview with author, April 2, 2000.

3 O'Brien FH, Dekaban AS. Maitland Baldwin, September 29, 1918 – February 9, 1970. *Neurology* 1971;21:872.

4 Ajmone-Marsan C. National Institute of Neurological Diseases and Stroke, National Institutes of Health: clinical neurophysiology and epilepsy in the first 25 years of its intramural program. *J Clin Neurophysiol* 1995;12:46-56.

5 Goldensohn EE. Interview with author, May 2000.

6 Karpati G, Mendell JR. *Neuromuscular Panorama: The Past, Present, and Prologue to the Future.* Education Program Syllabus 2FC.005, American Academy of Neurology, 2000.

CHAPTER THREE

DEVELOPMENT

A former director of NIH, James Wyngaarden,[1] once introduced an important review of NIH activities with a quotation from political columnist I.F. Stone:

"In government, the budget is the message."

In time, both the intramural and extramural programs at NINDS grew in parallel with NIH's budget.[2] This was not always true of other institutes, which were sometimes given much more of the Congressional allotment. This happened to the National Cancer Institute during the war on cancer in the 1970s.[3] NINDS, however, has never had that kind of particular attention, even during the Decade of the Brain; its budget rose and fell in parallel with that of NIH.

The dips in funding sometimes hit hard. For instance, NINDS and all the institutes suffered during the 1970s when budget cuts led to the abolition of training programs. This was accompanied by attacks on peer review, along with presidential directives to apply the results of basic research to patients and to target research, and also with the caustic remarks of presidential advisers who considered investigators "arrogant academics with the gimmees."[2]

Natalie Davis Spingarn, author of *Heartbeat: The Politics of Health Research*, believed that the Nixon staff was antipathetic to scientists and other academics who did not, in general, support the President's political program.[2]

Overall, however, the growth of all institutes has been a measure of the approval of the American people and of the officials they send to the Congress. The history of NINDS attests to this.

NINDB had its own budget for the first time in 1951, but it was a donation from NIMH and amounted to only $1,232,253. The first true Congressional budget came in 1954, at $4.5 million. Overall, the NINDS budget grew progressively and passed the $1 billion mark in fiscal 2000. The budget is directed primarily to the extramural program and investigator-initiated grants. The intramural program comes to about 10 percent of the total.

The Return of Mary Lasker

Mary Lasker was concerned with the budgets and activities of all of NIH through the years. She maintained the same methods of operation in battling for budgets as she had used so successfully earlier – even as the cast of supporting characters changed. Since by this time Senator Pepper had been defeated in his race for a Senate seat in 1950, her new friends in Congress became Senator Lister Hill and Representative John E. Fogarty.

NINDS Funding Compared to NIH Funding, 1951–2000
(dollars in thousands)

Fiscal Year	NINDS Appropriation	NIH Appropriation
1951	1,232	50,555
1952	1,562	47,115
1953	1,814	48,136
1954	4,500	59,058
1955	7,601	67,121
1956	9,861	80,457
1957	18,650	147,810
1958	21,387	171,966
1959	29,403	241,964
1960	41,487	331,910
1961	56,600	459,100
1962	70,812	629,459
1963	83,506	737,201
1964	87,675	730,379
1965	87,821	773,091
1966	101,153	873,931
1967	116,296	1,014,254
1968	128,633	1,076,461
1969	128,935	1,109,757
1970	97,315	1,061,007
1971	103,502	1,212,847
1972	116,732	1,506,156
1973	130,672	1,762,565
1974	121,358	1,790,425
1975	142,498	2,092,897
1976	144,446	2,302,126
1977	155,500	2,544,078
1978	178,438	2,842,936
1979	212,365	3,189,976
1980	241,966	3,428,935
1981	252,533	3,569,406
1982	265,901	3,641,875
1983	297,064	4,023,969
1984	335,883	4,493,588
1985	396,885	5,149,459
1986	414,727	5,262,211
1987	490,233	6,182,910
1988	534,692	6,666,693
1989	472,292	7,144,764
1990	490,409	7,576,352
1991	541,743	8,276,739
1992	959,082	8,921,687
1993	979,471	10,335,996
1994	1,065,583	10,955,773
1995	535,199	11,299,522
1996	1,168,483	11,927,562
1997	1,256,659	12,740,843
1998	1,351,655	13,647,843
1999	1,570,102	15,652,386
2000	1,798,038	17,813,587

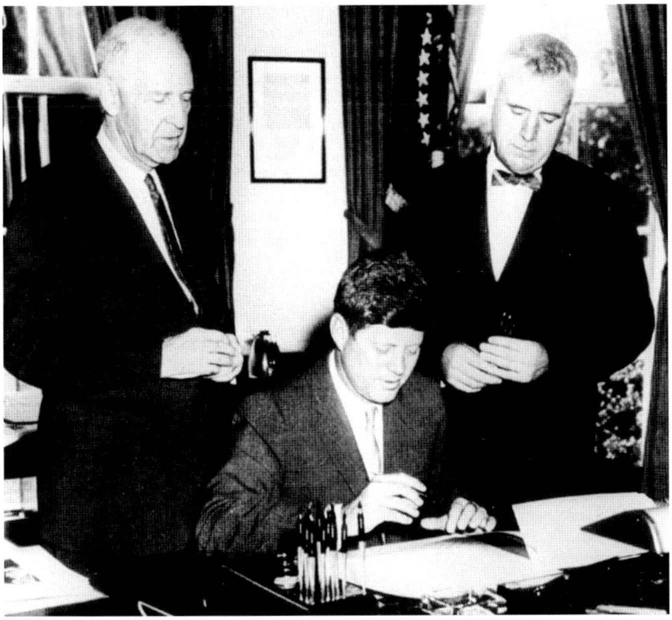

Representative John Fogarty (right), Senator Lister Hill (left), and President John F. Kennedy

Lister Hill came naturally to an interest in medical research. He was named after Joseph Lister, the father of antisepsis, and his own father was a surgeon. Early in his congressional career, Hill became known for the landmark Hill-Burton Act of 1946, which provided federal matching funds for construction and renovation of medical facilities, particularly in lower income areas.

In 1955, Hill became chair of the Subcommittee on Labor, Health, Education and Welfare Appropriations, and then chaired the Committee on Labor and Public Welfare. That is, he headed the two committees that were directly involved in deciding the annual budget for NIH. As a Senator, Hill exerted a great deal of influence over health legislation; not only did he shepherd bills through the approval process, but he was in a position to make sure they were actually funded. In his study of the politics of biomedical science, Steven Strickland[4] noted that "rare is the opportunity for a single senator to be able to write legislation that launches programs and then to control the pace of their progress by insuring provision of the necessary funds." Yet that is exactly what Hill did. When he retired 14 years later, he had sponsored 60 health laws.

Hill's opposite number in the House was John Fogarty. A former bricklayer and labor leader, the origin of Fogarty's interest in medical research was less obvious than Hill's. Nevertheless, Fogarty became as scientifically and politically adept a champion as Hill in guiding bipartisan support for NIH. He chaired the House Health Appropriations Subcommittee for 18 years.

In tandem, Hill and Fogarty would hold House and Senate hearings on the NIH budget. As she had done for the hearings to establish NIH (as described in Chapter 1), Lasker mobilized expert witnesses and helped write persuasive testimony. She now achieved this through her vigorous lobbyist, Mike Gorman, a former newspaper journalist and champion of mental health. He was responsible for writing the expert testimony. Mrs. Lasker's resolute partner, Florence Mahoney, moved from Miami to Washington to sustain her own interest in NIH.

Starting in 1955, just when Hill took over the committees, the Congress-Lasker axis acquired an additional asset when James Shannon became Director of NIH. He remained in that office until 1968, the longest term of any NIH Director and probably the most influential; his were the golden years of science at NIH. Under his direction, the scientific research at NIH itself and in the extramural programs ascended to new highs. And Shannon added an important force in dealing with Congress.

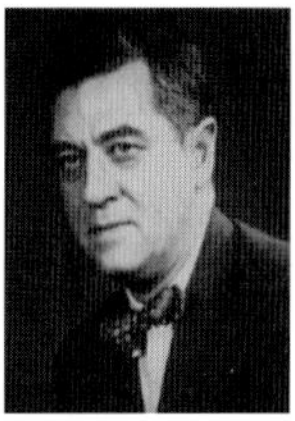

JAMES A. SHANNON, M.D., PH.D., WAS DIRECTOR OF NIH FROM 1955 TO 1968

Shannon had a distinguished research and administrative career even before he came to NIH. Born in 1904, he earned combined M.D. and Ph.D. degrees at New York University. He joined the NYU faculty and was an outstanding renal physiologist before World War II. In 1940 he was asked to head a military research program on malaria at the Goldwater Memorial Hospital in New York. There he assembled a team of brilliant young scientists, including Bernard Brodie, Sidney Udenfriend, and Julius Axelrod – who were all to play major research roles at NIH. Their malaria work was so successful that Shannon was given a Presidential Medal for Merit, the highest award at that time for civilian service in government. After the war, Shannon was Director of the Squibb Institute for Medical Research for three years. He moved to the National Heart Institute, then served as Associate Director of NIH from 1952 to 1955, before assuming leadership.

Shannon had many attributes that made him a natural leader. One was his ability to pick talent. He demonstrated that at Goldwater in choosing investigators. He then reassembled almost all of them at NIH and added new ones. Many of his recruits in different NIH institutes became famous themselves. Under his leadership, NIH flourished and grew rapidly. Fortunately for NIH, Shannon was also politically astute. Part of NIH's success stemmed from the Director's ability to work with Mary Lasker, Florence Mahoney, and their team of Gorman and physician experts. Like Lasker, Shannon also developed a close relationship with Senator Hill and Representative Fogarty.

Shannon, Lasker, and their allies prepared for congressional testimony. They were aided by Hill and Fogarty who surmounted the stricture that Institute Directors are members of the Executive Branch of the government and are expected to support – even defend – the President's budget. But Hill and Fogarty had no such limitations and would repeatedly ask the question: What would you do if we gave you more money? The testifying Director usually could take that clue and come up with sensible research proposals.

Shannon, Fogarty, and Hill, along with Mary Lasker, cooperated to orchestrate support for the budget, which increased by more than tenfold during the decade from 1955 to 1965.

Adding Stroke to the Institute's Name

Lasker became more impatient in 1962 when Joseph P. Kennedy, father of President John Kennedy, had a stroke. Mary Lasker contacted the President. She recalled:[5]

> ...strokes had always been overlooked by both the institute for neurology and blindness and the National Heart Institute. Cancer, heart disease, and strokes now cause 71 percent of all deaths in the U.S. I was really quite desperate about it, and I felt that, as I had had to do with the establishment of both [the Heart and Neurology Institutes]...
>
> I found that, somehow or another, stroke, which is a hardening of the arteries in the brain, mostly—sometimes hemorrhage, but mostly hardening of the arteries of the brain or of the carotid artery of the vein—was really being overlooked, and stroke victims, which both my parents had been, too, had really little help. Whether you recovered or not was really largely by chance. And I realized the President must be very frustrated by his father's illness, too. So in the early summer of '62, I finally got an appointment to see him....
>
> He looked very lively and very alert, and he always picked up everything that you said so quickly that it was a joy. I said, "I know what frustration you must have had finding that your father couldn't be really substantially helped through this struggle. And I want to tell you that this is a general thing for people, and that practically nothing is being done about it, and I think it would be wonderful if you would appoint a presidential commission on strokes." And he said, "Well, that sounds like a good idea. What do we do about it?"[6]

According to Mrs. Lasker, however, Theodore Sorensen, the President's counsel, had other ideas about the need for a presidential commission on stroke: She quoted him as saying:

> "Oh, we mustn't have any more commissions on any disease that affects the President's family because we've got a commission on retardation. So we shouldn't have a commission on strokes." Well, this dashed me terribly because I realized that, you know, this is just one point of view. And I really didn't know what to do.

> This all evolved, maybe, by July, and at the end of summer I went away for a vacation. In the early winter I came back, and I said, "Now, you know, really, we've got to do something about this because the President said he wanted it done." I remember sitting downstairs in the little dining room in the White House, and Sorensen, [Michael] Feldman, and Dr. [Sidney] Farber were there with me. Feldman said ... "Well, why don't we attach it to some other disease like cancer and heart and make it a commission on cancer, heart, and stroke?" I said, "That would be a wonderful idea. Fine, let's do it." All right, I took it up with the President; they took it up to the President; and the President said it was all right.

In Lasker's account, not much happened, despite her initiative, until she stepped in again:

> The year rolled around and it was '63, and I came again to see the President in his office. I said, "You know, Ted Sorensen and Feldman had this wonderful idea not just to have a stroke commission, but to have a commission on cancer, heart, and stroke. Don't you agree with them?" "Oh, yes," he said, "I think it's fine, and I think we should do it." He just was home from Berlin, and he was feeling very well and happy. I remember seeing a big German magazine with pictures of his triumphal visit to Berlin, probably around the first of July or so, on his sofa. And he said, "And I'll take it up with them." I said, "Fine, I'll take it up with them as soon as you have." I came back and Mike, by this time, was more interested in the thing and sort of decided, "Well, where are the papers? And who are we going to appoint? And who are they all, anyway? And who should be the chairman?" He wanted as chairman a Nobel Prize winner.
>
> Well, we fussed about the chairman quite a bit, and finally we decided that, on the whole, [Michael E.] Mike DeBakey would be the best.

The assassination of President Kennedy interrupted the process, but not for long, Lasker continued her saga:

> So I went immediately to Johnson—I went to him within 48 hours, really, I'm sure it was within 48 hours—and I said, "You know, one of the things President Kennedy was going to do was to appoint a commission on cancer, heart, and stroke." He said to me, "Don't tell me any more things the President was going to do; I've heard three hundred and fifty already." I said, "That's all very well, but this is about the main cause of death of the people in the United States. And Kennedy did promise to do this, and he was interested in it. And what's more, you're

surely interested in it, too." So he said, "Well, I guess you're right." So then he said, "Who is doing this?" And I said, "Mike Feldman." It was back on Mike Feldman again. "First," he said, "take it up with Abe Fortas." Well, I went to see Abe Fortas.

Fortas, an advisor to President Johnson and transient Supreme Court Justice, was interested, and so were others, including representatives from the American Heart Association, the American Cancer Society, and professional organizations such as the American Academy of Neurology. The President's Commission on Heart Disease, Cancer and Stroke was established in 1964, chaired by the famous heart surgeon, Michael DeBakey. The Commission report was submitted by the end of the year and President Johnson gave it high priority so that Congress passed the bill in 1965. As a result, Centers were established throughout the country for cancer, heart disease, and stroke. These Centers proved to have more of a demonstration function than one devoted to research. Authorities later doubted that they had much lasting impact on stroke theory or therapy.[7]

This episode illustrates Mrs. Lasker's access to Presidents, her boldness and perseverance, her influence with legislators, her use of expert commissions and fact-finding, her concern for particular diseases, and her desire to translate basic science into human treatments.

This episode also illustrates the tension between advocates of basic research and those who wanted immediate application. President Johnson and others wanted the fruits of basic research applied to people. Shannon and other scientists feared the premature application of incomplete knowledge. The cancer, heart, and stroke Centers raised awareness of the problems of these conditions, provided care for patients, and initiated clinical trials of treatment – but no cures emerged. Nevertheless, some of the Centers did clinical research in epidemiology and participated in therapeutic trials.

Naturally, however, there was criticism of the program from the outset. Some[8] questioned the expenditure on diseases of the elderly rather than the young, a view that seems to have disappeared soon thereafter, once the Aging Institute was established.

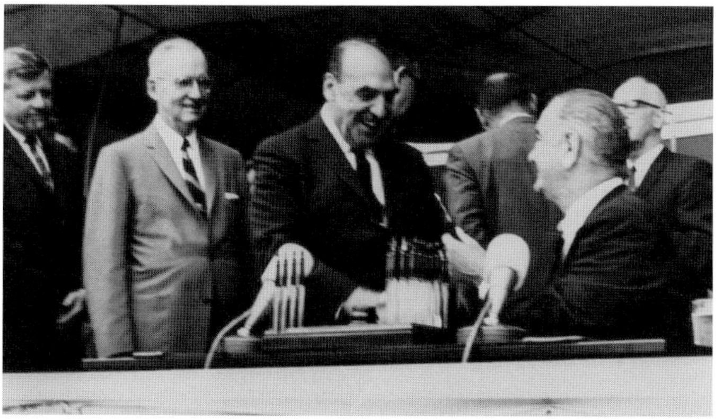

(from left) Luther Terry, M.D., Senator Lister Hill, and HEW Secretary Anthony Celebrezze greet President Lyndon B. Johnson during LBJ's visit to NIH in 1965

The tension between basic and applied research was manifest in other ways. Shannon had a bedrock belief in the importance of basic science and was distressed by what he perceived as a disease-of-the-month approach. Mary Lasker yearned for the swift application of scientific findings to therapeutic treatments. She found a natural ally in President Lyndon Johnson.

The differences between Shannon and Lasker became profound. For example, Shannon failed to credit Lasker in 1967 when he reviewed the 20-year history of NIH.[9] He paid homage to Hill, Fogarty, and Leonard A. Scheele, the Surgeon General who had appointed Shannon, but he did not even mention Mary Lasker.

The split between the Director and Lasker was only the first crack in the alliance. More trouble was yet to come. Fogarty died of a myocardial infarction in January 1967. The key NIH supporters, Lyndon Johnson and Lister Hill, both declined to run for re-election in 1968; Hill out of concern for his wife, who had developed parkinsonism. Shannon himself retired in 1968. Three of the four driving forces – NIH Director, Senator, and Representative – were gone, and Mary Lasker seemed to have lost her interest in stroke. The alliance that had done so much to build funding for NINDS fell apart.

After Hill and Fogarty left the scene, Senator Hill's committee chairs went to two research-supporting senior senators, Edward Kennedy and Warren Magnuson. However, the Nixon administration set a new tone of fiscal conservatism and a less favorable view toward research in general and NIH in particular. Shannon considered the years between 1967 and 1970 a time of "progressive constraints."[10] For some time the budgetary process was "chaotic," with "Presidential vetoes, overrides by Congress, proposed rescission of funds allocated, acceptance or rejection of these rescissions by Congress, impoundment of appropriations, and their later release by court action."

Subsequently, however, there came a long line of representatives and senators who became heroes at NIH and some saw their names emblazoned on campus buildings. In the House, Paul Rogers and John Porter were outstanding. In the Senate, Lowell Weicker, Mark Hatfield, Edward Kennedy, William Natcher, Thomas Harkin, and Arlen Specter became prominent supporters. Funding of NIH again ascended.

All institutes, including NINDS, shared the upward surge in appropriations for all NIH. But scrutiny by Congressional committees followed, as accountability became the operative word. The increases often did not exceed the rate of inflation. NIH officials and administrators during the 70s and 80s were constantly concerned about making ends meet, and they were not always sure they could meet commitments for grant awards. As recently as 1995, Harold Varmus, then Director of NIH, wrote about the impending steady state of the budgets.[11] He assumed that the era of constant increases would cease and that investigators could not expect increases ad infinitum. Scientists would have to live within a fixed budget (even though scientific opportunities were accelerating and more scientists were completing their training each year.)

But a few years later, Congressional friends responded to pressure from the voluntaries and professional organizations, which emphasized the enormous advances of the 1990s. Senators Arlen Specter and Tom Harkin successfully led the movement to double the NIH budget in five years. Their efforts took root and annual increases of 15 percent or more followed. The millennium was the second year of the road to doubling.

The latest increase has had its effect already. Investigator-initiated awards have always been protected to the extent possible, but with funds available now, requests for proposals (RFPs) give NINDS the opportunity to define research agendas with experts and advocates, and then to set aside money to initiate new programs. Nevertheless, in his analysis of the state of biomedical research, Shannon noted several problems that have persisted up to the present time, and which affect NINDS. One of the most serious has been the lack of integration between medical education and research in medical schools. This has tilted schools from teaching to research, with no reliably continuing renewal of clinical investigators.[12] This failure extended to the construction of new facilities, which have supported research but not buildings for education.

Shannon was also concerned about the budgetary process, which sometimes proceeded without participation of NIH except in reaction to proposals from the Executive Branch and the Bureau of the Budget. That pattern has persisted but became less of a problem when NIH budgets rose at the millennium. The question now is what will happen in future budgets. How long will the biomedical research expansion continue at NIH and in the universities where the research is carried out?

The tensions between those who favor more fundamental research and those who want immediate application are likely to persist. As important as Mrs. Lasker was to development of NINDS and other institutes, so she is still a somewhat controversial figure. The authoritative medical writer, Jerome Groopman, blames her for the "War on Cancer" of the 70s, which he now considers to have been an unmitigated disaster.[3] Sic transit gloria.

1 Wyngaarden JB. The National Institutes of Health in its centennial year. *Science* 1987;237:869-874, citing I.F., *Stone, Polemics and Prophecies 1967-1970*. New York: Random House, 1971.

2 Spingarn ND. *Heartbeat: The Politics of Health Research*. Washington-New York: Robert B. Luce, Inc.; 1976.

3 Groopman J. Annals of Medicine: the thirty years' war. *The New Yorker*, June 4, 2001:52-63.

4 Strickland SP. *Politics, Science and Dread Disease: A Short History of United States Medical Research Policy*. Cambridge, Mass.: Harvard University Press, 1972: 96.

5 *The Reminiscences of Mary Lasker* (April 16, 1966) in the Oral History Collection of Columbia University, New York; Series 1 (1965), pp. 14-17.

6 *Reminiscences of Mary Lasker*. Series 1 (1965), pp. 14-17.

7 Walker M. Interview with author, August 10, 2000; Marler J. Interview with author, April 25, 2000; and Tower DB. Interview with author, July 19, 2000.

8 Drew E. The health syndicate. *Atlantic Monthly*, December 1967:75-82.

9 Shannon JA. The advancement of medical research: a twenty-year view of the role of the National Institutes of Health. *J Med Edu* 1967;42:97-108.

10 Shannon JA. Federal support of biomedical sciences: development and academic impact. *J Med Edu* 1976;51:1-98.

11 Varmus H. Shattuck lecture: biomedical research enters the steady state. *N Engl J Med* 1995;333:811-815.

12 Seldin D. The intimate coupling of biomedical science and physician education. *Clin Res* 1975;23:280-286.

CELEBRATING 50 YEARS OF BRAIN RESEARCH

50th ANNIVERSARY

SECTION 2

CHAPTER FOUR

DIRECTORS OF NINDS

1951–1959	Pearce Bailey, M.D.
1959–1968	Richard L. Masland, M.D.
1968–1973	Edward F. MacNichol, Jr., M.D.
1973–	Robert Q. Marston, M.D., Acting
1973–1981	Donald B. Tower, M.D., Ph.D.
1981–1993	Murray Goldstein, D.O., M.P.H.
1993–1994	Patricia A. Grady, Ph.D., Acting
1994–1997	Zach W. Hall, Ph.D.
1997–1998	Audrey S. Penn, M.D., Acting
1998–2001	Gerald D. Fischbach, M.D.
2001–	Audrey S. Penn, M.D., Acting

Pearce Bailey, M.D.

Pearce Bailey was the founding director of NINDB and played a major role in setting the legislation. He had been Chief of Neurology for the Veterans Administration, an experience that proved to be important when NINDB established training and research programs throughout the country. Most medical schools used the funds to link training in both research and clinical neurology. VA hospitals were attached to universities and were also integrated into the program.

Bailey had another connection that proved invaluable in resolving one of his first challenges. "The voluntary health agencies backing the Institute during those early austerity years," wrote Bailey in his history of the Institute, "made a splintered and disjointed presentation to the members of the Congressional Appropriations Committee."[1] At the time he became Director of NINDB, he was also President of the American Academy of Neurology. He was therefore in a position to respond to prodding from Senator Lister Hill [Ala.], who asked him if there was a national organization of patient-advocates to assist him in setting priorities. He acknowledged there was no such organization.

Bailey's response was to call a meeting in July 1952, in which the energetic neurologist A.B. Baker of the University of Minnesota became chairman of the new National Committee for Research in

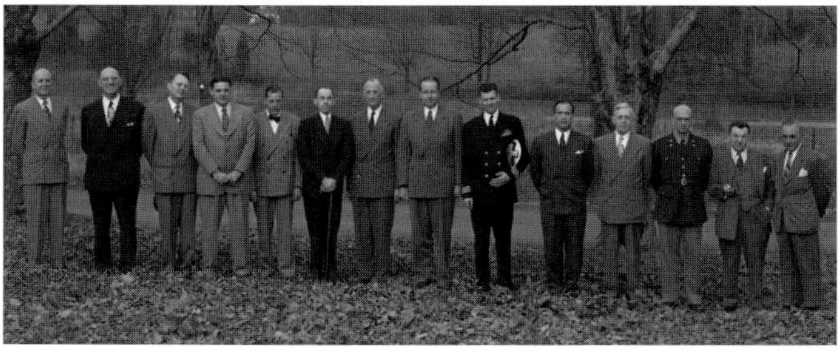

PEARCE BAILEY, M.D. (FIFTH FROM LEFT) WITH THE FIRST NINDB ADVISORY COUNCIL

Neurological Disorders. Baker continued in that position until 1970, when he was succeeded by Paul C. Bucy, a Chicago neurosurgeon and an equally determined champion of training and research. The Committee effectively linked professional and voluntary organizations for four decades. Over the years, a number of persons served as the Committee's Executive Director; Lawrence Hoffheimer, a Washington lawyer, became its last executive director in 1977 and served until the Committee ended sometime in the 1990s.

Bailey started the NINDB extramural grants programs. He also instituted field investigations for retrolental fibroplasia (identifying the cause as the exposure of low birth weight babies to excess oxygen), the geographic distribution of multiple sclerosis (directed by Leonard Kurland, chief of the Epidemiology Branch from 1955 to 1964), and the Western Pacific projects of Carleton Gajdusek. From the very start, Bailey appreciated the problem of mental retardation and cerebral palsy originating in the perinatal period. He determined to establish research in that area but it was not until Richard Masland was recruited to lead the perinatal program in 1958 that the pilot studies began in 1959. One indirect outcome of the perinatal project was documentation of the paucity of pediatric neurologists and the need to train more of them.

When Bailey's tenure as director ended in 1959, he transferred to an international NINDB program with offices in Belgium. In 1962 he became special assistant to William Windle, the director of an NINDB Primate Center in Puerto Rico and held that position until he retired in 1971. Bailey died in 1976.

Richard L. Masland, M.D.

Richard Masland became Director of NINDB in 1959 and served until 1968. The perinatal project became controversial and commanded much of his time,[2] but there were positive aspects. He gave Carleton Gajdusek and Joseph Gibbs their appointments in NINDB, sponsoring the field program that culminated in Gajdusek's Nobel prize-winning investigation of the devastating neurological disease of *kuru* in New Guinea.

Originally, Masland had proposed the use of the primate center in Puerto Rico for Gajdusek's and Gibbs' animal experiments with kuru and the related sheep disease of scrapie, but Joseph Smadel, the NIAID Associate Director and virologist who had recommended Gajdusek's hire at NINDB, opposed this because he feared that supervision of the animals would not be close enough. Smadel advocated use of a center in Laurel, Maryland, which led to diplomatic problems with the Department of Agriculture whose officials did not want scrapie in the neighborhood of their animals. Officials in Australia also objected to plans for roaming surveys in New Guinea by Gajdusek. That these problems were solved amicably and successfully and contributed so significantly to the advancement of

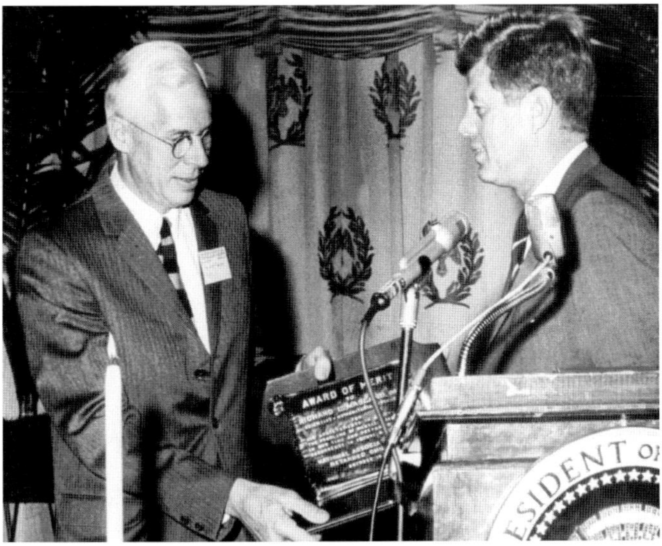

Richard L. Masland, M.D., receiving award of merit from President John F. Kennedy

science, was testament to Masland's ingenuity as well as his excellent interpersonal skills.

A pacifist Quaker, Masland nonetheless ended up in another contretemps. This one centered on John Sever, another NINDB virologist, who isolated the *rubella* (German measles) virus and prepared a vaccine – only to be challenged for priority claims by teams from Harvard University and Walter Read Army Hospital. Masland stood by Sever's side in what he called a "confrontation." All three reports were ultimately published more or less simultaneously. Sever made another major contribution in finding that vaccination for measles was commonly related to a severe encephalitis.

Masland established an epidemiology division with Leonard Kurland as chief. Kurland served from 1955 to 1964, when he left to direct epidemiology at the Mayo Clinic. In his time at NINDB, Kurland delineated the high incidence of ALS, dementia, and parkinsonism on Guam.

In 1961, NINDB established clinical research centers, first at the Albert Einstein College of Medicine at Yeshiva University, then at Columbia University. Within two years these initial outposts grew to fifteen centers and that number has continued to increase ever since, now under the rubric of program projects: teams of investigators working on related research. To the present time, there have been continuing questions about M.D.-investigators and clinical investigation, and these centers have provided practical demonstrations of the true possibilities.

To initiate a head injury program, Masland recruited William F. Caveness and, for an epilepsy program, J. Kiffin Penry. The epilepsy initiative comprised a basic science unit, epidemiology, and development of new drugs.

Ever the internationalist, Masland developed a concept of paired grants to assist neuroscientists in Poland, Yugoslavia, Romania, and other countries that needed aid. Originally, these poor countries could not pay for food they imported from the United States during World War II and after. The Department of Agriculture had set up the "PL-480" aid program to deal with the debts. Masland credits Representative John Fogarty [R.I.] with the idea of using the credits from that food program to support medical research. It was Masland's responsibility to find reliable investigators in Europe and the United States for neurology-oriented projects. NIH grants to centers in both countries facilitated the interchange, which included bidirectional travel and research cooperation.

When Milton Shy died in 1967, Masland was asked to head the neurology department at Columbia University. He accepted the invitation and served until 1973. Subsequently, he was president of the World Federation of Neurology from 1981 to 1989. At age 91, he is still vigorous.

Edward F. MacNichol, Jr., M.D.

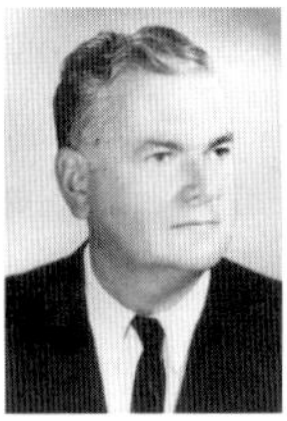

Edward F. MacNichol, Jr., M.D.

Edward MacNichol became director of NINDB in 1968, when the name of the neurology institute was changed to the National Institute of Neurological Diseases and Stroke. The name-change marked the creation of the independent National Eye Institute. Ironically, MacNichol was a biophysicist interested in vision, but he took over the Neurology Institute just as vision was leaving for its own home.

Harris[3] has described why and how the Eye Institute was formed. In the original enabling legislation for NINDB, Congress amalgamated the proposals for separate Institutes according to particular diseases. Rather than setting up numerous Institutes for neurological diseases, they gave one institute responsibility for all the different diseases of brain and nerves. The original bill made no mention of blindness. On July 10, 1950, Representative Andrew Biemiller proposed an amendment to the House bill to support research and training for blindness. The amendment was approved the same day.

In fiscal 1951, however, less than 7 percent of the NINDB budget was used for blindness and there was no intramural research on vision until 1955. The number of extramural grants on vision increased from 7 in 1951, 30 in 1952, 72 in 1954, to 84 in 1955.

In 1953, NINDB scheduled a conference on *retrolental fibroplasia*. At the time of the conference, one of the grantees reported a relationship to the use of extra oxygen in the neonatal period. A multi-center study was set up and confirmed the evidence, which was called the most outstanding discovery in ophthalmology in the fifties.

As the years went by, the Institute continued to give more attention to vision research. In 1956, 96 projects drew $1.0 million in support. A decade later, 337 projects cost $9.8 million. Nevertheless there was a feeling that vision research was not being supported adequately at NINDB.

A bill to establish an Eye Institute was prepared in 1967. Secretary of Health and Human Services, John Gardner, and his medical advisor, Philip Lee, opposed the new legislation. Additionally the Vietnam War was beginning. Nevertheless, the National Eye Institute was established in 1968 in an "eerie parallel to its parent institute," with no funding because of defense spending. Nevertheless, the new Institute has proven successful.

It is said that MacNichol was more interested in laboratory research than he was in administration, but MacNichol had to muster all the administrative skill he could during the difficult years of his directorship. He noted that his tenure marked the end of the initial "long period of NIH prosperity."[4] It was primarily a period of economizing and reevaluating existing programs. Clinical training programs were Congressionally terminated. The Puerto Rico primate center was closed. Funding of approved grants dropped below 10 percent. At a congressional hearing that established the national commission on multiple sclerosis, Representative Paul Rogers berated MacNichol because NINDS did not have anyone who served as a focus of activity for the disease. This gap was later remedied.

Yet there were achievements, too. Roscoe Brady's neurochemistry program investigating lipid related diseases was elevated to Branch status. King Engel and his associates found that prednisone was effective in the treatment of myasthenia gravis and acetazolamide prevented attacks of periodic paralysis. Creutzfeldt-Jakob disease was transmitted by inoculation into primates. The first equal employment opportunity programs were instituted. All in all, however, these years of financial insecurity may have been the most difficult time in the history of NINDS.

Donald B. Tower, M.D., Ph.D.

Donald Tower became acting director in 1973 and director of NINDS in 1974. His background was complex. In 1941, he graduated from Harvard cum laude, with a major in chemistry. He received his M.D. at Harvard in 1944 and then became a surgical intern in Minnesota. In 1945, he went on active duty in the U.S. Navy and served as a medical officer in the Philippines. In 1947, he became a research fellow in neurochemistry at the Montreal Neurological Institute, followed by a year as assistant resident in neurosurgery with Wilder Penfield. There followed more training in neurochemistry and a Ph.D. from McGill University in Montreal in 1951, after which he set up his own laboratory. In those years he was a pioneer in brain chemistry and began to investigate the biochemistry of the epileptic focus in excised brain tissue.

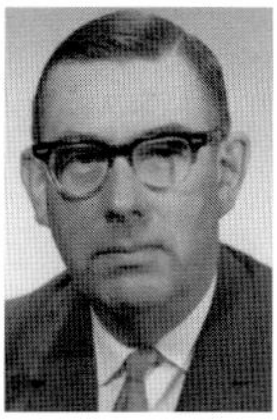

Donald B. Tower, M.D., Ph.D.

In 1953, he was offered a position at NINDB by his colleague from Montreal, Milton Shy. At first he was Chief of the Section of Clinical Neurochemistry. In 1963, he was Chief of the Laboratory of Neurochemistry. In 1967-1968 he was Acting Associate Director for Extramural Programs. Later he became NINDS Acting Director in 1973 and Director in 1974.

Fiscal austerity dominated Tower's term just as it had his predecessor. During his eight years, NINDS "kept losing money because of inflation."[5]

But that was not Tower's only problem as administrator of NINDS. He considered it his personal challenge to improve relations between NINDS and the director of NIH. He thought problems had originated because Masland had had direct relations with Congress, circumventing the chain of command, to the annoyance of NIH director Shannon and his staff. It was said that Fogarty or Hill "would call Masland directly to ask him how much he needed"[6] that year. Additionally, the NIH brass were not enamored of the perinatal project because it was considered to be too expensive and to be going in too many directions.

Tower has pointed out to the NIH that the perinatal project could not readily be terminated for administrative reasons. The staff included 300 with civil service tenure. Tower also found worthwhile features within the project

There were several changes in personnel during Tower's tenure. John Van Buren, the neurosurgeon, and Cosimo Ajmone-Marsan, in charge of the EEG division, left together for the University of Miami. Ayub Omaya, designer of a reservoir for the administration of drugs into the brain, left for private practice in neurosurgery. Tower credits Omaya with the first report of Hounsfield's development of computerized tomography (CT) in England.

DONALD TOWER WITH NINDB COUNCIL MEMBER JENNIFER JONES

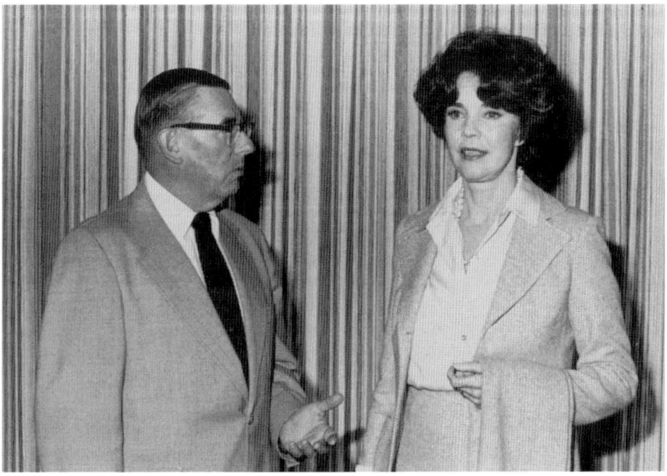

Tower considers J. Kiffin Penry's anticonvulsant drug development efforts one of the major successes of his tenure. It was a loss to the Institute when Penry moved to Bowman-Gray School of Medicine and a loss to all neurology when he died in 1996.

Gajdusek's Nobel Prize came during Tower's tenure. A national program in PET started when NINDS found itself with about 9 million unexpected dollars, enough to set up eight programs around the country. Giovanni DiChiro, head of intramural neuroradiology, provided input for that development. At the urging of Robert Katzman and Robert Terry, a workshop on Alzheimer disease led to the start of modern dementia research, with the National Institute on Aging becoming the "lead institute."

During Tower's term the Guam ALS-Dementia-Parkinson project mostly faded away. There had been a paucity of research on hearing and deafness. In 1975, therefore, the name of the neurology Institute was changed to the National Institute of Neurological and Communicative Disorders and Stroke to recognize this responsibility. Tower recruited several investigators and a national effort was made to improve cochlear implants, with particular urging from Senator Barry Goldwater.

Murray Goldstein, D.O., M.P.H.

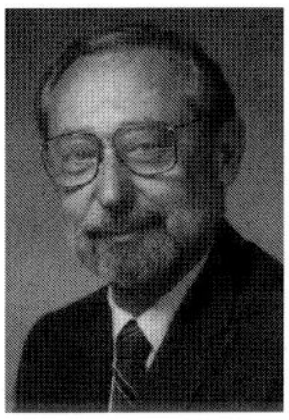

Murray Goldstein, D.O., M.P.H.

Murray Goldstein was director of NINCDS from 1982 to 1993. He had served as acting director a year earlier and, before that, as deputy director since 1978. His service at the Institute extended even farther back; he had been director of extramural programs from 1961 to 1976 and director of the stroke and trauma program from 1976 to 1978. No other head of the Institute has served as long as extramural director and few have had administrative experience comparable to Goldstein's. He was a major force in NINDS for 32 years.

Goldstein is also the only director of an institute in the history of NIH to hold an osteopathic, rather than a medical, degree. In a roundabout way, his degree was directly responsible for his appointment.

Goldstein grew up in Brooklyn and attended New York University but had to interrupt his college studies to serve in the Army from 1943 to 1946 during World War II. He returned to NYU to finish his senior year and graduated in 1947. Goldstein wanted to go to medical school but the competition from other returning veterans was fierce. A friend told him about osteopathic schools and he applied successfully to one in Des Moines. There he found that the practicing osteopaths were good teachers. He graduated and started residency training in internal medicine.

One day the president of the school told Goldstein he wanted him to take a written examination for the United States Public Health Service because no D.O. had ever been appointed as a medical officer in a federal uniformed service and he thought Goldstein could do well on the exam. Goldstein was just completing a residency in general internal medicine at the Des Moines College Hospital and performed well on licensure examinations in New York and Iowa, so he did not mind taking one more. Soon he was invited by the Surgeon General to come to Washington for an interview.

Immediately on arrival, he was ushered into the office of James Shannon, then head of the intramural program of NIH, but not yet Director of NIH. He asked: "Goldstein, how much experience have you had in research?" The reply came swiftly: "Absolutely none sir." They discussed Goldstein's interest in hypertension and Shannon referred him to a research lab, but since the lab had no space for another fellow, Shannon offered Goldstein a position within the extramural grants program.

When Goldstein returned to Iowa, the president of the school explained the real story behind why he had been sent to Bethesda. As the president explained it, the American Medical Association (AMA) still considered osteopathy a cult and blocked any attempt by a uniformed service to appoint a doctor of osteopathy (D.O.). Now the osteopaths had their opportunity with Goldstein. They had already presented Goldstein's credentials to the Secretary of Health and Human Services, Nelson Rockefeller, who had taken them to President Eisenhower. Goldstein's attributes included military service, a Silver Star medal for valor in combat, a Purple Heart medal for a war injury, and top performance on the examination. Eisenhower was said to have commented personally: "Appoint him. I will handle the AMA." "So, Murray," said the osteopathic school president, "everybody is going to be very disappointed if you walk away."

In November of 1953, Goldstein arrived in the office of Frank Yeager's NIH extramural program, to serve as the clinician on the three-person staff, covering the entire heart research program. He served in that office until 1957, when he took a year off to train in epidemiology at the University of California before he returned to NIH to work on hypertension and stroke.

The Director of the Heart Institute told Goldstein that if he was interested in stroke, he would be better off in the Neurology Institute. Richard Masland had just been installed and he referred Goldstein to Leonard Kurland, who had begun an epidemiology program. Goldstein joined NINDB and initiated a stroke epidemiology project. Then Masland induced him, first, to take charge of the perinatal project, and then, to administer the grants program for two years. In fact, Goldstein ended up heading the extramural program from 1961 to 1976.

At mid-point during that experience, in 1968, Goldstein asked for permission to work at the Mayo Clinic as a clinical resident to gain experience in neurology. He had been at the Mayo Clinic for nine months when he received a phone call from James Shannon, who had become Director of NIH. Shannon informed Goldstein that Masland was resigning to move to Columbia as chair of neurology and that his return was needed to provide some continuity and stability. By the time Goldstein returned three months later, Edward MacNichol had been appointed director of the Institute, followed five years later by Donald Tower.

In 1976, Tower reorganized the administrative structure of NINCDS and Goldstein became head of the Stroke and Trauma program, including both grants and contracts. That did not last long, however, because in 1978 Tower asked Goldstein to transfer the Stroke and Trauma program to Michael Walker so that he could be appointed as deputy director of NINDS.

When Tower retired in 1981, Goldstein became acting director of the Institute. There was some opposition to appointing him director because of his osteopathic degree, but Goldstein had the support of neurologists and neurosurgeons. He also had the support of NIH director, James Wyngaarden.

Asked about his proudest achievement as director, Goldstein cited the training programs. When NINDS started, he recalled, there were 53 training positions in the entire country. He credits A.B. Baker of Minnesota with the energetic push to develop training programs. Baker had been active in founding NINDB, had led an Institute committee on training, and had chaired the committee of voluntary agencies that worked with Congress to promote adequate budgets for NINDB.

In contrast to other Institutes at NIH, only neurology and mental health could give grant money to a department to support teachers, not just stipends for fellows. That is, they were able to build departments rather than support only individual trainees. In retrospect, this philosophy can be considered the basis for the expansion of neurology in the United States. However, this practice became an administrative difficulty for Goldstein. His first major problem was Shannon, who emphasized research and instructed both NIMH and NINDB to terminate the "clinical training programs."

Goldstein responded that "we don't have a clinical training program, we have an academic training program. All the people we train are preparing for careers in academic medicine. We don't prepare people to go out into the hinterlands, and I can show you the data... Here are our trainees and here is what they are doing now. They are the future of American academia."

Shannon said: "You can give stipends after somebody finishes their residency, or if they spin out. Then they come in for research fellowship awards." Goldstein thought Shannon was concerned with the public image. "This was a research NIH. We were not to be in clinical medicine."

NINDS compromised, "if a Fellow wanted to rotate out for a year during his residency or if the third year of his residency for what was, in fact, research, we would provide the funds. By that time, of course, the Departments had been built and were relatively strong."

But the same conflict had some serious fallout – the secession of NIMH. In Goldstein's words, Shannon "was dedicated to getting clinical activities of any kind out of NIH. Which is why the National Institute of Mental Health left NIH. Bob Felix was Director of NIMH, took NIMH out of NIH. It left this organization, physically and legally." Years later, NIMH returned to NIH.

Goldstein's second major problem was the competition between advocacy groups to earmark funds for specific diseases or conditions. When the Institute was small, Congress did not pay much attention to individual programs. When the budget passed $500 million, however, scrutiny became more intense. As it did so, the coalition of voluntary agencies each became more protective of its own field – multiple sclerosis, stroke, or head injury. Leadership of the National Committee for Research in Neurological Disorders (the organization that had done so much in the past to unify and empower the efforts of the advocacy groups) had passed from Abe Baker and Paul Bucy to officers of the individual groups. So Goldstein had to spend time with each of the organized coalitions to convince them that presenting a unified front was better for the advancement of their own cause than turf wars that wasted time and effort. Goldstein thought earmarking was a terrible idea. He said he "fought that battle right until the day I retired."

He argued that neurology was visible and neuroscience was exploding. People were paying attention. "We weren't just one of those Institutes any longer. And the organized patient groups were getting more and more powerful. And more independent of each other; and going their own way. They said 'We want money for spinal cord injury.' I tried to finesse that into what we need is money for trauma of the nervous system, whether it is head injury or spinal cord. We are looking at the same problem, how the nervous system reacts to injury, what neuroprotective agents can do during the acute period and restitution of function after injury. Whether it is the brain or the spinal cord, it is just a model. I fought, and fought. That was my second biggest problem."

His third problem was internal – "how to keep the Institute from splitting up into little pieces of earmarked dollars. I had a stroke and trauma program, a degenerative disease program, and an epilepsy program." Each one had a director. He was grateful to Jack Brinley, Mike Walker, Gene Streicher, and Carl Leventhal, but had to keep them from competing with each other for money. Weekly staff meetings were effective in keeping them together.

Another concern was problem number four: the spin-off of both the Eye and the Ear Institutes. Although vision research had proceeded apace in NINDB, ophthalmologists did not want to be in an institute run by neurologists. Stroke became part of the name in 1968, when vision left NINDB and communicative disorders became part of the institutional name. At that time stroke was also added to the title because, as Goldstein put it, Mary Lasker "spun it right in. It was one of the last things Mary Lasker did in a real political sense. We needed a stroke identify and she did it." Stroke has remained part of the name ever since. Communicative disorders was dropped when hearing developed its own institute in 1988.

Goldstein also had to manage the boycott of NINDB by neurosurgeons led by the renowned and highly respected Henry Schwartz, head of neurosurgery at Washington University in St. Louis, who, according to Goldstein, thought that "once neurosurgery became dependent on government money, government would control neurosurgery. In a very nice, open, non-hostile way, Henry fought that battle all along. The opposite of Henry," said Goldstein, "was Arthur Ward at the University of Washington in Seattle who was all for government support of medical research training."

Goldstein worked persistently with the neurosurgical community, meeting with their leaders, adding some to the NINDS Council. He was even elected an honorary member of a major neurosurgical society.

The Decade of the Brain initiative was a particular challenge during Goldstein's tenure. The concept and the label originated in one of Goldstein's staff sessions with Leventhal, Walker, and Brinley. Representative Silvio O. Conte of Massachusetts, who had been contacted by Goldstein, picked it up. Despite a lack of harmony with NIMH in planning and implementing the idea, program projects were implemented to propel basic and clinical neurosciences forward into the future with spectacular results.

In the initial years, sizeable additional funds were appropriated to the NINDS, leading to new initiatives such as the establishment of the nationwide program of PET centers and the development of the clinical trials program.

In addition, Goldstein brought clinical trials into neurology and neurosurgery. Neurology began to focus on therapeutic trials and neurosurgery divided into subspecialties as techniques evolved. Thanks to Goldstein's cooperation, there are now tumor neurosurgeons, spine neurosurgeons, base-of-the-skull neurosurgeons, vascular surgeons, pain neurosurgeons, and functional neurosurgeons (for implanting stimulating devices or for recording electric activity during treatment for movement disorders and epilepsy).

The matter of paying for clinical trials was a critical issue that Goldstein had to face. An attempt to share costs for a surgical trial led to negotiations with the Health Care Financing Administration (HCFA) to work out a policy for Medicare reimbursement. HCFA was resistant to paying for surgery of unproven value. An evaluation had been initiated to evaluate the stroke-preventing surgical procedure. But even though the operation was being used frequently throughout the country, HCFA remained unconvinced and would not share costs.

As for the disappearance of the clinical investigator, Goldstein had experience with one aspect of the remedy. When training grants were ascendant, it was feasible for NINDS to pay salaries of the faculty and, in the process, provide stable financial support for junior faculty. At one point this was so prevalent in neurology, Goldstein quipped, there were two kinds of universities in the United States – state schools and federal schools.

Basic neuroscientists could benefit from a similar program, and Goldstein would have it incorporate teaching because longstanding opposition from the AMA made it impossible for NIH or any other federal agency to provide direct aid to medical schools, including construction of facilities.

In 1993, after 40 years of service at NIH and 33 at NINDS, Murray Goldstein retired to become medical director and chief operating officer of the United Cerebral Palsy Research and Educational Foundation. He is still involved in stimulating fundamental neuroscience and developmental neurobiology with the goal of ameliorating or preventing human disability.

Patricia A. Grady, Ph.D.

Patricia Grady became Acting Director of the Institute in 1993 when Goldstein retired. She was the first woman and the first former nurse to be a director of NINDS. She received her diploma in nursing at Hartford in 1964, taught at the University of Maryland School of Nursing for twenty years and, in the process, gained a Ph.D. in cerebrovascular research. Her association with NINDS started in 1988 when she became a health scientist administrator in the division of stroke and trauma. In 1992, she was appointed assistant director of the Institute, then acting director and, after the arrival of Zach Hall, deputy director. By that time her multitalented experience made her the ideal choice to head the newly created National Institute of Nursing Research in 1995, a position she still holds.

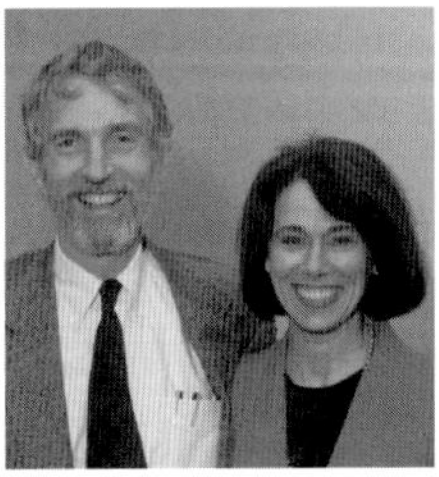

Zach W. Hall, Ph.D., and Patricia A. Grady, Ph.D.

Zach W. Hall, Ph.D.

Zach Hall was the first among the directors in three critical characteristics. He was the first director of NINDS since Pearce Bailey who had not matured within the Institute. He was also the first director who did not have a medical degree, and the first DNA-era molecular neuroscientist.

Hall came from Atlanta. He received his B.A. in English at Yale in 1958, and then registered in the medical school at Emory. His instincts led him to research and his career was determined by a summer course at the Marine Biological Laboratories in Woods Hole, Massachusetts. He was not only persuaded by the science he experienced there, but he also became friends with Ed Fuhrspan, one of the original members of the new neurobiology department led by Stephen Kuffler at Harvard. Hall became their first graduate student and received his Ph.D. in 1966. His next experience, as a postdoctoral fellow at Stanford, was equally exhilarating. Hall returned to Harvard for a faculty position in Physiology in 1968 and became known for his research on the neuromuscular junction. In 1976 he was recruited to become Chair of Physiology at the University of California in San Francisco.

At UCSF, Hall became an adroit administrator as well as a scientist. In addition to the Physiology Department, he headed the graduate programs in neuroscience and biomedical sciences. He also became a Saturday afternoon runner and, by chance, his partner was Harold Varmus. The two shared scientific as well as athletic interests. Soon after Varmus became the director of NIH, Goldstein retired as NINDS director and a search committee was established to fill the vacancy. Independently of Varmus, but also surely welcomed by him, the committee selected Hall and the pair of science leaders was reunited.

Varmus emphasized basic science over targeted research, just as Shannon had earlier. This approach suited Zach Hall, too, as he tried to invigorate the intramural program. Coming from a university, he was concerned that the appointment process and tenure system at NINDS had become ingrown. In a university, there is ongoing renewal as new positions are subject to search committees and tenure appointments are scrutinized with zealous care – sometimes too zealous, according to critics. At NINDS, Hall found, appointments were often made to foster the research of a branch chief and then, after years of service, the investigators would be given tenure because they had devoted years of service, not because they were, or could be, independent investigators.

Pointing this out led to some vigorous debates with established staff. In a recent interview, Hall noted:[7] "A difficulty with the NIH system is that it is built in the European mode. The money goes to the Chiefs who then distribute it to people under them. The genius of the extramural awards program is that money goes directly to young people if they have good ideas. It is funny that what the NIH recognizes so well with its extramural hand it did not seem to recognize so well with its intramural hand." The problem was general within NIH, not particular to NINDS.

Hall's first new appointments were applauded. Story Landis came from Case-Western Reserve to be scientific director, in charge of the intramural program. Audrey Penn, an established neuroimmunologist at Columbia University, was named deputy director. Kenneth

Fischbeck was recruited from the University of Pennsylvania to head a new neurogenetics laboratory in the intramural program. Hall told Fischbeck that although he was the target of recruiters from universities throughout the country, if he came to NINDS, he could be "saved from becoming a departmental chair. There is a wonderful opportunity at NINDS if you want to do research."

Administration of the extramural program also came under scrutiny. Hall was concerned about the concentration of power in the division directors' offices and so he began to set up a system in which there would be a larger number of program directors, chosen by a national search, who would themselves be experienced investigators and not beholden to division chiefs. Hall's first new appointments made with this approach were Arlene Chiu, Alan Willard, and Gabrielle Leblanc. All of them were experienced lab scientists.

In addition to the tensions that arose from attempts to reorganize the programs, Hall's era was one of "austere budgets." This led to conflicts between the need to do basic research and the need to support researchers whose research problems were more immediate or closer to significant findings. Hall was faced with the archetypal top-down versus bottom-up quandary. "Some problems are ripe for solution," he explained, "and some are not ready, no matter how much money you pour in." Which doesn't necessarily mean they should not be supported. "Science is unpredictable," said Hall. "We don't know where our next help is going to come from."

As an example, Hall cited the late Senator William Proxmire, who gave bogus Congressional Awards for those who wasted public money on "the most ridiculous research grants. You could almost hear him chuckle: 'Can you imagine spending money for an award to study the sex life of bacteria?' But what Proxmire failed to note [in this case] was if that research by Joshua Lederberg had not been done fifty years ago, there would have been no Human Genome Project."

But Hall's concerns were not restricted to basic research. He knew that NINDS and its researchers couldn't simply "turn our backs on people who are sick. Five hundred thousand people in the United States have a stroke every year. You cannot simply walk away and say there is nothing we can do. You have an obligation to try to help."

"Even if there is not a really good new idea in the field, we are going to spend some money here and help. [But] If you do only that, you are going to get only better and better iron lungs. You are not going to find out the real cause or effective prevention. The place that this came up – more than anything else when I was there – was Parkinson disease. That brings us to patient advocacy and the whole politics of science – what biomedical research is supported by the public and we have a responsibility to the public, not just future generations, but to those who are here, now. I was enormously impressed by the patient advocacy groups."

Hall's three years as Director had a lasting impact on the Institute. His time would undoubtedly have continued had it not been for family and other considerations that lured him back to San Francisco, where he became Associate Dean in 1997 and then, the next year, Vice Chancellor for Research at UCSF.

Audrey S. Penn, M.D.

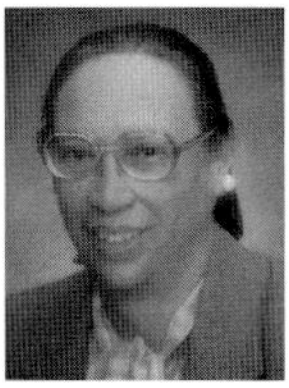

Audrey S. Penn, M.D.

Audrey Penn became Acting Director when Hall left. She grew up in New York City, received her B.A. from Swarthmore College and her M.D. from Columbia. She interned at the Bronx Municipal Hospital Center of the Albert Einstein College of Medicine of Yeshiva University and returned to Columbia for training in neurology. With postdoctoral training, she became a skilled investigator in the biochemistry and immunology of human muscle diseases, especially muscular dystrophies – diseases that lead to the excretion of myoglobin in the urine – and myasthenia gravis. (Myoglobin is the protein that imparts a red color to muscle or steak; when muscle is severely affected by disease, the pigment is released into the blood and thence into the urine. Myasthenia gravis is a disease in which there is a failure of messages from nerve to muscle; it is probably the best understood of all human autoimmune diseases.)

One of Dr. Penn's special interests was how therapeutic drugs could induce an autoimmune disease; for instance, a drug called penicillamine had been used to treat collagen-vascular diseases but some patients developed myasthenia gravis while using the drug which disappeared when the drug was stopped.

For 13 years before she came to NINDS, Dr. Penn had been a Professor of Neurology at Columbia University. In 1995, she was recruited by Zach Hall as a model clinical scientist to become Deputy Director of NINDS. That position had become open when Dr. Grady was appointed Director of the Nursing Institute.

As a public servant, Dr. Penn had been a member of the Board of Managers of Swarthmore, a member of the Council on the Education of Women at Yale, chair of international meetings on myasthenia, chair of the Review Panel for Research Training Fellowships for Medical Students of the Howard Hughes Medical Institute, President of the American Neurological Association, and a member of the Council of NINDS. In many of these positions, Dr. Penn was the first woman, the first African American, or both. The combination of clinical, research, and administrative experience made her an ideal choice for leadership at NINDS.

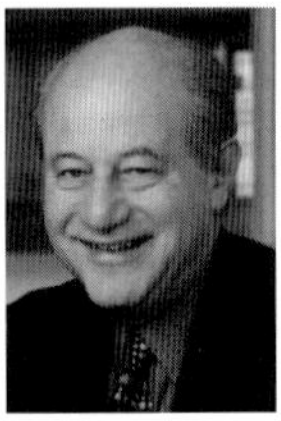

Gerald D.
Fischbach, M.D.

Gerald D. Fischbach, M.D.

Gerry Fischbach became the seventh director of NINDS in 1998. His interests in molecular neuroscience and the neuromuscular junction were much like Hall's and he also had a distinguished academic record. At Colgate College, he had aimed for medicine, which he considered an avenue to biological research.[8] Fischbach then attended Cornell for medical school and took advantage of an NIH fellowship for research midway in the curriculum.

At Cornell, Fischbach worked with Walter Riker and learned the tools of the trade sufficiently well to win a prize for the best research by a student. By the time he graduated, he was set for a research career but instead interned in medicine at the University of Washington in Seattle. He came to NIH in 1966 to work in the NINDB spinal cord section headed by Karl Frank with assistance from Wade Marshall's laboratory of neurophysiobiology at NIMH.

Fischbach enjoyed the research environment and kept postponing a return to neurological residency. After eight years of spinal cord and motor neuron research, he finally abandoned any thoughts he had about clinical practice in favor of neuroscience research. He moved to Harvard Medical School where he spent seven years in the Pharmacology Department. In 1981 he moved to Washington University in St. Louis, where he chaired the Department of Anatomy and Neurobiology for ten years. There his scientific productivity continued and he also became attracted to administration, creating a stimulating environment for investigators and making strategic recruitments. In 1990, personal reasons led him to accept the Chair of Neurobiology at Harvard, including a university-wide project on Mind, Brain, and Behavior.

In 1998, Fischbach was asked to become director of NINDS. He had been happy in Boston but he was lured by the "sense of renewal at NIH. Harold Varmus had done a magnificent job in bringing science to the forefront of the institutes' goals." Fischbach said. "I felt that neuroscience should have a tremendously prominent role in that, and that the fields of neuroscience and neurology had evolved so that there were many exciting new ventures that could be undertaken."

Although Fischbach did not know it when he accepted the position, the financial status of NINDS was about to change. Instead of the traditional, almost level, funding, annual increases of 15 percent or more were in the offing, making it "possible not just to think about the advances of neuroscience but to try and do something about it."

Fischbach acted on the belief that applying advances in basic science to treatments for neurological disorders and diseases would be the biggest challenge in the neurosciences. The excitement about stem cell research was revolutionary. Having additional funds made it possible for NINDS to be a facilitator, not just a funder. Through program announcements or requests for applications or contracts, Fischbach believed that the institute could call for research in areas that the staff and extramural advisors thought were either particularly opportune or particularly needy, or on the verge of a breakthrough.

Fischbach also sensed that the Institute could not only steer research but also set standards through conferences and workshops. Additional money raised the funding level from the traditional 15 percent of approved grants to 35 percent, making it possible to steer the direction of research projects without jeopardizing investigator-initiated research.

Fischbach had strong feelings about the intramural program, thinking it shouldn't be "just another neuroscience department or just another neurology department." Fischbach thought there were unique things that could be done at NINDS that were translationally oriented or mission-oriented research, but along very broad themes, and not necessarily pinpointed to one disease.

Fischbach made several other contributions to the evolution of NINDS as a research institution. First, he continued the hiring of scientist program directors for the extramural program, and grouped the programs into overlapping clusters: Neurodegeneration, Systems and Cognitive Neuroscience, Channels, Synapses and Circuits, Repair and Plasticity, Neural Environment, Neurogenetics, Special Programs, Clinical Trials, Technology Development, and a Scientific Review Branch.

Fischbach also made intense efforts to interact with the voluntary agencies by organizing workshops that could be organized by NINDS staff members with consultants from the voluntary agencies and interested universities. These workshops brought together experts to discuss research opportunities and obstacles, hammering out requests for proposals for investigator-initiated research or program projects.[9] Neurodegenerative diseases, epilepsy, and stroke benefited greatly from this approach.

Fischbach worked closely with scientific director Story Landis to bolster the intramural basic science program. He enticed Guy McKhann, the former chair of neurology at Johns Hopkins University, to review and invigorate clinical intramural research.

Fischbach also tackled the problem of the disappearing clinical investigator as described in the section on training (Chapter 8). A major concern of his is the late age at which neuroscientists finish their training, because new ideas are often the attributes of young investigators.

Fischbach worked closely with Steven Hyman, Director of NIMH, and other Institute Directors to conceive a new National

Neuroscience Center on the campus. This new building will house neuroscientists from any NIH institute in a way that will foster interaction and collaboration.

In less than three years, Fischbach restored a sense of renewal within the Institute that encompassed both intramural and extramural affairs. Fischbach had done such a good job that, in the spring of 2000, Donna Shalala, Secretary of Health and Human Services, announced her support for him as the candidate to replace Harold Varmus as director of NIH. His nomination, however, fell by the wayside because of the inherent uncertainties of a presidential election year. In February 2001, Fischbach left NINDS to become Columbia University's Vice-President for Health and Biomedical Sciences, Dean of the Faculty of Health Sciences, and Dean of the Faculty of Medicine.

Once again, Audrey Penn became Acting Director of NINDS and a search committee was established to find a new director. At a time of unparalleled promise for neuroscience research, the leader of NINDS will have more opportunities than ever before.

1 Bailey P. National Institute of Neurological Diseases and Blindness: origins, founding, and early years (1950–1959). In Brady RO, ed. *The Basic Neurosciences*. vol. 1 of Tower DB. *The Nervous System: A Three-Volume Work Commemorating the 25th Anniversary of the National Institute of Neurological and Communicative Disorders and Stroke*. New York: Raven Press,1975: xxi-xxxii.

2 Masland RL. National Institute of Neurological Diseases and Blindness: development and growth (1960–1968). In Tower DB, ed. *The Basic Neurosciences*: xxxiii-lii.

3 Harris RR. A Brief History of the National Eye Institute. *Govt Publications Rev* 1985;12:427-448.

4 MacNichol EF, Jr. National Institute of Neurological Diseases and Stroke (1968–1973). In Brady RO, ed. *The Basic Neurosciences*: xlvii-lii.

5 Tower, DB. Interview with author, July 19, 2000.

6 Tower, DB. Interview with author, July 19, 2000.

7 Hall, Z. Interview with author, May 4, 2000.

8 Fischbach, G. Interview with author, April 21, 2001.

9 Fischbach also brought in voluntaries and outside scientists to discuss the institute's efforts to plan programs and set priorities.

CHAPTER FIVE

THE SCIENTIFIC DIRECTORS

From the time NINDS commenced, a scientist has been in charge of the institute's intramural research program. Sometimes, responsibilities were split between a clinical and a basic science chief; at other times, one was fully in charge of both divisions. From 1951 until 1974, there were eight scientific directors. Since 1974, there have been only three. The views and actions of these three modern scientific directors have differed, partly because times change, and partly because they differ in their personal ideas about how the intramural program should be organized.

Thomas N. Chase, M.D.

Thomas Chase was first of the three modern scientific directors, and a neurologist with a deep and abiding interest in neurotherapeutics. He grew up in the environs of New York City, expressed an early interest in science, and was an undergraduate student at the Massachusetts Institute of Technology. He decided later to prepare for medicine, which he did at Columbia University.

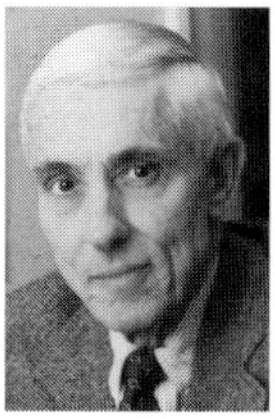

THOMAS N. CHASE, M.D., WAS THE FIRST SCIENTIFIC DIRECTOR AT NINDB

Chase then went to Yale Medical School and had his neurological training at the Massachusetts General Hospital with Raymond D. Adams. Once, in a hallway meeting, Adams asked Chase about his plans for the future. Chase replied that neurology was bereft of effective drug therapy; he wanted to do that kind of research. Adams advised him to try NIH.

Chase had just heard Kety give a lecture at Harvard on tricyclic drugs. Before long, in 1966, Chase spoke to Seymour Kety and was assigned to Irwin Kopin's laboratory. After a few years in the laboratory he felt the yen of a clinician for patient-oriented research and he was allowed a few NIMH beds in the Clinical Center. His clinical service and laboratory operation grew together.[1]

One day in 1974, NINDS director Donald Tower phoned Chase to ask if he would consider being the NINDS's scientific director. Chase again expressed his view that the dearth of neurotherapeutics was a major problem for neurology. He thought drug therapy for epilepsy was moving along, but Alzheimer and Parkinson diseases were being ignored.

Tower made the opportunity more attractive. If Chase took on the administrative role, he could also make 12 staff appointments to set up an Alzheimer-Parkinson disease research program. With that assurance, Chase moved from NIMH to NINDS.

Chase's life as scientific director naturally focused on his own research. He covered a broad range, delineating the changes in monoamine blood and cerebrospinal fluid levels when patients were treated with levodopa. With that information he could modify the timing of dosage or make dietary adjustments to optimize treatment. He reported the first case of a condition that differed from parkinsonism clinically but also improved with levodopa treatment ("dopa-responsive dystonia"). The eponym for that disease is "Segawa syndrome," named after the neurologist, Masaya Segawa, who studied it thoroughly.

Chase was one of the first researchers to use PET to delineate brain abnormalities in Alzheimer disease and Tourette syndrome. He documented the use of prolonged-acting preparations of levodopa, including slow-release forms and combinations with drugs that inhibit the enzymes terminating the action of levodopa. He developed clinical trials to evaluate 21 new drugs for neurodegenerative diseases. Now he uses the methods of molecular biology to study mechanisms of cell death in neurodegenerative diseases, aiming to develop therapeutic interventions. Chase also conducts therapeutic trials in Alzheimer and Parkinson diseases.

As scientific director, Chase sponsored large meetings of investigators to encourage research where there had been almost none. For instance, he organized one on Huntington disease in 1972, at a time when most thought there was almost no worthwhile research going on. By the time Chase and the other organizers finished scouring the world for participants, however, they had 100 speakers. He edited the proceedings, which proved to be a landmark publication. There had been few literature citations to Huntington disease research before that meeting but afterward there was a sharp rise. A few years later, Chase had similar success with a meeting on Tourette syndrome.

One other result of that Huntington meeting was Chase's introduction to Nancy Wexler. He recommended her for the position of director of the Congressional Commission for the Control of Huntington's Disease and Its Consequences. Later, he was instrumental in helping her start the Lake Maracaibo field project that has done so much for the investigation of Huntington disease.

Chase considers one of his major achievements to be the expansion of NINDS – in three ways. During his tenure, the budget almost doubled, laboratory space almost doubled, and the number of investigators increased almost as much. His first new investigator, Dale McFarlin (who had been hired by Donald Tower) and putting the neuroimmunology branch together became Chase's first responsibilities.

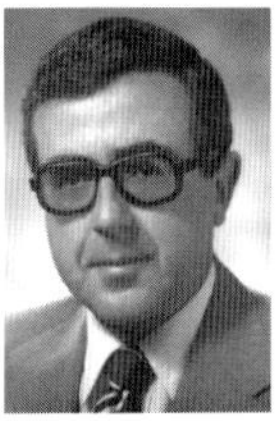

Donald Calne, M.D.

Chase was faced with reorganizing the clinical research programs.[2] Medical neurology was largely restricted to neuromuscular disease and surgical neurology to temporal lobe epilepsy. To add to these programs, Chase hired Donald Calne, a British neurologist, whose main interest was in Parkinson disease. Calne introduced bromocriptine, the first effective dopamine receptor agonist, and opened research in that area. Calne, in turn, recruited a basic scientist, John Kebabian, who discovered that there were multiple dopamine receptors.

In time, Calne became director of the medical neurology program and Richard Irwin, a neurophysiologist, headed the basic program.

Chase also expanded epilepsy research, which, until then, had been restricted to experimental surgery for temporal lobe epilepsy. Cosimo Ajmone-Marsan, who had been responsible for the EEG laboratory at NINDS for the past two decades, was soon to retire. Chase therefore hired J. Kiffin Penry to develop a medical epilepsy program. Penry had a unique dual role, working in both the extramural and intramural programs. He, in turn, recruited Roger Porter and they worked with industry to develop new antiepileptic drugs.

Neurosurgery was also revitalized when Paul Kornblith arrived. His main interest was in developing chemotherapy for gliomas by growing tumor cells in culture and exposing them to candidate drugs.

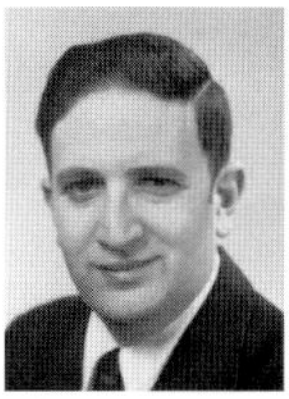

Paul Kornblith, M.D.

Not every effort succeeded. Chase saw the need and opportunity to develop an intramural PET program but it proved to be too difficult for the several interested NIH institutes to collaborate adequately. The development of PET was turned over to the extramural program. He saw the need to develop closer relations with pharmaceutical companies for drug development, an effort that was thwarted by the ethical complexities of federal guidelines.

All in all, the nine years of Chase's tenure brought new talents and new organization to NINDS.

Irwin J. Kopin, M.D.

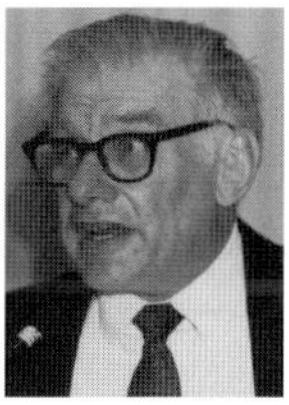

Irwin J. Kopin, M.D., was scientific director of NINDS from 1983 to 1994

Irwin Kopin is one of the few people who, like Tom Chase, served in both NIMH and NINDS. He was scientific director of NINDS from 1983 to 1994 and had covered a lot of research en route.

Kopin grew up in The Bronx, New York City, and graduated from The Bronx High School of Science in 1946. He then attended City College for 2 years, switching to get his degree from McGill University in Montreal. He stayed there for medical school, graduated in 1955, and then trained in internal medicine at the Boston City Hospital.

In the second year of his residency, he was notified that he was about to be drafted into the U.S. Army. He was already married and had children, so he tried to avoid a period of unemployment. He checked with the Army and Navy and neither had a convenient opening. When he learned that the Public Health Service could take him immediately, he volunteered and was assigned to a tuberculosis research section because someone noticed that he had taken mathematics courses in college and thought he might serve well as a statistician. When Kopin told them he was not a mathematician he lost that job, but found another as a research associate in Kety's Laboratory of Clinical Science in NIMH.[3]

That was in 1957, when NIMH and NINDS were still sharing their laboratories. Seymour Kety was seeking a physician to conduct physicals on a group of schizophrenic patients who were part of a study he had initiated looking for hereditary factors in the disease. It was Kopin's job to determine that the patients were free of any physical diseases.

Kopin was pleased to do the examinations but he saw another opportunity. Serotonin had just been discovered in carcinoid tumors by Albert Sjoerdsma in the Heart Institute and had been discovered in the brain by Parkhurst Shore in Bernard Brodie's laboratory. That made serotonin a target for psychiatric research. Kopin became interested in serotonin and sought advice from Marian Kies, then head of the NINDS-NIMH Laboratory of Biochemistry. He was already doing lumbar punctures on the schizophrenic patients to exclude neurosyphilis and would have access to samples of cerebrospinal fluid (CSF), but he needed a more sensitive method to measure the low levels of serotonin, so he developed one.

Kopin's training in biochemistry consisted of an Honors Biochemistry course at McGill University, but he had started to work in laboratories in high school. When he applied to CSF the method for 5-HIAA, the major metabolite of serotonin, Kety asked him to synthesize radioactive tryptophan for a study in patients. That effort in organic chemistry was also successful and led to more biochemistry.

At the same time, Axelrod was in the Laboratory of Clinical Science at NIMH-NINDS and had just discovered catechol-O-methyl transferase (COMT), which modified epinephrine by adding a methyl group. The question then arose about which was more important in terminating the action of epinephrine metabolism: COMT or monoamine oxidase? Kopin conceived an experiment that could decide. Metanephrine, a product of epinephrine metabolism, would be synthesized with a carbon-radiolabel in the methyl group and another isotope (tritium) would be used to label the norepinephrine or epinephrine. Then, by measuring the ratios of the two compounds, it would be possible to determine how much of the titrated compound was being converted to the carbon-labeled one.

At the time, Axelrod was not interested in doing the study. Finally, Kety told Kopin to do the experiment himself. It worked. COMT was the more important of the two enzymes in terminating the action of catecholamines, but re-uptake of the inhibitor was more important than either enzyme. Kopin wrote the paper without Kety; Kety declined to be co-author because he thought that inclusion of his name might detract from the credit Kopin deserved for a major innovation.

As these experiments went forward, Axelrod eventually became involved and Kopin worked with him, participating actively in Axelrod's experiments on re-uptake of transmitter in the heart and the salivary gland (as described in Chapter 20).

Another success was evidence for the "false transmitter" theory that explains the action of some drugs, especially the widely used monoamine oxidase (MAO) inhibitors. For instance, a derivative of norepinephrine may be formed from a drug action; then the new compound may substitute for norepinephrine in the nerve terminals and, with less effect of its own, it may diminish or even block the actions of the true transmitter. The formation and accumulation in sympathetic neurons of octopamine as a result of MAO inhibition explained why MAO inhibitors lower blood pressure and may cause orthostatic hypotension. Kopin's group showed that a positron-emitting false transmitter, ^{18}F-6-fluorodopamine, could be used for imaging peripheral sympathetic nerves. This led to the direct demonstration of degeneration of sympathetic nerves in peripheral autonomic failure and to the discovery that in most patients with parkinsonism, there is degeneration of cardiac sympathetic nerves.

Amidst these investigations, Kopin went to the Columbia-Presbyterian Medical Center for one year to finish his medical residency, returning immediately to NIMH. First, he served as a clinician-scientist in the Laboratory of Clinical Science at NIMH, starting in 1963. In 1968, Kety left for Harvard and the position of lab chief opened. Louis Sokoloff and Edward Evarts were already chiefs of their own laboratories and Axelrod did not want administrative obligations. Kopin was made acting chief for one year and then, in 1969, he was appointed lab chief, a position he held until 1983.

After 1965, Kopin's published papers included the names of his students, many of whom became well-known themselves: William Bunney, Frederick Goodwin, Ross Baldessarini, Richard Wurtman, Menach Goldstein, Joseph Schildkraut, Tom Chase, Richard Katz, George Wooten, and Alan Faden. His students came from diverse specialties – neuroscience, psychiatry, neurology, cardiology, and anesthesiology. By the time Kopin moved to NINDS, he and his associates had published 432 peer-reviewed papers that included research on drugs of abuse, high blood pressure, antipsychosis medication, familial dysautonomia, schizophrenia, and Parkinson disease – all related chemically. By the turn of the century he had published 710 papers.

Still at NIMH, Kopin had a major neurological research opportunity. He studied the very first person to develop parkinsonism as the result of taking the chemical MPTP–1-methyl-4-phenyl-1,2,5,6-tetrahydropyridine – that had contaminated his homemade version of meperidine (Demerol). The patient was a young man who lived in the shadow of NIH and whose frozen appearance was first thought to be catatonic schizophrenia. But he improved when given levodopa. When Kopin and his associates gave the drug to a monkey by injection into one carotid artery, only one hemisphere of the brain was affected and only one side of the body became parkinsonian – an important step in proving that the chemical could cause parkinsonism and was a link to neurology for Kopin.

In 1983, Murray Goldstein became director of NINDS and invited Kopin to become scientific director for the intramural program. In 2001, he said he served with only one NINDS director, Murray Goldstein, and never had to face a change in administration.[4]

Kopin reorganized the intramural program. In 1984, he brought Mark Hallett from the Peter Bent Brigham Hospital in Boston to serve as clinical director. In 1990, Kopin went to the Institute for Child Health to recruit Harold Gainer as director of the basic neurosciences program. With his actions, he led as part of a triumvirate. Both of his associates had outstanding qualifications.

Kopin is proud of numerous recruitments during his tenure. He brought John Hallenbeck from the U.S. Naval Hospital to start a stroke program. Because the NIH Clinical Center is a research hospital with no emergency room, it was necessary to seek a hospital that could provide access to stroke patients. As the program unfolded, Bethesda's Suburban Hospital became the venue for stroke clinical trials at NIH.

A search committee found Ronald McKay, who initiated a stem cell research program. J. Craig Venter came to study neurotransmitter receptors, which occupied his attention until he became interested in expressed sequence tags as a marker in gene searches. Joan Schwartz worked in Kopin's laboratory and then became an ethicist; she now works in the Office of the Director, NIH. Another recruit was James Battey, a neurophysiologist who is now the scientific director of the National Institute of Child Health and Human Development.

Kopin said that his biggest problem was finding space for a faculty that had to grow because of the combined policies of investigator tenure and the prohibition against a mandatory age for retirement. In 1994, Zach Hall became director of NINDS and Kopin retired for two reasons. First, he thought the new director should have the option of choosing his own scientific director. Second, Kopin was then 70 years old and it was time to retire. He still collaborates with members of his old laboratory and his CV is still growing.

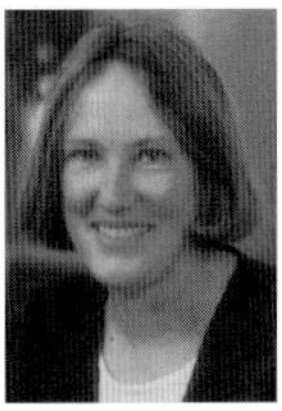

Story Landis, Ph.D., is the current scientific director of NINDS

Story C. Landis, Ph.D.

Story Landis became scientific director in 1995, having been recruited by Zach Hall. She had received her Bachelor's degree at Wellesley College and then, in 1973, she gained her Ph.D. at Harvard, where she worked with Richard Sidman on mutations that affected development of the cerebellum in mice. From the outset, she was interested in cellular morphology and she was a postdoctoral fellow with a series of illustrious neuroscientists – Floyd Bloom, David Potter, and Ed Fuhrspan. She explored the neuronal cell biology of the mutant mice in great detail and with diverse techniques of modern neuroscience. She ascended the academic ladder at Harvard and became an associate professor of neurobiology in 1984. The next year she moved to Case-Western Reserve University in Cleveland and, in 1988, became director of its Center for Neurosciences. In 1990, she was appointed chair of the Department of Neurosciences.

One of Dr. Landis's research themes is neuronal plasticity as manifested by changes in neurotransmitter responses in the process of development. It is important to understand how the functional characteristics of a nerve cell change with changing circumstances. For instance, the sympathetic neurons that innervate sweat glands first show the characteristics of cells that make norepinephrine. Later, however, through the actions of a soluble signal from the target tissue. the neurons acquire the properties of cells that make acetylcholine. Signals from the sweat glands are needed for development of the nerve cells.

Reciprocally, neuronal activity is needed for the targets to develop. That is, the effects are seen in both directions. Without activity of the neuronal signals, the sweat glands do not develop the cellular features that characterize secretory cells. She has found similar transformations in other targets, including the periosteum, the membrane that encloses bone. These changes depend in part on the presence of growth factors that are carried back from the target to the neuron. Dr. Landis's laboratory is busily engaged in determining how the several growth factors exert their effects.

Dr. Landis has garnered many honors. She was an established investigator of the American Heart Association and a Javits Investigator from NINDS. She has given a Presidential Lecture and a Special Lecture at the Society for Neuroscience and she held a MacKnight Senior Investigator Award.

Landis came to NINDS as scientific director at the invitation of Zach Hall. Like former directors Hall and Gerry Fischbach, she has not given up her own research career. She maintains a laboratory at NINDS in addition to taking on more administrative responsibility. Her reasons for moving to NINDS were straightforward:

> The intramural programs at NIH have extraordinary resources and extraordinary resources mean extraordinary opportunities. There was also a tradition of excellent neuroscience in the clinical arena and the basic science arena. Which made it clear that you could do very special things here that would be difficult to do in the extramural community.[5]

Landis is proud that she has been able to attract 12 new investigators, including those in Kenneth Fischbeck's neurogenetics branch, Alan Koretsky's experimental magnetic resonance imaging group, and Steven Warach's stroke diagnostic and therapeutic program (which, for acute studies, he is developing off-campus at the nearby Suburban Hospital). These additions enable Dr. Landis to get closer to her goal: "outstanding clinical, translational, and basic neuroscience."

In her ideal, there would be no separation of basic and clinical neuroscience, and investigators would communicate and collaborate seamlessly to bring the fruits of basic science research to the bedside. Consider her comments that scientific leaders should strive:

> . . . to try to meld people with very different ways of thinking about the nervous system and very different tools to study the nervous system into a community that can answer questions about function and dysfunction in the most effective possible way.

Or, to put it another way:

> . . . if you want neuroscience to go forward and things to get translated from people doing basic research to clinical diagnostics and therapeutics, you don't split the two groups into two different divisions with different people running them. You try to integrate and not divide.

Attaining that goal, however, means overcoming some traditional restraints. At the NIH she has found that laboratories tended to be isolated:

> Each lab or branch was like a mini-department. Not only was it a mini-department, but in some cases small enough not to be psychologically . . . to have complicated interactions. Each of them was a unit unto itself with none of the glue that would hold a university community together. Each lab or branch ran its own seminar series. They didn't get together and run a joint seminar series. Each lab or branch had its own shared equipment, but they didn't share equipment with other labs or branches.

To overcome that separateness, she has a clear vision that merges with her desire to meld basic and clinical neurosciences:

> You need to have developed mutual respect between the practitioners of each discipline. So, for example, we have a senior clinical investigator in the institute who, for whatever sets of reasons, feels that no Ph.D. can offer anything useful to his patient-based program. Now, obviously, this person is not going to seek out a basic scientist and say, "I have this interesting clinical problem, can you offer me any insights?" Similarly, I think the basic scientists we hire need to recognize that they can learn from clinicians and that ultimately what they are doing

> needs to be translated. We get money, not because we want to figure out how potassium channels work but, if we know how potassium channels work, we might be able to do something for epilepsy, or learning and memory.

With these thoughts in mind, Landis has set out to reorganize the intramural program. An opportunity to do that came in 2000. After 16 years as clinical director, Mark Hallett decided to concentrate on his research by relinquishing his administrative responsibilities as clinical director. Hallett is one of the world leaders among clinical investigators of movement disorders and the plasticity of the human brain – how the brain adapts after stroke or other injury – and he has been honored many times for his work. He is past president of the Movement Disorder Society and an editor-in-chief of the journal *Clinical Neurophysiology*. In 1999, he was designated Physician Researcher of the Year by the Public Health Service.

After Hallett changed positions, Landis and NINDS director Fischbach brought Guy McKhann of Johns Hopkins University to serve temporarily as clinical director. McKhann brought years of experience as a highly respected leader at Hopkins and as an advisor to The Dana Foundation. McKhann returned to his university in mid-2001. Any formal reorganization of the clinical programs, however, will probably await the arrival of the next NINDS director.

Dr. Landis has become an ardent advocate of the new John Edward Porter Neuroscience Research Center, which has been planned by former NINDS director Fischbach and NIMH director Steve Hyman. She explains:

> ...those faculties won't be distributed in terms of space by institutes, but actually by interest area. You could imagine a collection of people who work on glial cells, a collection that works on neurodegeneration, and a collection of people who work on systems and circuits – together, independent of their institutes, and with as many of the clinical investigators as possible from Building 10 having their main labs at the new center.

The clinical investigators might be doing disease-oriented research but not the kind that requires the patients themselves, for that kind of research would be more appropriate for the Clinical Center.

Landis has a view about recruiting young M.D.-investigators, the kind of physicians who populated all of NIH during the first two decades and who are now, with the disappearance of the military draft – and for other reasons, too – in short supply. Loan-repayment is part of the solution, because medical students have such huge debts upon graduating. But debt forgiveness alone cannot suffice because that has been tried as part of the National Health Service Program (which included service at the NIH); even with that program, physician-investigators did not flock to NIH. Building up the science at NIH is more feasible, and more likely to attract them once again.

Having an outstanding basic scientist at the helm is a major asset for NINDS, especially if she thinks so clearly about clinical opportunities, too.

1 Chase TN. Interview with author, June 23, 2000.
2 Chase TN. Telephone interview with author, June 3, 2001.
3 Kopin IJ. Interview with author, November 21, 2000.
4 Kopin IJ. Interview with author, November 21, 2000.
5 Landis S. Interview with author, March 26, 2000.

CHAPTER SIX

INTRAMURAL PROGRAM

The budget for the intramural program of NINDS, like that of other NIH institutes, fluctuates from year to year. However, even with administrative costs included, the intramural portion does not exceed 10 percent of the total institutional allotment. The impact of the Bethesda campus program is vastly greater than this small proportion of the budget might suggest.

The intramural program is highly visible – and not just because local investigators have won Nobel and other prizes. Visiting investigators come for short or long periods of collaboration. Some of them return to their countries where they became leaders of the next generation of biomedical scientists. For decades after World War II, a generation of young researchers came to NIH to discharge military obligations and to take advantage of an unparalleled opportunity to work with talented mentors in a setting of unbounded research opportunities. Those junior partners are now senior investigators who are among the leaders of clinical and basic neuroscience throughout the country.

The intramural NINDS research programs have been numerous and diverse. Some have been laboratory programs on the Bethesda campus. Others have been linked to extramural programs, as in the antiepileptic drug development program. Some have been part of Collaborative and Field Operations, such as the kuru studies in

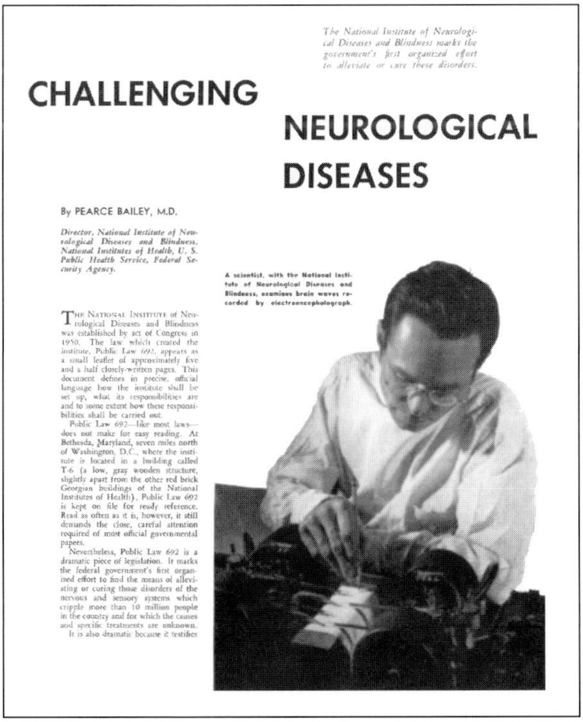

The National Institute of Neurological Diseases and Blindness marks the government's first organized effort to alleviate or cure these disorders.

CHALLENGING NEUROLOGICAL DISEASES

By PEARCE BAILEY, M.D.

Director, National Institute of Neurological Diseases and Blindness, National Institutes of Health, U. S. Public Health Service, Federal Security Agency.

THE NATIONAL INSTITUTE of Neurological Diseases and Blindness was established by act of Congress in 1950. The law which created the institute, Public Law 692, appears as a small leaflet of approximately five and a half closely-written pages. This document defines in precise, official language how the institute shall be set up, what its responsibilities are and to some extent how these responsibilities shall be carried out.

Public Law 692—like most laws—does not make for easy reading. At Bethesda, Maryland, seven miles north of Washington, D.C., where the institute is located in a building called T-6 (a low, gray wooden structure, slightly apart from the other red brick Georgian buildings of the National Institutes of Health), Public Law 692 is kept on file for ready reference. Read as often as it is, however, it still demands the close, careful attention required of most official governmental papers.

Nevertheless, Public Law 692 is a dramatic piece of legislation. It marks the federal government's first organized effort to find the means of alleviating or curing those disorders of the nervous and sensory systems which cripple more than 10 million people in the country and for which the causes and specific treatments are unknown.

It is also dramatic because it testifies

A scientist, with the National Institute of Neurological Diseases and Blindness, examines brain waves recorded by electroencephalograph.

EARLY NINDB PUBLICATION, CIRCA 1950s

New Guinea (Chapter 17) or the Lake Maracaibo investigations of Huntington disease (Chapter 15). We will now present others. In so doing, we have had to omit much interesting research, a situation that warrants apology to those investigators whose work has not been included.

Multiple Sclerosis

Few intramural programs have survived the half-century since the founding of NINDB. One is an emphasis on neuromuscular disease, a legacy of Milton Shy. Others have been intermittently prominent, such as epilepsy and multiple sclerosis (MS). MS provides a good example of the appearance, disappearance, and re-emergence of a field.

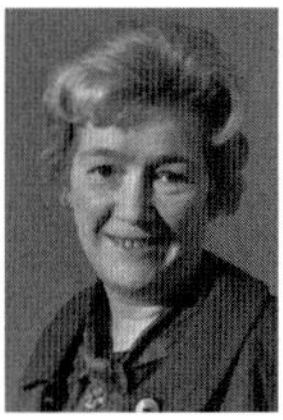

MARIAN KIES, PH.D., WAS AN EARLY MULTIPLE SCLEROSIS RESEARCHER

The origins of MS research at NINDB are uncertain. The confusion has to do with the earliest days of NIMH. It was widely believed that Seymour Kety made the very first assignments to the scientific staff. For instance, a key appointment was Marian Kies, Ph.D., who worked on an animal model of MS.

Perhaps Kety, seeking a biological explanation for schizophrenia, was willing to entertain any reasonable theory, including autoimmunity. Not so, said Louis Sokoloff.[1] He claims that Norman Goldstein had appointed Kies. Since the three principal people – Kies, Kety, and Goldstein – are now deceased, direct inquiry is not feasible, but we have some clues left behind by Goldstein.

Goldstein was well known as a clinical neurologist at the Mayo Clinic. He served at NINDB for only two years, 1953 to 1955, when he was the head of the Laboratory of Clinical Science in NIMH. That was the laboratory Kety himself headed after 1956, the same laboratory that became the incubator for so many neuroscience leaders.

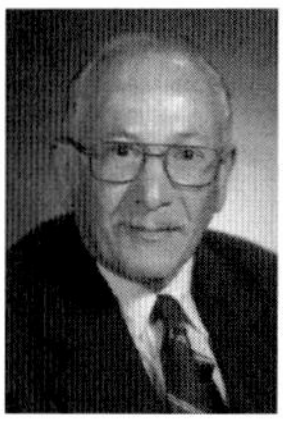

NORMAN GOLDSTEIN, M.D.

Goldstein, born in Brooklyn, New York, went to undergraduate school for three years at New York University but finished and received his B.A. and M.D. degrees at George Washington University during the World War II years. He interned at Mt. Sinai Hospital in New York and was then a Fellow, sequentially, in both medicine and psychiatry at the Mayo Clinic. He completed the six-year program at the Mayo in 1953 and then came to NINDB, like so many others, to fulfill his uniformed service obligations.

In between undergraduate and medical school, he received an M.A. degree, which must have been in biochemistry because he published two papers on serum lipids in 1943 and seven more by 1949. He published his first paper on experimental allergic encephalomyelitis (EAE) in 1953, and in the following years, would publish several more on the subject with Marian Kies. Among his co-authors from the Mayo Clinic was Lawrence J. Kolb, a neuropsychiatrist who was in charge of intramural research at NIMH between 1948 and 1950,[2] as well as being one of several founders of

NINDB. If Kety did not appoint Goldstein, the choice must have been that of Robert Felix, the first Director of NIMH, perhaps with the guidance of Kolb.

After two years at George Washington University, he returned to the Mayo Clinic in 1955 as a consultant and teacher in neurology. After retiring from Mayo in 1983, he consulted for the Federal Medical Center in Rochester, Minnesota. He died in 1994.[3] Like several others who served NIMH at the time, Goldstein claimed credit for having appointed Julius Axelrod.[4]

Another MS investigator of the same two years, 1953–1955, was Ellsworth C. Alvord, Jr., M.D., Chief of the Clinical Neuropathology Section in NINDB. Like some other staff members, Pearce Bailey appointed Alvord before Milton Shy arrived. Bailey was referred to Alvord through Lewis Stevenson, a neuropathologist at Cornell who had been mentor for both of them – at different times. Forty-six years later,[5] Alvord remarked that he had not been Shy's first choice; Shy would have preferred Jerzy Olszewski (whose name was recorded in the eponym Steele-Richardson-Olszewski syndrome, now known as progressive supranuclear bulbar palsy). Alvord left NINDB for a faculty appointment in Pathology at Baylor University and then moved to the University of Washington. In 2001, Alvord is still actively doing research and teaching in Seattle.

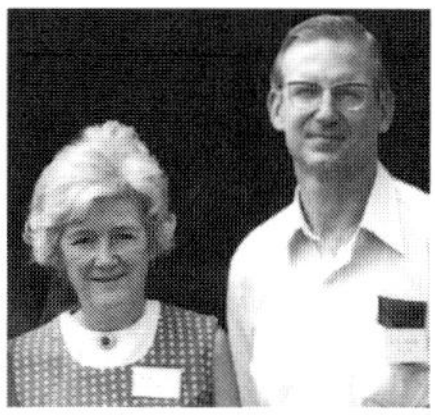

Marian Kies, Ph.D., and Ellsworth C. Alvord, Jr., M.D.

The central figure in this group of MS researchers was Marian Kies, but we have little information about her other than one obituary[6] and two written messages from Alvord.[5]

Kies had been working in the Department of Agriculture before she arrived at NINDB. As Alvord related the story, Goldstein had asked her to confirm one of his findings about the cause of EAE. "She needed a pathologist and I was delighted to have a biochemist to pick up where I had left it in 1948 with Jordi Folch-Pi's 'total lipid extract' and Elvin Kabat's admonition to quantify the extraction. So Marian extracted and injected titrations and I read the pathology and we soon discovered it was not lipid but protein."[5]

Folch-Pi was an investigator of lipids in the brain at Harvard and Elvin Kabat, at Columbia University, was one of the pioneers in quantitative immunochemistry. In 1948, Kabat had discovered that the level of gamma globulin in cerebrospinal fluid was abnormally high in more than half of the patients with MS. He had also earlier found that the gamma globulin fraction in the blood contained antibodies, so his discovery about the spinal fluid was a major support for the autoimmune theory of MS.

Alvord continued his story:

> Another biochemist at Georgetown was Elizabeth Roboz [later Roboz-Einstein, when she married a son of Albert Einstein] . . . . She had an apparatus for the electrophoretic preparation of proteins and discovered a basic protein in abundance and wanted

> to know what, if anything, it did – and Marian offered to test it – and it worked. It was the same protein that Marian had found to be encephalitogenic, but it was probably in a more pure form, so we joined forces.

In the process they had discovered *myelin basic protein*, a key protein in the sheath that provides a kind of insulation for the nerve fibers that convey electric messages in the CNS and in peripheral nerves. It has been the most-studied compound in the creation of this animal model of MS. Kies elucidated the interaction between antibodies and T-cells, including factors that determined susceptibility and resistance to EAE.

Marian Kies was not only a prominent researcher at NINDS; she was also one of the highest ranking women at NIH and was featured in a book about the ten most admired women in scientific research. Outside the institute, she devoted time and effort to nurturing and supporting women in biochemistry research. She was a founding member, along with Seymour Kety, Louis Sokoloff, and Jordi Folch-Pi, of the American Society of Neurochemists. Kies worked on EAE until her death in 1988.

Leonard Kurland was another MS investigator during those early years. Bailey recruited him to set up an epidemiology unit in NINDB. Kurland arrived in 1955. He had graduated from medical school at the University of Maryland in 1945 and was already well known for research that gained him a master's degree from the Harvard School of Public Health in 1948 and a doctorate in public health from Johns Hopkins in 1951. He then went to the Mayo Clinic for training in neurology.

Kurland's doctoral research interest was the epidemiology of multiple sclerosis. He had found that the incidence was much higher in Canada than in southern United States, just as it was much higher in Scandinavia than in the south of France and in Italy.[7] This distribution suggested that an environmental agent played an important role, which augmented evidence that CSF levels of gamma globulin were abnormally high in patients with MS. These two observations suggested that the triggering event might be a viral infection.

At NINDS, Kurland continued his work on MS and also began a study of amyotrophic lateral sclerosis in Guam. He completed studies comparing MS prevalence in different countries.[8] Kurland left NIH in 1964 to take advantage of the unique patient record system at the Mayo Clinic, where every person in Olmstead County, Minnesota, is registered. Under Kurland's direction the epidemiology of many major diseases has been analyzed there. Kurland's work in both Bethesda and Rochester, Minnesota, established him as the father of neuroepidemiology.

After Kurland's departure, the epidemiology of MS became an extramural program for NINDS. In neuropathology, Igor Klatzo, who recorded the pathology of spongiform encephalopathies and was interested in cerebral edema – but not especially in multiple sclerosis – followed Alvord. MS research was now in the hands of Marian Kies and she continued to work on EAE for 25 years.

Modern MS research in the intramural program began in the mid-70s. According to one apocryphal story, the director of NINDS was testifying before a Congressional committee for the institute's annual budget. At one point, a Senator asked: "Do you have one person in charge of multiple sclerosis research?" To his chagrin, the Director had to admit there was no such person, and the Senator inquired, "Don't you think you ought to get one?"

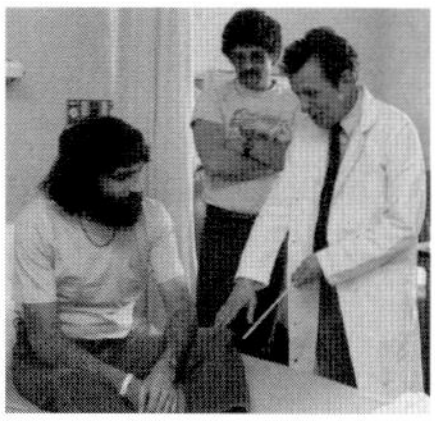

Dale E. McFarlin, M.D., served as Neuroimmunology Branch Chief from 1975 to 1994

That episode seems to have led to the recruitment of Dale E. McFarlin, who returned to NINCDS for the second time in 1975 to serve as a Neuroimmunology Branch Chief. McFarlin had graduated from medical school at Vanderbilt University, was trained in neurology at the University of Rochester, and was a Clinical Associate at NINDB in 1963-1965. By that time, his interests in the immunology of neurological diseases were firm. He went to Harvard for neurological training in 1965 and then returned to join the staff of NINDB in 1967. He became known for research on myasthenia gravis and several other disorders. In 1969, he was a Guest Worker in the laboratory of George Humphrey at Mill Hill, London, and became expert in cellular immunology. He was an Assistant Professor of Medicine at Emory University from 1971 until 1975, when he came back to NINCDS as a branch chief. He also published his first paper on allergic encephalomyelitis that year. At NINDS, he continued to make contributions to both myasthenia and multiple sclerosis. He analyzed the role of T-cells and B-cells and studied the HLA immune system as a susceptibility factor in patients with MS.

Back in 1973, McFarlin had attended a scientific meeting and was assigned to room with Henry McFarland. Linked by friendship, common research interests, and confusingly similar surnames, they joined forces at NINCDS as related by McFarland, who now leads the NINDS research program in MS.[9]

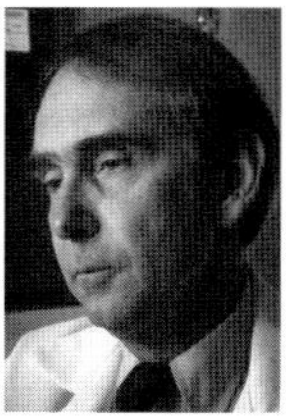

Henry McFarland, M.D., is the current Neuroimmunology Branch Chief

McFarland, the son of an ophthalmologist, spent his formative years in Phoenix, graduated from the University of Arizona, and from medical school at the University of Colorado. While in medical school he did some biochemical research on myelin lipids that led to discovery of the pathology of MS. During his neurology residency at Jefferson Medical College in Philadelphia, he researched EAE and his first paper was published in the prestigious *Proceedings of the National Academy of Sciences.*

As so often happens, a single episode changed his life.

> ...during the Academy meeting, I was in Washington and I heard [neurologist] Dick Johnson give a talk on lymphocytic choriomeningitis. I was absolutely convinced at that point...it

> was like a conversion, that this was the direction that I wanted to go. It was such a fascinating model that you have a viral induced immunopathological disease. I talked to Dick and Dick took me. I started in 1970 and the next three years [at Johns Hopkins] were probably the best years of my life . . . . [9]

After that he spent another three years as a fellow in immunology with Martin Raff in London and then returned for a faculty appointment at Johns Hopkins. In 1973 he met McFarlin and one year later, when Donald Tower invited McFarlin to set up a new neuroimmunology branch, McFarlin became its Branch Chief and invited McFarland to be Deputy Branch Chief. When they started in 1975, Marian Kies was still active and the world of MS research centered on EAE; patient-oriented research was meager at the time.

McFarlin focused on EAE in rodents, and McFarland was interested in human immune reactions. They were both concerned with the possible role that viruses might play in causing MS, especially measles virus. They had a working relationship with Kies and Sever, whose laboratories were in the same building. For nearly 20 years the two had a successful collaboration, until tragedy struck in 1994, when McFarlin died in his sleep at age 58, unexpectedly and inexplicably – presumably a myocardial infarct or arrhythmia.

Henry McFarland became Branch Chief at that point. Asked recently to consider his major achievements, he responded:

> Probably the biggest achievements have been over the last 10 or 12 years in redefining the natural history of the disease using MRI. I think we were probably the first ones that did that. I think it brought a new concept to our understanding of the disease. Prior to that time, we used to think that the disease – the relapsing-remitting course – was inactive between attacks. We know that is probably not the case, at least in the majority of patients; the disease is active from the very beginning.
>
> A second thing is that this sort of data has given us new treatment paradigms: how to test new experimental treatments. I think that has been extremely effective in quickly determining whether treatments can modify the disease process.
>
> Over the last five years the thing that has really given me the greatest satisfaction, is seeing the entire branch flourish. I think this branch is unique in the Institute. Each scientist has a fair amount of independence, but we actually function as a cohesive unit with a common interest – approaching problems in different ways and asking different questions. The whole is greater than the sum of the parts.
>
> There are probably only one or two groups in the world that are doing immunology at the level of what we're doing here.

> Tying it in with the MRI has been a tremendously helpful process.... it lets us correlate changes immunologically with a more precise measurement of disease activity. We can go through and look at immunological events and immunological measurements and correlate them when disease activity is high versus when disease activity is low. If one just tries to do that using clinical measurements, you really aren't coordinating it with the real disease process.
>
> We are studying the frequency of T cells, the activation of T cells, cytokine levels, gene expression using a cDNA microarray to see if we can find different gene expression when there are periods of increased disease activity versus lower disease activity. You combine the increasing power of the immunological tools with the ability to really closely monitor the disease. It is unique.[9]

With these major changes during McFarland's tenure as Branch Chief, MS research has shifted from a focus on immunology and MRI to patient research and therapeutic trials. The treatments being studied by Dr. Roland Martin and his group were developed by altering the structure of myelin basic protein and adding synthetic peptides (known as *ligands*) derived from this protein. Depending on the nature of the ligand, immunization of the patient led to different effects on MRI activity of the MS and also on the nature of the T-cell response. William Biddison has contributed to descriptions of the structure of the receptors for these peptide ligands. New antigens involve the oligodendroglia, supporting cells of the nervous system. New effects involve the nerve axons, not only myelin, so that current MS research overlaps with that on neurodegenerative diseases.

On the virus front, scientists have explored many different viruses. One focus now is on human herpes virus type 6. The field is bubbling and new therapeutic opportunities are numerous: altering the immune response by immunization or immunosuppressive drugs, repelling particular viruses, or coping with cell degeneration – among others.

In 1998, McFarland won the John Jay Dystel Prize, which is awarded annually by the American Academy of Neurology and the National Multiple Sclerosis Society.

McFarland knows that other laboratories are expert in similar MRI studies and some are outstanding in human MS immunology, but they mostly do one or the other research: only the NINDS program does both. The world of MS research has been changed immeasurably in the last 25 years because of the techniques spearheaded by McFarland and because new immunologic treatments have proven effective as measured by MRI in therapeutic trials. The extramural program of NINDS has sponsored much of that research. But the treatment is incomplete, and the search for both understanding of pathogenesis and more effective treatment goes on. Just as past research has depended on new and unexpected advances in technology – especially MRI and microarrays, as well as new chemical immunology – so can we expect more results now, not in some remote future.

From Kies to Alvord to McFarlin to McFarland, NIH has been prominent in MS-related research.

Epilepsy

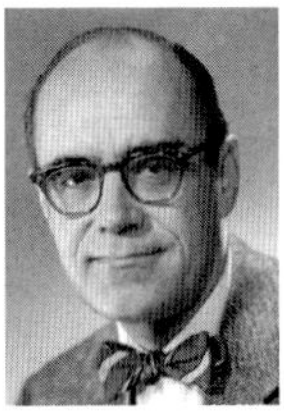

John van Buren, M.D., directed epilepsy research during the intramural program's early years

Maitland Baldwin, a neurosurgeon, and his successor, John Van Buren, drove the original epilepsy research during the intramural program's early years. Throughout their time, advances in medical epilepsy proceeded through the extramural program. This division of research changed in 1966, when Richard Masland, then Director of NINDB, invited J. Kiffin Penry to become Chief of the Epilepsy Section.[10]

J. Kiffin Penry, M.D.

Masland and Penry had known each other earlier because Penry started his neurology training at the Bowman Gray School of Medicine when Masland was head of the department. Penry finished his training with Derek E. Denny-Brown at the Boston City Hospital and then served in the U.S. Air Force until he moved to NIH. Penry was at NINDB and NINCDS for 13 years and he left a remarkable record. Roger Porter,[10] another epilepsy expert, wrote that Penry "became *the* national and international force for accomplishment in epilepsy and epilepsy research" in time.

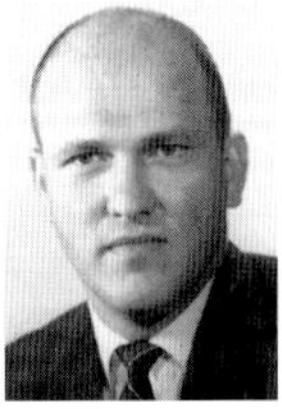

J. Kiffin Penry, M.D., headed the epilepsy program from 1966 to 1979

Although the Bethesda campus was his venue, Penry's activities were part of the Collaborative and Field Research Program, which had both intramural and extramural components. His first project was achieved through interaction with universities to develop therapeutic trials. To that end, it was necessary at the time – for both industry and academia – to use contracts.

One of the first arrangements was one with Fritz Dreifuss at the University of Virginia, a project concerned with an analysis of automatisms and petit mal seizures using then-new simultaneous recording of the clinical seizure by video and EEG activity. Because the efficacy of some drugs depends on the nature of the seizures, this documentation proved to be a major advance in developing antiepileptic medications. Until then there were only three drugs – phenobarbital, phenytoin, and succinimide – and the proportion of all seizure patients who achieved seizure control was not satisfactory.

As the program developed, other kinds of seizures were similarly approached to verify the attacks and document the characteristics. Penry prodded pharmaceutical companies to develop new drugs, then organized clinical trials. He found that many physicians treating patients with seizures did not have access to the literature and he introduced new computer programs to provide abstracts, a forerunner of Medline. He set up intramural and extramural programs to measure blood levels of the drugs and to modify dosing schedules according to the results.

Penry's work led to FDA approval of the new drugs, clonazepam and valproate. When he learned that carbamazepine was available in Europe but not in the United States, he organized the trials that led to its approval by the FDA. He also headed an international effort to refine the classification of seizures.

In the early 1970s, as Epilepsy Branch Chief, Penry established the Anticonvulsant Drug Development program, which was intended to speed up the search for new treatments. He developed a screening program that allowed academic or drug company scientists to submit compounds for tests of efficacy and toxicology in rodents. He assisted foreign companies with toxicology studies that were needed for FDA approval of their products.

Because more basic science was needed, Penry developed a grant program that stimulated extramural research and hired Harvey J. Kupferberg for an intramural screening program in the laboratory.[11] Kupferberg's research included toxicology, metabolism, and methods of action of the drugs. Altogether they screened more than 23,000 compounds and 25 were deemed promising enough for clinical studies.

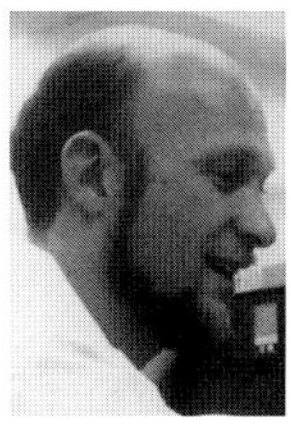

HARVEY J. KUPFERBERG, PH.D., CHIEF OF THE PRECLINICAL PHARMACOLOGY SECTION IN THE EPILEPSY BRANCH FROM 1982 TO 2001

Kupferberg had received his Ph.D. in Pharmacology from the University of California in San Francisco. He was appointed to an NINDS staff position in 1971 and became Chief of the Preclinical Pharmacology Section in the Epilepsy Branch in 1982. He was honored by several epilepsy societies and at a national epilepsy conference organized just before he retired in 2000.[12]

Throughout the early period, Penry was engaged in research. As a measure of the esteem he commanded at NINDS, Penry was eventually designated as Director of the Extramural Neurological

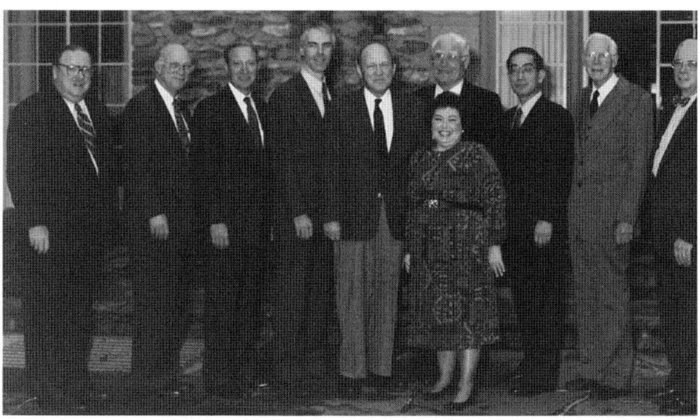

J. KIFFIN PENRY AND COLLEAGUES AT BOWMAN GRAY MEDICAL SCHOOL SYMPOSIUM IN 1995 HONORING PENRY'S CONTRIBUTIONS TO THE FIELD OF EPILEPSY RESEARCH. *FROM LEFT TO RIGHT:* THOMAS R. BROWNE, M.D., HARVEY J. KUPFERBERG, PH.D., ROGER J. PORTER, M.D., BRUCE L. EHRENBERG, M.D., J. KIFFIN PENRY, M.D., JAMES J. CEREGHINO, M.D., BETTY JEAN HESSIE, SUSUMU SATO, M.D., RICHARD L. MASLAND, M.D., AND LAWRENCE SMITH

Disorders Program, where he was responsible for Alzheimer and Parkinson disease research as well as epilepsy and other conditions.

In 1979, Penry returned to Bowman Gray as Professor of Neurology and Associate Dean for Research Development. Although he had broader administrative responsibilities, epilepsy was still his passion. In a "minifellowship" program he developed, physicians treating patients would come to Penry for several days or weeks to learn current theories and practice. Penry died in 1996, at age 67, as a result of complications of diabetes. He had been treated with dialysis for several years and had a stroke. In a memorial article, Roger Porter concluded, "Dr. Penry touched the lives of millions of people with epilepsy in a most positive way."

Roger J. Porter, M.D.

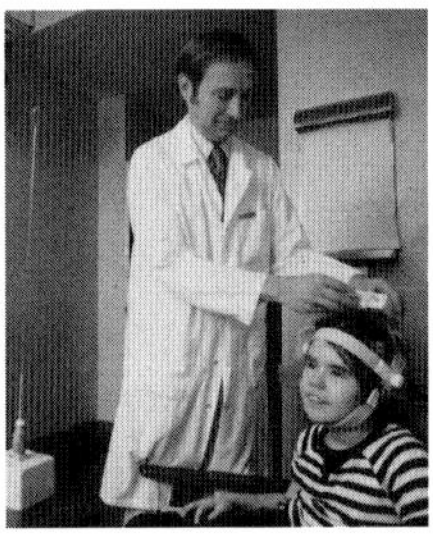

ROGER J. PORTER, M.D., AND PATIENT

After Penry left NIH in 1979, Roger Porter assumed responsibility for the epilepsy programs.[13] As a medical student at Duke, Porter had faced the draft. While still in medical school he did an elective rotation with Penry. Later he spent two years with Penry at NIH from 1969 to 1971. Porter "had an interesting time" but left with no intention of returning.

While still a resident in neurology at the University of California, San Francisco, Porter worked with Robert Layzer on phenytoin metabolism. Then Penry offered Porter a position in the Epilepsy Program. When he arrived in 1974, there was still an epilepsy surgical program. Van Buren's tenure as director of the Epilepsy Program was winding down.

A year after Porter arrived, Van Buren retired and left five epilepsy research beds in the Clinical Center. Penry was still nominally the Chief of the intramural Epilepsy Program but he delegated to Porter management of those beds.

After a few years, the collaboration of Penry and Porter was terminated in 1979 by Penry's departure. Porter became the Chief of the Epilepsy Branch in the extramural program and then also Chief of the Clinical Epilepsy Section of the intramural program. In 1984 he left the extramural program to become Chief of the Medical Neurology Branch and continued to head the intramural epilepsy section.

Porter's greatest interest was in the Drug Development Program. He also ran the clinical trials so that the system created by Penry moved smoothly. When Penry started there had been few investigators who knew how to conduct a trial and Penry himself had to learn. Porter stimulated academic centers by initiating four multicenter trials of four new drugs in two years. By the mid-1980s, clinical trialists were numerous and NIH stimulation was less necessary. Also, pharmaceutical companies had become more active in sponsoring trials.

In the intramural program, pharmacologic investigations included documentation of the limited efficacy of phensuximide and the efficacy of magnesium valproate. He and his associates studied the interaction of two popular drugs – phenobarbital and valproate – and they pioneered non-sedative combinations. EEG-video monitoring defined several types of seizures, including those that were psychogenic. With William Theodore, and using one of the first PET scanners, they documented the increased cerebral glucose metabolism during a seizure.

Porter extended other programs that had started with Penry. When Porter took over, there were six Comprehensive Epilepsy Centers. He vigorously increased the number to 40. He also added to the basic science program by hiring Michael Rogawski as a physiological pharmacologist. Rogawski received his M.D. and Ph.D. degrees at Yale, and was trained as a neurologist at Johns Hopkins. He arrived at NINDS in 1986 to establish a laboratory studying the role of ion channels in epilepsy, using cultured neurons, brain slices, and other models of epilepsy. Rogawski now heads the intramural Neuronal Excitability Section.

In 1987, Katherine Bick moved from being Deputy Director of NINDS to work in the NIH Director's office. Porter succeeded her as Deputy Director. Among his other responsibilities in that position he was active in the Decade of the Brain campaign. He and his colleague at NIMH, Alan Leshner, worked to coordinate institutional activities. Porter made the initial contact with Congressman Silvio Conte, who led congressional actions.

Porter and Leshner also interacted with James Wyngaarden, the former Director of NIH, who was then working in the White House Office of Science and Technology Policy where the President's Science Advisor was stationed. They coordinated the Decade of the Brain effort with all the other government agencies.[14] Porter judged it "the most exciting bureaucratic work I did."

In 1989, Porter took a sabbatical leave to work at the Association of American Medical Colleges and to write a book on the relations between academia and the pharmaceutical industry. That book presaged an impending change of his own. In 1992, he left NIH to become Vice-President for Clinical Pharmacology at Wyeth-Ayerst, located near Philadelphia, where he continues his interest in developing antiepileptic drugs.

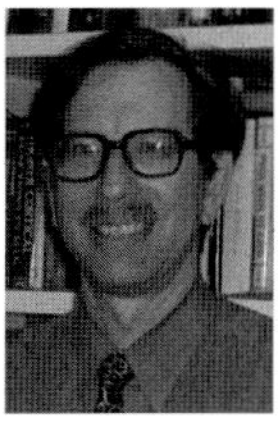

William H. Theodore, M.D., is the current chief of the Clinical Epilepsy Section

William H. Theodore, M.D.

William H. Theodore, who had been a Fellow with Porter a decade earlier, took responsibility for the epilepsy programs when Porter left. Porter had encouraged Theodore to use PET and he became one of the world's experts on neuroimaging in epilepsy.

Theodore did his undergraduate work at Harvard and received his medical degree from Columbia. He trained in neurology at Mt. Sinai and was appointed Chief of the Clinical Epilepsy Section at NINDS in 1988, where he remains. He and his associates have concentrated on treating uncontrolled epilepsy using noninvasive methods of diagnosis for the localization of epileptic foci and for cognitive mapping. The methods include video-EEG, magnetic stimulation, PET, functional MRI and MR spectroscopy, including the co-registration or simultaneous use of more than one of these methods. Pre-operative localization of language functions is a major goal. Theodore has been honored with an Outstanding Clinical Investigator Award from the American Epilepsy Society.

The national burden of epilepsy is a major problem. More than 2 million people in the United States – about 1 in 100 – have either experienced an unprovoked seizure or been diagnosed with epilepsy. Most seizures can be controlled with modern medicines and surgical techniques, but some people continue to have seizures even with the best available treatment. Improved diagnosis, treatment, and quality of life for patients are all continuing goals of both the intramural and extramural programs of NINDS.

Clinical Neurophysiology

Mark Hallett, M.D.

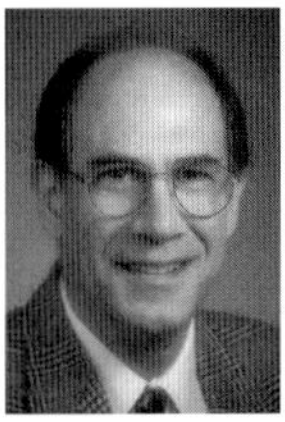

MARK HALLETT, M.D., IS THE CURRENT CHIEF OF THE MEDICAL NEUROLOGY BRANCH

Mark Hallett's interest in the brain started when he took a high school course in psychology. When he went to Harvard as an undergraduate, astronomy attracted him transiently. By the end of his sophomore year, however, he was more interested in biology and had decided on a premedical curriculum, with the aim of going into psychiatry, neurology, or neurosurgery. His course was set by the time he was a senior. Hallett still recalls a lecture by the renowned Norman Geschwind, a student of language disorders after brain injury.

In medical school at Harvard, during the summer after his freshman year, he worked with Hubel and Wiesel on the sensory cortex of the cat. After his sophomore year, he spent the summer with Geschwind. Gradually his three clinical interests became one, as he focused on neurology. His decision was cemented by a rotation with C. Miller Fisher, another master teacher.

An internship at the Peter Bent Brigham Hospital (now Brigham and Women's Hospital) followed and he was accepted for neurology training at the Massachusetts General Hospital. The military draft of physicians loomed and he discharged his service obligations at NIH by working for two years with Ichiji Tasaki, the biophysical physiologist who contributed to knowledge of the nerve impulse. While Hallett was there, Edward Evarts and a visitor from Sweden, Ragnar Granit, gave a year-long series of seminars on motor control, a subject far removed from Tasaki's focus on peripheral nerves. Granit focused his lectures on how the brain is involved in planning and executing body movements through a complex set of physiological mechanisms. The impact of these lectures and discussions on

Hallett was permanent; he was to make it a central theme of his own research.

After his residency, he secured a traveling fellowship to London and joined a young British investigator, C. David Marsden, who was then virtually unknown in the world of clinical investigation but ultimately became pre-eminent in all aspects of movement disorders, including motor control. Hallett returned to Boston as director of the clinical neurophysiology laboratories at the Peter Bent Brigham Hospital, a position he held from 1976 to 1984.

The next step in his career involved spousal appointments in academia. Hallett's wife, Judith, is a philologist of classic languages and she accepted a tenured position at the University of Maryland. Mark sought a position nearby. Donald Calne had just left NINDS as Clinical Director, so that line was open. Hallett knew NIH well from his earlier experience. The opportunity to emphasize research (as opposed to patient care and teaching) was a powerful attraction.

When Hallett started working at NIH, he was not only Clinical Director but also Chief of the Human Motor Control Section, a creation of his own that conformed to his research activities. Later, when Roger Porter became Deputy Director of NINDS, Hallett became Chief of the Medical Neurology Branch.

His administrative challenges were multiple: providing diagnostic electromyography and electroencephalography for the entire Clinical Center; providing an effective clinical consultation service for the other institutes; and managing the demand for the 40 research beds allotted to NINDB, which were under considerable pressure from several research protocols to study brain tumors, parkinsonism, multiple sclerosis, epilepsy, neuromuscular diseases, and lipid storage diseases. At first, otolaryngology was included. Those administrative tasks commanded about half of his time.

But Hallett's greatest satisfaction has come from his research as he and his team have advanced understanding of brain plasticity and, in particular, how the brain adapts to carry out essential functions after brain injury has interfered with the normal pathways. For instance, using PET and functional MRI, he found that sightless people read Braille with their fingers, not only by using the sensory cortex to evaluate what they feel, but also by using the occipital cortex, which is ordinarily involved in vision. The process of going from one mode to the other is called *transmodal plasticity*.

Other forms of plasticity are also open to analysis. For instance, what happens to the brain after a limb is amputated and the motor cortex is no longer connected to the limb it formerly controlled? Does the brain develop new functions for parts of the body that remain or does it become silent? In fact, Hallett found that the motor cortex reorganizes to innervate parts of the body that were not originally under its control.

Another example of brain plasticity is seen in motor learning. For instance, learning to play a simple tune on the piano alters the excitability of the motor cortex.

Hallett has been a pioneer in developing new methods of clinical neurophysiology in order to analyze voluntary and involuntary movements. He aimed to analyze the origin of myoclonus, the sudden involuntary jerk of a limb. In one form of myoclonus, electrical activity is seen over the motor cortex – preceding the muscle contraction. That is, the brain activity is transmitted down through the brain to the motor neurons in the spinal cord. The muscle contracts when these motor neurons are activated.

In another form, however, the anticipated brain activity is not so obvious, so Hallett and his colleagues used a method of "back averaging." They recorded many jerks electronically, lined up the records of the muscle activity and the simultaneously recorded electroencephalogram. When they did that, the ups and downs of the normal brain waves cancelled each other to create a flatter average background thus reducing the "noise." As a result, the discharge over the motor cortex emerged and they saw a change in the brain activity just preceding the muscle jerk.

The same back-averaging method can be applied to other normal or abnormal movements. In some disorders, these abrupt movements are easily evoked by sensory stimuli – a loud and unexpected noise or a tap on the limb suffices. The sensory cortex is hyperactive and the stimulus rapidly spreads to the motor cortex before the jerk appears.

Hallett has also pioneered the use of transcranial magnetic stimulation to study disorders of movement. He was one of the first to use botulinum toxin to treat the sustained movements called dystonia. His team has evaluated the physiology of different kinds of involuntary movements, the slowness of movement in parkinsonism (*bradykinesia*), and the unsteady ataxic gaits of people with cerebellar disorders.

However, the competing pulls between administration and research finally took a toll. In 2001, after 17 years in his multiple roles, Hallett stepped aside as Clinical Director to focus more on his research. His successor has not yet been selected.

With a record like Hallett's, it is no surprise that he is internationally prominent. He has been Chief Editor of *Clinical Neurophysiology*, the leading journal in the field. He is in broad demand as a lecturer, has been elected an honorary member of the Australian Neurological Society, and has been President of the Movement Disorders Society and the American Association of Electrodiagnostic Medicine. Hallett's trainees now lead their own departments throughout the world.

Neurosurgery

Edward H. Oldfield, M.D.

Edward Oldfield arrived at NIH in 1981 and began a new era of intramural neurosurgery at NINDS. Until then, the surgeons' main interest was the treatment of focal epilepsies and the opportunities those operations gave for exploring the human brain. The first NINDS neurosurgeon, Maitland Baldwin, was a student of Wilder Penfield, whose studies had originated the field at the Montreal Neurological Institute in the 1930s and 1940s. Baldwin's successor was John Van Buren, who continued the focus on epilepsy surgery. Ayub Omaya was more interested in cerebrospinal fluid and left his name in the eponym for a plastic reservoir that is used for repeated delivery of drugs into the ventricular cerebrospinal fluid. Omaya was followed in 1978 by Paul Kornblith, who was interested in the chemotherapy of gliomas. But from 1953 into the 1980s, throughout the years of these excursions into other aspects of neurosurgery, epilepsy surgery still remained a dominating specialty at NINDS.

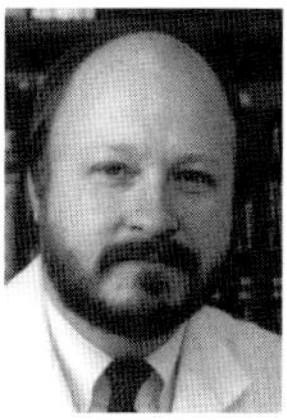

EDWARD H. OLDFIELD, M.D., IS CURRENT CHIEF OF THE SURGICAL NEUROLOGY BRANCH

Oldfield[15] majored in Physics at the University of Kentucky, but never received his undergraduate degree because he entered the university's medical school after finishing his junior year. As an undergraduate, he and his friends participated in a psychological questionnaire to make some money for their fraternity. Afterwards, Oldfield was told that the test results were clear. His personality and interests pointed toward surgery. In medical school, charismatic teachers, including David Clark and Horace Norrell, led him to see that the nervous system was a field ripe for new discoveries.

After medical school, Oldfield moved to Vanderbilt University for training in general surgery, followed by a year of neurology at the National Hospital at Queen Square in London, England. This experience solidified his neurological interests before he returned to neurosurgical residency at Vanderbilt. He spent one year in private practice in Lexington, Kentucky, and then contacted Paul Kornblith (who was then head of NINDS neurosurgery) to learn that one of the staff members had just left and there was an open position. They needed someone who had a clinical interest in surgery because Kornblith was more laboratory-oriented. Oldfield's goal was to work a year or two to gain some academic credentials and then return to a medical school.

As a Senior Staff Fellow, Oldfield was free to develop his own projects. He worked with endocrinologists and made pituitary tumors a specialty. He worked in cellular immunology, which he applied to brain tumors. With Robert Dedrick, a bioengineer, he explored systems for drug delivery to the brain. His goal became the translation of biological advances into effective treatments and protein therapy and gene therapy.

Oldfield became Deputy Chief of the Surgical Neurology Branch in 1983 and Chief three years later. He has remained at NIH because he feels the need to probe for new knowledge and is convinced that NIH is an ideal environment for that.

Oldfield's surgical interests have been broad – pituitary tumors, brain tumors, arteriovenous malformations, the vascular tumors of familial von Hippel-Lindau syndrome, and the dynamics of syringomyelia, or cysts, within the spinal cord.

As a result of his interest in pituitary tumors, he has become involved in the molecular genetics of the disorder called *multiple endocrine neoplasia.* His interest in vascular tumors of the nervous system has led him to participate in research on the molecular genetics of von Hippel-Lindau syndrome.

Oldfield's group has pioneered the use of novel approaches to therapy for *gliomas*, a major challenge. The tumors are common and survival is little better now than it was 25 or 50 years ago. Oldfield's group combines gene therapy and immunotoxins with ingenious methods to deliver the treatment.

He and his associates, Douglas Laske and Richard Youle, have taken advantage of the need of tumor cells for iron, which is transported into cells by being attached to a protein called *transferrin.* In normal brain, receptors for transferrin are found only on the cells of the smallest blood vessels. In contrast, however, tumor cell surfaces are loaded with these receptors.

To take advantage of this mechanism, Oldfield and Youle conjugated normal transferrin to a genetically engineered diphtheria toxin. Then they circumvented the normal CNS barriers to entry of large molecules by using a high-flow interstitial infusion technique (a new drug delivery approach discovered at NINDS by Oldfield, Dedrick, and their colleagues) to deliver the treatment directly to the tumor.

Nine of 15 patients showed significant response, and the tumor disappeared in two patients. With this excellent progress, Oldfield and his colleagues are working to improve all aspects of the experimental treatment delivery. He sees a bright future for this kind of "biological surgery."

Oldfield has also pioneered new approaches to syringomyelia, a cystic abnormality of the spinal cord that affects more than 21,000 people in the United States. Long regarded as a congenital abnormality that has defied treatment, Oldfield's team has applied diverse modern imaging methods to study the associated malformation of the cerebellum, the flow and pressure changes of cerebrospinal fluid, and the deformity of the spinal cord. The methods include MRI, ultrasonography, and pressure measures. Oldfield and his researchers have found evidence that the disorder is acquired, not congenital, and that it can be corrected with a relatively simple operation.

Oldfield looks forward to endoscopic, robotic, miniaturized neurosurgery. He expects that what is now called "minimally invasive surgery" will become even less invasive. And he sees impending benefit for the brain by advances in procedures outside the head when cardiac surgery improves with the introduction of a synchronized and resonating imaging system to support robotized operations. With achievement of that, there would be no need to stop the heart and clamp the aorta during surgery, thus reducing the likelihood of cerebral emboli and providing a form of brain protection.

Epilepsy surgery, too, is taking new turns as the localization of seizure foci improves and it becomes possible to perfuse the area of seizure outset with drugs that can determine how large an area the discharging cells cover (an important conceptual and therapeutic issue in epilepsy) and how the electric seizures can be controlled, temporarily at first and then permanently. This new treatment approach would not require surgical excision.

This heavenly vision of the future of neurosurgery is marred by one development. One of Oldfield's goals has always been to provide biological research training for neurosurgical residents from medical centers throughout the country. He has done this for many years but the system is now threatened by the economics of medical practice – the need of academic departments to operate on more patients to make up for the disappearing money. The result? Residents cannot be spared for the once-hallowed two years of research training.

Oldfield is much in demand as a lecturer throughout the world, perhaps the most revealing measure of admiration from his peers in neurosurgery, cancer research, and endocrinology. He is more than a model of the modern clinical investigator; his clinical service is an example of what patient-oriented research can be in the intramural program.

Nerve Structure Determines Function

Thomas S. Reese, M.D.

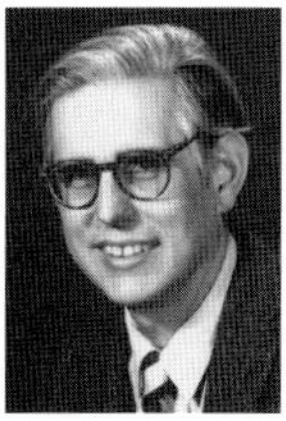

THOMAS S. REESE, M.D., IS CURRENT CHIEF OF THE LABORATORY OF NEUROBIOLOGY

Tom Reese became smitten with the brain when he was an undergraduate at Harvard. There he encountered the Psycho-Acoustic Laboratory, which included Nobelist Georg von Békésy, the physiologist of hearing, and B.F. Skinner, the behavioral psychologist – and still others. Reese intended to go to graduate school but was convinced by several family members who were doctors that a medical degree would give him more flexibility. At Columbia University College of Physicians and Surgeons, however, Reese was bored with the rote instruction of his first year in medical school.

Independently, he began to study olfactory receptor neurons. Cell biologists at Columbia – Margaret Murray, George Pappas, and Stanley Crain – advised him in his attempt to separate functional cells from the brain. He succeeded but his scientific knowledge had not yet matured enough to put them to good purpose.

When the clinical years of medical school arrived, he found that scientific principles could be applied to clinical problems, and, his interest piqued, he thought he might become a neurologist. He went to the Boston City Hospital for his internship and then, faced with the physician draft, came to NIH for advice. His interest in neurology proved to be an asset because he had read a book on cranial nerves by the Swedish neuroanatomist Alf Brodal. In fact, he had done more than read it; he knew it by heart.

On the day he visited NIH, he was taken to meet Milton Shy who was conducting rounds on a patient with a cranial nerve problem. In his usual manner, Shy was teaching dramatically by grilling his clinical associates about the relevant anatomy. None of them knew the answers, and so Shy turned to the unknown visitor and asked him. Reese had the answers down cold.

Shy was impressed and asked Reese to come to his office so they could talk, and introduced him to several investigators. Reese ended up speaking with Keith Richardson, an NINDB scientist who had developed staining methods to study synapses in the brain.

This led to an offer of a postdoctoral fellowship at NINDB after his internship ended. Reese arrived in Richardson's laboratory and went to work on the olfactory cells. Before long he had interesting photographs of the surface of those cells. Richardson suggested he use the electron microscope, which he did. The results were published and impressed the renowned cell biologist Keith Porter, who included Reese's pictures in a new atlas.

With only a few months of his postdoctoral fellowship remaining at NINDB, Reese used electron microscopy (EM) to study the olfactory cells in the brain. In that effort, he was aided by NIMH researcher Sanford Palay, one of the pioneers of ultrastructural study of the brain. Milton Brightman, of the same laboratory, joined Reese. Their observations seemed to contradict a major theory of the day, which held that the creation of synapses was based on differences in the structure of axons (nerve fibers leaving the cell) and dendrites (fibers entering the cells). It was thought that the only way for messages to be transmitted was from an axon to a dendrite. The physical characteristics of dendrites would presumably prevent passage of a message between two dendrites. But that is just what Reese found, *dendro-dendritic synapses.*

That was a major contribution. More were in the offing.

When his two-year stint ended, Reese returned to Harvard where he worked with Don Fawcett, again doing his own research. When Manfred Karnovsky lectured on peroxidase, Reese recognized the value of the new approach. Peroxidase is a protein large enough and easy to stain so that it can be used as a marker of any cell that contains it. Reese recognized that it could be used to analyze an important unsolved characteristic of the brain – the blood-brain barrier – a term used to describe the failure of large proteins and chemicals to enter the brain from the blood. It explains why administered antibodies (large proteins) or some chemicals used for chemotherapy and some antibiotics do not enter the brain. Instead of giving them by mouth or intravenously, it is necessary to inject these compounds into the cerebrospinal fluid, which is not only cumbersome but also inefficient and sometimes ineffective.

According to one contemporary theory, the barrier was created by tight junctions between the glial cells that lay just outside the small blood vessels of the brain. The close packing made it impossible for large molecules to pass. Reese reasoned that giving peroxidase could prove that theory. However, the experiment failed. Peroxidase could not be seen in the EM preparations.

Reese thought the failure might be related to the methods used to preserve the structure of the brain, which involved giving intra-arterial injections of fixative; the process is called "perfusion fixation." He thought he might get around that by excising a piece of brain tissue and dropping it into the fixative. When he did that, the answer was clear. The peroxidase was blocked from leaving the blood vessels by tight junctions of the cells lining the blood vessels, not by the glia that lay outside the vessels.

To prove the point, Reese studied vessels in kidney and muscle, where the cellular structures differed and so did permeability to peroxidase. The brain barrier was unique among the organs. The observation was put to some practical use when it was shown that the injection of highly concentrated (hypertonic) solutions into the carotid artery could open these junctions in preparation for the injection of chemotherapeutic drugs. The observation also accounted for some of the adverse effects of carotid angiography, a diagnostic procedure in which radio-opaque material is injected directly into the carotid artery to visualize the blood vessels of the brain. Since these injections were hypertonic, they often had ill effects on the brain because the barrier was opened to iodine-containing solutions. In time, the injections were made by way of a catheter that could be placed in a more advantageous position without directly puncturing the carotid artery.

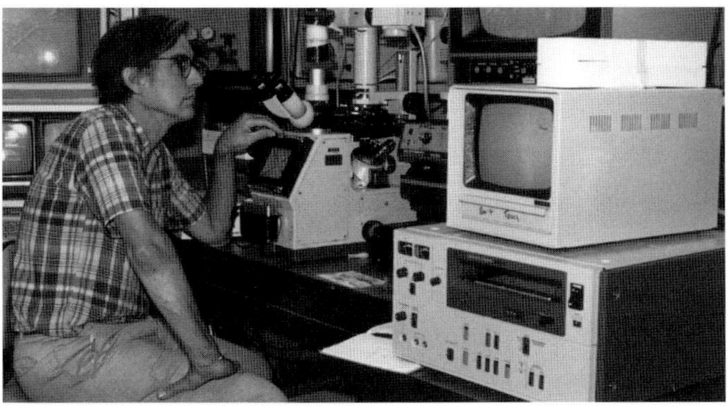

Tom Reese at the Marine Biology Laboratory at Woods Hole, 1984

As Reese's postdoctoral experience at Harvard ended, he looked for a permanent position and considered several before he ended up in 1966 as a Research Medical Officer in the Laboratory of Neuropathology and Neuroanatomical Sciences in NINDB. He has worked at NINDS ever since. He became a Section Chief in 1970, and then a Laboratory Chief in 1983, a title he still holds.

When he returned to NIH, Reese rejoined Brightman in working on the blood-brain barrier. One day, Reese's supervisor, Igor Klatzo came and said he had a young investigator – John Heuser – he wanted to add to Reese's staff. On that historic occasion one of the great teams of investigators was created, but that, too, took time to mature.

Heuser had come from the laboratory of Sir Bernard Katz and Ricardo Miledi in London. Like so many others, he came to NIH to cover his public service obligation under the physician draft. According to Reese's custom, he would allow postdoctoral fellows to do their own work instead of providing them with a specific problem. Soon, Heuser announced that his methods for preparing tissues were better than Reese's. Reese said they should do a comparative study of frog muscle, which showed unequivocally that Heuser, the student, was correct.

Together, Reese and Heuser tried to see what happened at the synapse when they stimulated the nerve. They already knew that the nerve terminals were packed with tiny bags or *vesicles* that were enclosed by a coating of complex structure. Quickly they found that, after a single stimulus, there were more of these "coated" vesicles that contained the neurotransmitter. The membranes of these little packages fused with the surface membranes, turned inside out, discharged their contents, and filled again in a recycling process.

Heuser later went to the University of California in San Francisco and Reese made several trips to join him there temporarily as they constructed a new apparatus for rapidly freezing the tissue specimens they needed for EM studies. It took some time before they succeeded with a technique using liquid helium as the freezing agent.

With rapid freezing possible they could learn how the recycling was achieved by stimulating the nerve just once. If the stimulus was given just once 2.5 milliseconds (msec) before the tissue was frozen, there was no difference in the number or appearance of the vesicles. A period of 2.5 msec is almost a thousand times shorter than a second. If the interval was a tiny bit longer, 3.5 msec, they could see the vesicles fusing with the surface membrane and releasing their contents. They found that the number of vesicles involved was proportionate to those discovered physiologically by Katz and his colleagues, who found that the transmitter acetylcholine is released at the neuromuscular junction in "quanta" or packets of specified amounts, not larger or smaller. The anatomic EM observations of Reese and Heuser proved the quantal theory.

The discovery of recycling vesicles was a major contribution. The phenomenon recalls the recycling of neurotransmitters found by Axelrod and Carlsson, but differs in an important respect. Reese and Heuser were concerned with the package's membranes, not the neurotransmitters they contained.

That is, Axelrod had found that transmitters epinephrine and norepinephrine were recycled and Carlsson had found that dopamine and other catecholamines were recycled. However, Heuser and Reese were analyzing the mechanisms of the neuromuscular junction. There the transmitter is acetylcholine and the process differs from that involving the catecholamines. Instead of being recaptured by re-uptake, this transmitter is destroyed by enzymes at the junction. The products of the reaction are choline and acetate, which re-enter the nerve, are re-combined by local synthetic enzymes, and the product re-enters the vesicles at the post-synaptic membrane.

Reese also analyzed the role of calcium in the nerve impulse, using fast freezing methods and X-ray microscopy to demonstrate that membrane structures within the axon (the endoplasmic reticulum) accumulate calcium during the impulse. The methods they used gave a measure of the total amount of calcium involved. In contrast to more popular dyes used to determine the amount of "free" or unbound calcium, Reese's methods measured total calcium.

Later, Reese turned his attention to another major problem, how neurotransmitters and other functional chemicals are synthesized in the cell body of a neuron and carried down the long axon to the terminals. The process is called axonal transport, which comprises both fast and slow transport, and moves in either of two directions, from the cell body to the terminals (anterograde transport) or the reverse (retrograde transport). In either direction the substance moves along fixed structures of what is called the *cytoskeleton*. What is the motor that propels the process? Reese found that a protein called *kinesin* is responsible for anterograde transport. Others found that another protein, *dynein*, is responsible for retrograde transport. The anterograde process is continuous; the retrograde process is intermittent. The mechanism is – naturally – complex and is now known to involve multiple forms of kinesin.

This is an impressive list of achievements: dendro-dendritic synapses, the blood-brain barrier, recycling vesicles, the role of calcium in transmitting the nerve impulse, and the role of kinesis. Reese is now directing his attention to the post-synaptic apparatus, how it works in transmission. We can be certain that more advances are in the offing.

Tom Reese was elected to the National Academy of Sciences in 1987.

Neurogenetics

Kenneth H. Fischbeck, M.D.

Kenneth Fischbeck is called Kurt by all who know him. His interest in neuroscience was kindled when he was in high school. Irving Cooper, a charismatic neurosurgeon with a flair for the dramatic, came to give a lecture on his achievements in treating Parkinson disease by making lesions in the thalamus or other structures in the basal ganglia. About the same time in the mid-1960s, George Cotzias made headlines when he described the dramatic effects of levodopa treatment of parkinsonism. Fischbeck was "struck by what could be done by understanding normal brain function and treating patients" with neurological disease. "If you knew something about the pathogenesis of a disease, you could devise a rational treatment."[16]

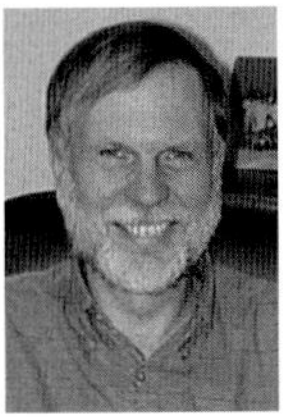

KENNETH H. FISCHBECK, M.D., IS CURRENT CHIEF OF THE NEUROGENETICS BRANCH

That thought remained subliminal as Fischbeck went through undergraduate years at Harvard and took courses in neuroscience. When he graduated, he took a year as a graduate student with Jack McMahon in the Neurobiology Department at Harvard Medical School and learned the benefits of working with simple systems; there, he worked on the neuromuscular junction. Next came medical school at Johns Hopkins, where he did research with Daniel Drachman. James Patrick and Jon Lindstrom had just discovered antibodies to the acetylcholine receptor, so the atmosphere was charged in Drachman's myasthenia research laboratory. After graduation Fischbeck did a year of medicine at Case-Western Reserve and then had his neurology residency at the University of California, San Francisco, under the tutelage of Robert Fishman.

In 1980, while in his third year of residency, Fischbeck attended the annual meeting of the American Academy of Neurology, held that year in New Orleans. A chance encounter on the homeward flight had an even more dramatic effect on his life than Cooper's lecture.

"I sat next to Stan Prusiner," said Fischbeck. "During that flight from New Orleans to San Francisco he laid out for me the whole idea of positional cloning. He told me if I wanted to find the cause of Duchenne muscular dystrophy, don't look at the muscle plasma membrane; look on the X chromosome. This was a new idea back then."

The first chromosomal marker had just been identified a few years previously and the key theoretical paper of Botstein, White, and Davis had not yet been published – but Prusiner had heard it at a meeting. By that time, Fischbeck had already signed on for a post-residency fellowship with Donald Schotland at the University of Pennsylvania. He had intended to study muscle surface membranes in Duchenne muscular dystrophy. When he arrived he did do the morphological work, but he also worked with Roy Schmickel of the Genetics Department to learn the fundamentals of positional cloning. He also served as clinical collaborator for the laboratories directed by

Louis Kunkel and Ronald Whorton, collecting blood from hundreds of patients and having a close relationship with the trials and tribulations of early gene mapping.

By now, Fischbeck's course was set. He was appointed to the Penn faculty, given a laboratory, and supported in part by an NINDS program project grant on neuromuscular disease. He continued to work on Duchenne dystrophy and spent time in laboratories in the Netherlands working on the project.

Duchenne dystrophy is an X-linked recessive disease and Fischbeck became interested in other neurological diseases encoded on the X-chromosome. One of them was Kennedy syndrome, a form of motor neuron disease that causes weakness of limb muscles and difficulty speaking; its formal name is "X-linked spinobulbar muscular atrophy." In 1991, Fischbeck and his colleagues reported that the affected gene encoded the androgen receptor, a report that achieved landmark status for several reasons, not the least because an important endocrine gene was involved.

Perhaps more important for neurology, it was the first disease in which the mutation was not a deletion or a change of an amino acid. Instead, there was an expansion of a *trinucleotide repeat*, a normal structure in the genome until it exceeds a certain size. The list of these diseases, a subset of which are called "polyglutamine diseases," includes fragile X syndrome, myotonic dystrophy, Huntington disease, Friedreich ataxia, and several different familial ataxias. These diseases provided explanations for old genetic observations. The greater the expansion number, the earlier symptoms of the disease appeared ("*anticipation*") and the more severe the symptoms were ("*potentiation*"). Then it was found that in the polyglutamine diseases the affected protein – a different one in each of the several disorders – tends to aggregate in the nerve cells; the aggregates seem toxic to the cells or at least represent a toxic property of the mutant protein. Toxic proteins prone to aggregations probably play a role in other neurodegenerative diseases too – not just the polyglutamine disorders but also Alzheimer disease, Parkinson disease, and ALS.

In 1998, Fischbeck moved to head a newly created Neurogenetics Branch in the intramural program. He enlarged his program by setting up one laboratory for the study of neurodevelopmental disorders and another to reproduce neurodegenerative diseases in *Drosophila*, the fruit fly. He has continued to work on the Kennedy syndrome and another X-linked disease, a peripheral neuropathy. He has also assumed new activities in the world of muscular dystrophy, attempting to modify gene transcription favorably by giving an antibiotic, gentamicin.

At NIH, Fischbeck has also become more closely involved with voluntary health agencies and with the extramural program directors who deal with the grant programs relevant to the genetics of neurologic disease. In recognition of his achievements, Fischbeck was elected to the Institute of Medicine of the National Academy of Sciences in 1999.

The Wonder of Stem Cells

Ronald D.G. McKay, Ph.D.

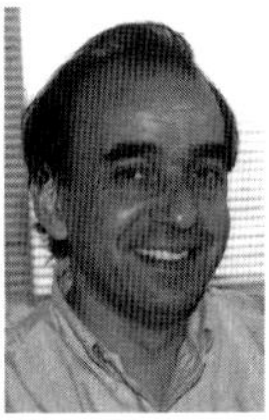

RONALD D.G. MCKAY, PH.D., IS CURRENT CHIEF OF THE LABORATORY OF MOLECULAR BIOLOGY

Ron McKay evinced an interest in science as an adolescent. One of his favorite writers was Charles Darwin. He graduated from the University of Edinburgh in 1971. For his Ph.D., he worked with DNA pioneer Edward Southern (of Southern blot fame, a key method for the analysis of DNA and encoded proteins). Then, as a postdoctoral student, he mapped genes with another noted geneticist, Walter Bodmer at Oxford University. They were in one of two laboratories that worked on restriction fragment polymorphisms, the DNA markers that paved the way to gene mapping. McKay and his group analyzed the Y-chromosome and, in 1978, found the first human polymorphisms, akin to the smooth or wrinkled peas of Mendel.

McKay came to the United States in 1978 to join the Cold Spring Harbor Laboratory, where he first worked on DNA-protein interactions. He also began to work on the organization of the nervous system, especially the chemical events in development that had attracted Roger Sperry. There, he first tried to identify different neurons with monoclonal antibodies. James Watson recognized the importance of McKay's ideas and encouraged his nascent interest in neuroscience.

He continued as a neurobiologist when he moved to the Massachusetts Institute of Technology in 1984. At MIT, he came to take another approach, as he described it:[17]

> That was the place where my work became almost completely focused on this issue of stem cells. That emerged very naturally from the discovery that the nervous system was so complex. Milstein discovered the hybridoma method and I realized you could use that now to ask whether the nervous system was very complicated. In 1980, we were the first people to show that – which was widely recognized as being important. It was out of that work that I realized that the molecular complexity of the nervous system exceeded all the current tools we had available to understand molecular functions. There were so many differences among neurons that we had to develop a new technology to understand how molecules act together to carry out high-level functions. That made me start looking for the cell that gave rise to neurons. We knew about work from Europe that was already advanced by the 1950s, and then work from Seymour Benzer in *Drosophila* that was published in the

> mid-1970s, that there was a plastic multipotential precursor to neurons in both flies and vertebrates. So we went looking for that cell and tried to understand how that cell operated – and to create a technology that intervened so that it would be one level up from genes and proteins.[17]

In 1993, Ernst Freese died and left open the position of Chief of the NINDS Laboratory of Molecular Biology. Marshall Nirenberg, the first NIH Nobel laureate, suggested McKay for the open position, and Hal Gainer led the search that ended in the choice of McKay. As a measure of the paltry turnover of some major positions at NIH, McKay was told that he was the first lab chief to be recruited from outside in 15 years.

McKay is grateful for the opportunity to work at NINDS. "We could not have done this and made this field the way it is" without the kind of support NIH provides. "It requires a different combination of skills from the traditional molecular biology." He also amplified his view about genetic analysis:

> What people were beginning to realize is that you could not do what you wanted to do simply with genes. Remember, this is why I got into the problem in the first place. There are too many genes. You are just never going to figure it out looking at it one gene at a time.

By the mid-1990s, McKay's stem cell research had advanced. The year 1998 proved to be a crucial year in the development of interest. Papers by John Gearhart and James Thomson announced that human embryonal stem cells could be grown. Following McKay's earlier demonstration that stem cells really exist in the rat, the 1998 reports stimulated wide interest.

The extraordinary developmental potential of stem cells is one of the central discoveries of the field. In a series of experiments, McKay and his group demonstrated that nervous system stem cells would differentiate to many new fates. In one set of experiments, they engrafted cells into the cerebral vesicles while the receipient was still in the uterus. The donor cells entered the host brain and proliferated in the tens of thousands and differentiated appropriately into neurons in new locations.

The ability to manipulate stem cells suggested that these new tools might be used to treat disorders of the nervous system. To that end, they developed techniques to derive a precursor of oligodendroglial cells – the supporting cells that make myelin – from embryonic stem cells. They implanted these cells in transgenic mice lacking proteolipid protein, an essential component of the myelin sheath, which covers and insulates nerves in the brain as well as peripherally.[18] In this mouse model, the protein was lacking, just as it is in Pelizaeus-Merzbacher disease, a rare human inherited disease in which brain myelin is defective. Transplanting stem cells into these mice had spectacular effects. The stem cells proliferated, migrated to the proper sites, enveloped the naked axons, and synthesized myelin. This was one of the first demonstrations that embryonic stem cells might be turned into useful cells of the nervous system.

That experiment was one of several advancing the possibility that stem cell therapy may be effective in many human diseases. McKay and his group have now generated brain cells that make the neurotransmitters dopamine or serotonin, which might be applied to Parkinson disease or psychiatric disorders. In many studies they identify early nerve cells by using antibodies to a protein called *nestin*, an acronym for *n*euro-*e*pithelial *st*em cells.

When the same marker protein was found in pancreatic islet cells, they found that embryonal stem cells could differentiate into organelles resembling pancreatic islets and produce insulin, the hormone missing in 16 million Americans with diabetes mellitus.[19] Similarly, a team including McKay and other NIH researchers found that bone marrow-derived stem cells could repair degenerated muscle in experimental heart attacks brought on by tying off blood vessels.[20]

There is a huge chasm between stem cells and human therapy but the discoveries of this NIH team have become an important part of contemporary medicine. McKay's work is as basic as it can be, trying to understand how nerve cells arise and develop. At the same time, the research is surely disease-oriented, giving promise of radically new treatments. This research also illuminates the unexpected value of research in one area for quite a different set of problems, and illustrates how "fortune favors the prepared mind."

Passing Through; en Route to Fame

J. Craig Venter, Ph.D.

Craig Venter is a genuine world celebrity. His face appears on the cover of Time and other magazines. He is often seen on television screens. His comments appear in popular and scholarly publications. He is a star of both genomic science and biotech commerce; his history has therefore been told many times.[21]

But not many people know that Venter worked at NINDS from 1984 to 1992, a time of personal transition for him and a transition that was of prime importance in the history of biomedical science.

Venter was 19 years old when he entered the U.S. Navy Medical Corps and served in Vietnam from 1965 to 1968. He had declined to enter college in favor of swimming and surfing but the horrors of the war injuries he witnessed led him to think seriously about his future. He returned to the University of California, San Diego, where he majored in biochemistry. He became a graduate student there under Nathan O. Kaplan, the noted enzymologist, and received his Ph.D. in 1975.

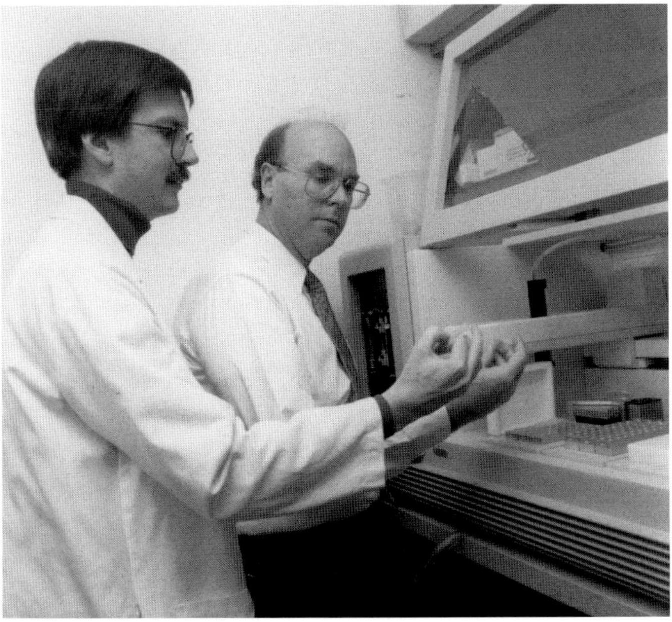

J. CRAIG VENTER, PH.D., AND MARK ADAMS IN THE LAB, SOMETIME IN THE 1980S

From 1976 to 1984, he rose through the ranks at the State University of New York at Buffalo. He investigated enzymes immobilized on glass beads or other inert surfaces and then studied adrenergic receptors. In 1982 he wrote a review of the use of monoclonal antibodies to isolate receptors for neurotransmitters. Dopaminergic and muscarinic receptors fell into his purview. By 1983, he was on the editorial boards of relevant journals.

In 1984, he came to NINDS as Chief of the Section of Receptor Biochemistry. By 1987, he was Co-Director of the Laboratory of Molecular and Cellular Neurobiology and, in 1990, Chief of that laboratory.

During this period, his many publications were all about membrane receptors. Then, at the end of 1990, he was the author of a summary of a conference on genome sequencing. Early in 1991, his personal world and the world of biomedical research changed with the publication of a paper on expressed sequence tags and the human genome project, a new method to map genomes. With that contribution he became totally immersed in genomics. His last paper on receptors was published in 1991. The next year he described the sequence identification of human brain genes. From then on, his productivity continued, all directed to unraveling the genomes of many species.

The transition was not as abrupt as it might seem on the surface. In a telephone interview, Venter explained how it came about.[22]

For ten years before he came to NINDS, Venter's interest in neurotransmitter receptors had led him to understand the need for molecular biology so he and his staff were all retrained for the new approach. He arrived at NINDS in 1984 and they completed the cloning and sequencing of genes for the beta-adrenergic receptor and the muscarinic cholinergic receptor in human brain. That feat was achieved by "manual sequencing," the mode of the day.

Manual sequencing was dull, laborious, and painfully slow. Sydney Brenner, an early champion of mapping the genome, advocated the use of manual sequencing as a punishment for prisoners, "the more heinous the crime, the bigger the chromosome they would have to decipher."[23]

In February 1987, Venter read a paper describing an automatic sequencer for the analysis of DNA. Later that year he and his associates reported on the very first genes to have been sequenced by automated methods. They had leaped from taking a decade for one gene to a few months for the task of cloning and sequencing. The introduction to the paper included the understatement that the "technique will have a considerable impact on DNA sequencing."[24]

At the time, discussions and debates were starting about the advisability of sequencing the human genome. The estimated time was ten to 15 years – and they had taken ten years for a single gene – so his new techniques would be important. Shortening the time would also have an impact on the billions of dollars the project would cost.

Venter thinks he was the first biochemist to enter genomic research. Situated in a neurological institute, it seemed reasonable for Venter to seek some relevant genes and he went after two, the Huntington disease gene and the myotonic muscular dystrophy gene. To do that required the sequencing of large stretches of DNA and it seemed as though it would be faster to sequence the entire genome than to isolate genes one by one. That led him "straight to the genome."

To interpret the sequence data, they had to analyze the "complementary" DNA or cDNA, which was obtained by matching pieces of DNA to messenger RNA (mRNA). In the process of "transcription," RNA is produced from a DNA template. In other words, going backwards from mRNA to cDNA was a way to identify pieces of genes, a process of gene discovery. In one paper, they described 2,375 new genes in the human brain;[25] that single paper doubled the total number of known human genes (although the function of those genes was still unknown).

The process of identifying those pieces of cDNA led to the term "expressed sequence tag" or EST, which – according to Venter – has become the "dominant method for gene discovery." ESTs are areas of DNA that are expressed; they are selected from whole DNA because they are expressed genes and do not include the large portions of DNA that do not serve as genes. Millions of genes in different species have been found that way but it was this experience that led Venter to the genome.

For this opportunity, Venter is grateful for his experience at NINDS.

Venter left NIH in 1992 to found the first of three genomic companies. One result was a productive competition between his "private" company and the public consortium – productive in the sense that Venter's results prodded everyone involved to accelerate the completion of the human genome project by 2000. In the process, NINDS was the incubator for a brilliant scientist whose career is a clear example of the importance of allowing scientists to follow leads, not orders.

An Overall View

These examples of work in the intramural laboratories of NINDS complement those of the prize winners in Section III. As Roscoe Brady has said, "NIH is, and ought to be, a place for high-risk research of uncertain outcome that may take years to complete." It is also an institution where brilliant investigators in many institutes interact fruitfully. It may appear to be a cumbersome elephant of a structure but its positive attributes have withstood the rigors of the first 50 years.

1 Sokoloff L. Conversation with author, April 2001.

2 Kurland L, Brody JA. The development and application of epidemiologic methods to neurology: a historical perspective. In Chase TN, ed. *The Clinical Neurosciences,* vol. 2 of Tower DB, *The Nervous System: A Three-Volume Work Commemorating the 25th Anniversary of the National Institute of Neurological and Communicative Disorders and Stroke.* New York: Raven Press, 1975:5-23.

3 Anonymous. Obituary. Norman Goldstein, *Post-Bulletin* (Rochester, Minn.) October 20, 1994.

4 Windebank AJ (Dean, Mayo Medical School) to author, May 1, 2001; Whisnant J. Conversation with author, May 10, 2001.

5 Alvord EC. E-mail Communication to author, May 2 and July 31, 2001.

6 Lisak RP. Obituary for Marian Kies. *J Neuroimmunol* 1989; 23: 91-92.

7 Kurland LT. The frequency and geographic distribution of Multiple Sclerosis as indicated by mortality statistics and morbidity surveys in the United States and Canada. *Am J Hyg* 1952;55:457-476.

8 Goldberg ID, Kurland LT. Mortality in 33 countries from diseases of the nervous system. *World Neurol* 1962;3:444-465.

9 McFarland H. Interview with author, March 27, 2001.

10 Porter R. James Kiffin Penry (1929-1996). *Neurology* 1996;47:1345-1356.

11 Garnett SE. NINDS's Kupferberg Retires. *The NIH Record,* Aug. 8, 2000.

12 Frazin N. Epilepsy conference emphasizes "no seizures, no side effects." *The NIH Record,* May 16, 2000.

13 Porter RJ. Telephone Interview with author, June 5, 2001.

14 *Maximizing Human Potential. Decade of the Brain, 1990-2000.* Report of Subcommittee on Brain and Behavioral Sciences. Office of Science and Technology Policy, Federal Coordinating Council for Science, Engineering, and Technology, Committee on Life Sciences and Health, April, 1991.

15 Oldfield EH. Interview with author, October 2, 2000.

16 Fischbeck KH. Recorded Telephone Interview with author, July 6, 2001.

17 McKay RDG. The origins of cellular diversity in the mammalian central nervous system. *Cell* 1989;58:815-821.

18 Brustle O, Jones KN, Learish RD, Karram K, Choudhary K, Wiestler OD, Duncan ID, McKay RD. Embryonic stem-cell derived glial precursors: a source of myelinating transplants. *Science* 1999;285:754-756.

19 Lumelsky N, Blondel O, Laeng P, Velasco I, Ravin R, McKay R. Differentiation of embryonic stem cells to insulin-secreting structures similar to pancreatic islets. *Science* 2001;292:1389-1394.

20 Orlic D, Katjstura J. Chimenti S, Jakoniuk I, Anderson, SM, Li B, Pickel J. McKay R, Nadal-Ginard B, Bodine DM, Leri A, Anversa P. Bone marrow cells regenerate infracted myocardium. *Nature* 2001;410:701-705.

21 Davies K. Cracking the Genome: Inside the Race to Unlock Human DNA. New York: The Free Press, 2001.

22 Venter JC. Telephone Interview with author, June 22, 2001.

23 Roberts L. The human genome: news, controversial from the start. *Science* 2001; 291:1182-1188.

24 Gokayne J, Robinson DA, Fitzgerald MG, Chung F-Z, Kervalage AR, Lentes K-U, Lai J, Wang C-D, Fraser DM, Venter JC. Primary structure of rat cardiac ß-adrenergic and muscarinic cholinergic receptors obtained by automated DNA sequence analysis: further evidence for a multigene family. *Proc Natl Acad Sci* USA 1987;84:8296-8300.

25 Adams M, Dubnick M, Kerlavage A, Moreno R, Kelley J, Utterback T, Nagle J, Fields C, Venter JC. Sequence identification of 2375 human brain genes. *Nature* 1992;355:632-634.

CHAPTER SEVEN

EXTRAMURAL PROGRAM

The extramural program of NINDS is the motor that propels most research in clinical neuroscience and much of basic neuroscience in the United States. As a proportion of the total NINDS budget, the extramural program varies but has averaged more than 80 percent over the years.

NINDS is not the sole source of research support at NIH for the neurosciences. NIMH supports basic neuroscience research and has its own clinical programs. The National Institute on Aging and the National Institute of Child Health and Human Development support clinical research for dementias, developmental disorders, and some forms of epilepsy. The National Cancer Institute, the National Institute of Allergy and Infectious Diseases, the National Institute of Environmental Health Sciences, and the National Institute of Arthritis and Musculoskeletal and Skin Diseases have shares. The National Institute of Dental and Craniofacial Research supports pain research. The National Eye Institute and the National Institute on Deafness and Other Communication Disorders accommodate their fields. A few other institutes also support smaller grants.

The pharmaceutical industry's support of research has been increasing for all brain disorders, and voluntary health agencies contribute as well. These multiple sources of funding make it difficult to calculate the percent of the total costs attributable to NINDS, but in the year 2000, the extramural NINDS expenses came to $902,000,000 or 88 percent of the total budget.

How NINDS distributes the money depends on the choices made from among a glittering array of vehicles – individual research grants, training awards, contracts, and small business awards. In large measure the individual institute directors and their staffs make the choices. But the whole NIH and its history also determine the process and the guidelines for each institute. The two dominant principles guiding these choices have been the priority of investigator-initiated grant applications – as opposed to centrally planned research – and peer review. In turn, peer review involves "study sections," as explained by former NINDS director Murray Goldstein.

32 Years at the Extramural Helm: Murray Goldstein

The modern story of extramural NINDS activity has to begin with Murray Goldstein because he was director of all NINDS extramural programs from 1961 to 1976 and led the extramural stroke and trauma program from 1976 to 1978. Then he was, successively, deputy director for two years, acting director for one year, and director of NINDS from 1982 to 1993. Therefore, Goldstein – explicitly or indirectly – was responsible for the extramural program for 32 consecutive years.

NINDS Extramural Funding, 1951–2000
(dollars in thousands)

Fiscal Year	Total Funding	Extramural Funding	Extramural as % of Total
1951	—	1,232	—
1952	—	1,562	—
1953	—	1,814	—
1954	3,354	4,500	75%
1955	5,054	7,600	67%
1956	6,300	9,861	64%
1957	14,280	18,650	77%
1958	16,250	21,387	76%
1959	23,166	29,403	79%
1960	33,908	41,487	82%
1961	47,867	56,600	85%
1962	56,240	70,812	79%
1963	67,022	83,506	80%
1964	74,241	87,675	85%
1965	73,147	87,821	83%
1966	84,800	101,153	84%
1967	96,130	116,296	83%
1968	107,001	128,633	83%
1969	101,151	128,934	78%
1970	72,857	97,315	75%
1971	75,884	103,502	73%
1972	86,683	116,731	74%
1973	99,640	130,672	76%
1974	97,209	121,358	80%
1975	112,353	142,498	79%
1976	113,548	144,446	79%
1977	118,244	155,500	76%
1978	133,472	178,438	75%
1979	162,678	212,365	77%
1980	189,934	241,966	78%
1981	198,438	252,533	79%
1982	207,387	265,901	78%
1983	236,290	297,064	80%
1984	271,160	335,883	81%
1985	328,238	396,885	83%
1986	350,510	414,727	85%
1987	417,235	490,233	85%
1988	455,353	534,692	85%
1989	390,786	472,095	83%
1990	405,878	490,409	83%
1991	444,762	541,743	82%
1992	476,335	577,938	82%
1993	495,589	600,078	83%
1994	528,067	630,650	84%
1995	547,130	649,786	84%
1996	575,104	680,902	84%
1997	618,816	726,407	85%
1998	669,553	780,713	86%
1999	781,603	902,680	81%
2000	901,961	1,029,376	88%

In 1987, the medical historian, Stephen Strickland, interviewed Goldstein[1] and asked him to explain the origin of study sections. Goldstein replied:

> When the grant system was first evolving at NIH... the law established the National Advisory Cancer Council to make decisions about cancer grants, and the National Advisory Health Council, to make decisions about everything else. The original thought was that the Council itself would have the technical expertise to make the scientific judgments and to make appropriate recommendations. So the authority was vested in these Councils.... At the first few Council meetings, the Council was handling this. Then, with the sudden growth of the grant program, and the diversity of the kinds of applications that were being presented to the Council, particularly the Cancer Council, [it] recognized that it did not have expertise in certain specific areas. [Members of the Cancer Council] therefore asked that expert review committees be set up to advise it . . . the first scientific review panels . . . were the Councils themselves. This was vested in the law.
>
> Occasionally there were applications that *no* member of a Council could have an informed opinion about, or only one member knew something about, and the Council had to rely entirely on that [individual]. Nobody was comfortable with this. So, the study sections were formed, and they began in the context of the Cancer Institute.

By the time Goldstein arrived at NIH, the Division of Research Grants (DRG; now the Center for Scientific Review) was supervising the study sections.

> Not only did the study sections advise the Councils on scientific merit, but they were also charged with taking steps themselves to have an overview of their fields, to present reports about the status of research...and to take steps to stimulate needed research in biophysics by holding research workshops and conferences and other ways . . . . Sections then were program development organizations, moving ahead vigorously . . . to help build a science at the same time that they were judging individual applications . . . . The rather sharp lines that have evolved in the recent years between the responsibilities of the institutes for program development and the responsibilities of the scientific review committees were very blurred...in my opinion rightfully so.
>
> NIH was expanding rapidly. It was trying to learn from the scientific community what the best opportunities were, and how the NIH could usefully and legally aid and abet in this development . . . .

> Then the persons involved in the scientific merit review were to be divorced completely from program development. The study sections were told: 'Your only responsibility is scientific merit review.' It was thought that it was not appropriate for the same person who was developing the grants to also be reviewing the grants.

Goldstein summarized the change in the late 1950s that lasted for the next three decades:

> The study sections essentially started as subcommittees of the councils, advising the Councils, at the request of the Councils. They evolved...into independent bodies having absolutely nothing to do with either the institute or the Council, functioning as if they were in a completely different organization.

After 1954, for years the ample budgets permitted funding of all approved grants. To assure quality, NIH Director James Shannon decided that applications in the lower 10 percent would not be funded and it became the function of study sections to identify those applications – to determine which applications would *not* be supported.

Over the years, the study sections remained part of the DRG, distinctly separate from the institutes. The DRG in turn depended on and set rules for the whole NIH, not the individual institutes. Although the study sections were supposed to be concerned with merit review only – and not program development – their priority scores determined which fields of research were to be supported and which were not. Eventually, they determined which grants were to be funded. In lean years, funding rates fell below 20 percent of approved grants and the system was severely stressed.

Extramural programs were administered at first by generalists who were assigned to the study sections to monitor the process. Gradually that practice changed and program directors became specialists in, for example, stroke or Parkinson disease, and they found themselves in competition with each other. To accommodate the need for program development outside the study sections, the institute took 20 percent of the extramural budget and set it aside for decisions outside the priority score system. This policy was greeted warmly by the scientists and by the Congress. As Goldstein explained, the 20 percent rule permitted support for "young researchers, for exploratory fields, for newly evolving fields, and for the kooky application which we think is approvable."

The Councils made the ultimate determinations. Individual members were urged to consider the whole institute, not just their specific fields. At first, that included hearing and vision research, but the pressures ultimately led the staffs, scientists, and the patient advocates of those fields to secede and form their own institutes.

There are now multitudinous study sections for neuroscience grant applications. Sometimes different study sections consider the same kinds of applications. One section is called Neurology A and another Neurology B. As Goldstein put it, applicants may sometimes complain that they were put in the wrong study section and that their application would have received "more sympathy" if it had been put in the other. Or the beef may be that a clinical research proposal was sent to a basic study section that included no M.D.s. In fact, however, the approval rate for applications by M.D.s and Ph.D.s is about equal.

In addition to describing the study sections, Goldstein also traced the origin of program projects, which are different from individual investigator's grants. Program projects began with the development of general clinical research centers in medical institutions. At first, these clinical facilities consisted only of the hospital beds supported for research and the laboratories in which the research was done. After that, came the specialized centers, including neurological clinical research centers. When the basic scientists wanted a similarly large bolus of funds because, for instance, they needed an electron microscope (which could not be justified by a single research project) there had to be a funding mechanism as well. Goldstein's response was to say, "But all we've got is project authority and they are looking for program support. Hey – why don't we give them program projects?"

And that is how the term "program project" was born in the late 50s. They were reviewed by special institute-based committees, not by DRG study sections. Similarly, institute-reviewing committees were formed for training applications.

By the time of the Strickland interview in 1987, Goldstein had recognized several continuing problems that have continued to this day. This first was competition between institutes for specific grant applications about a particular disease of interest to more than one. That problem has become more widespread with the proliferation of institutes dealing with neuroscience.

The second problem concerns the peer review process, which has had difficulty keeping pace with the growing number of applications. Are applications receiving adequate review or are they being over-reviewed?

The third problem is financial instability, which is created by fluctuations in funding that range from 40 percent in some years to less than 15 percent in others. This has been less of a problem in the last three years because of Congress' assent to double the NIH budget over a five year span. But the warning signs are up because there seems to be little likelihood that there will be another doubling after 2003 when the current expansion will end.[2]

A fourth problem facing the extramural grant program has been a shift in the relationship between universities and government. At first, NIH financial support came in the form of "grants-in-aid."

The money was intended to support research in the university. Gradually, however, the term became "government-supported research" as universities requested salary support in proportion to faculty time spent on a research project. Then indirect costs were added. Goldstein asked:

> Are the research grants supposed to underpin the operation of universities? If that is true, why shouldn't they just become federal universities, as exist in other countries of the world? Then we would run them. But they do not want it like that and neither do we.

This last conundrum leads to one more: the use of the contract mechanism. The federal guideline is that a contract supports research determined by the government, whereas grants are supposed to be an *assistance* program for investigator-initiated research.

Goldstein concluded that, despite all the persistent problems:

> The system is the envy of the world; every nation and every committee that has been selected has said it is a magnificent system in that it permits people to enter the system. It gives them an opportunity to compete. It is a benevolent system that is responsive to science, and yet also responsive to the needs of the public. If one were to sit down in the abstract and design this system to meet those objectives, it would probably look like the NIH.
>
> NIH was not designed to be the way it is today – it evolved. It evolved in what I consider to be the best interrelationship between the government, the public, and science.

Some of these problems are experienced by all of the institutes within NIH, and are not to be resolved within NINDS alone. For instance, William Landau was, for 21 years, head of the research-oriented department of neurology at Washington University in St. Louis. He is still concerned with the inclusion of faculty salaries on NIH research grants, which he considers an abrogation of university responsibility for choosing and paying for its own professors.[3] However, there seems little likelihood that paying partial salaries by way of research grants can be changed at this late date – even if it were deemed desirable. In 1967, Thomas Turner, then Dean at Johns Hopkins, proposed an alternative plan for federal funds to support faculty salaries through grants to the university – but that never materialized.[4]

Three Decades, Four Division Directors

Murray Goldstein was not the only long-term leader of the extramural program. Four division directors also served for more than 30 years. They were Eugene Streicher, Jack Brinley, Carl Leventhal, and Michael Walker. Unlike the administrative structure in place today where there is one Director for Extramural Research (Constance Atwell) who supervises a large number of program directors, these four all reported directly to the NINDS Director, Murray Goldstein, and supervised groups of program directors.

The first of these was Eugene Streicher, who had been trained in neurochemistry with Ralph Gerard, the University of Chicago neurophysiologist who is credited with being one of the founders of the Society for Neuroscience. Streicher came to NIH in 1954 to work on drug sensitivity in the rat brain as part of an early aging study in the laboratory of Jack Birren, a psychologist hired by Seymour Kety. When that program terminated, Streicher worked on experimental brain edema in the neuropathology laboratory of Igor Klatzo. His research was to measure the biochemical effects of the edema. When pressure was applied to make that laboratory take on more diagnostic responsibility Streicher saw another closure looming.

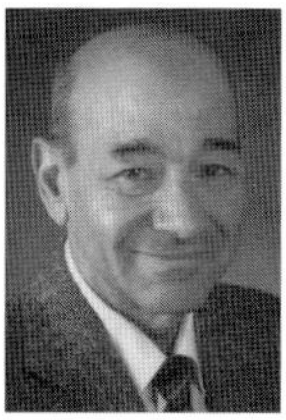

Eugene Streicher, M.D.

He moved to NINDS administration in 1964, recruited by Richard Masland. He started with the training committee under the direction of Elizabeth Hartman and, after two years, he moved to basic science grants management. He continued in the extramural program for a total of 43 years, which may be a record for institutional longevity.

In time, Streicher headed the Division of Fundamental Neurosciences where his responsibilities were diverse. Among the achievements of the time was the development of the cochlear implant (an auditory prosthesis) which was done by Terry Hambrecht – before hearing research moved to its own institute in 1988.

Streicher described the relationship of the program directors to Murray Goldstein:[5]

> This was a one-man institute. Murray was the institute. We served him. Whenever there was something to be taken up with Murray, or he had something he wanted to discuss, the four division directors would hash it out first. We'd spend as much time as it took to put together the pros and the cons, the influences and so on, so that it could be laid out in a very efficient way. "You asked about this; we think this or we think that. These are the pros and these are the cons."
>
> Instead of attacking each administrative issue or each new one out of the blue…it had a place to really get taken up in great detail.
>
> So we basically took these problems of various kinds that Murray was concerned with and, for as much time as it took, got the thing ground out. We may have disagreed, but at least we got down to the essence of the problem and the consequences or potential consequences of each procedure. Also, it was a way of passing on to Murray – not that he needed it, his ear was to

the ground more than anybody else's – the information that we might have gotten from friends in other institutes or from other people. We basically gave him a fair amount of stuff to worry about, or to chose from.

I think that it was valuable because it educated us. Educating us in turn, it educated our HSAs [health science administrators, now program directors]. What was coming down the road? If there were certain things that we felt Murray would be interested in or information we needed, we would ask our people in terms of their grantees, or other people, if there was any information they had about something that would be passed on to Murray at these meetings.

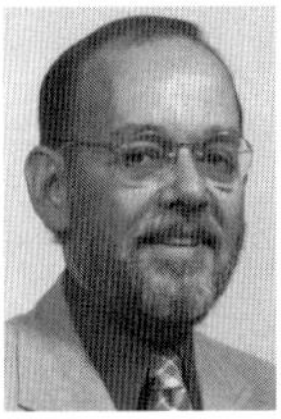

CARL LEVENTHAL, M.D.

Carl Leventhal, M.D., also started to work at the neurology institute in 1964 as an officer in the Public Health Service and remained at the institute until he retired in 1996. He had graduated from Harvard and then the University of Rochester Medical School. After training in medicine at Johns Hopkins, he was a neurology resident at the Massachusetts General Hospital. There he became interested in neuropathology through his admiration for E. Pierson Richardson. He first applied to NIH for military service and was assigned to a neuropathology laboratory that was part of the Perinatal Project.[6] That experience was not very productive so he moved to the Cancer Institute where, with Mike Walker, they set up a national program in brain tumor chemotherapy.

At the time, brain tumors were a joint subject for the Cancer and Neurology Institutes and Leventhal came to know Murray Goldstein, who was then head of the NINDS extramural program. Leventhal had a chance to work in the office of the NIH Director, James Shannon, starting in 1966, just before Shannon retired. Then came the difficult political years in the Director's office during the Nixon Presidency. Several outstanding members of Shannon's staff left NIH in the disputes and Leventhal was at loose ends. One day in 1981, he met Murray Goldstein in the cafeteria; at lunch, Goldstein said, "Carl, come home." He did and his assignment was to relieve Jack Brinley, who had accumulated too many grants. Leventhal became director of the Division of Demyelinating, Atrophic, and Dementing Disorders. Formally, Brinley's charge was the Division of Convulsive, Developmental, and Neuromuscular Disorders (DCDND), still a formidable collection.

The high points of Leventhal's participation were related to Huntington disease: his role in the Lake Maracaibo project led by Nancy Wexler; the establishment of the two Huntington Disease Centers Without Walls; and the mapping of the Huntington disease gene by James Gusella and the group in the Center at Massachusetts General Hospital led by Joseph Martin.

Another achievement was the collaboration he achieved with Byron Waksman and Steve Reingold of the New York chapter of the National Multiple Sclerosis Society, which he considered "one of the best examples of close interaction with a voluntary society." Parkinson disease was also in Leventhal's portfolio and so was neuro-AIDS.

In 1994, Leventhal lost his wife to carcinoma of the colon and he lost his close administrative friend when Murray Goldstein retired as NINDS Director. Two years later, after 32 years at NIH, Leventhal retired.

While Donald Tower was Director of NINCDS in 1978, he asked Goldstein to be Deputy Director, leaving open the position of Director of the Stroke and Trauma Program. To fill that gap, they recruited Michael Walker, M.D., who had been trained as a neurosurgeon and came to NIH for research training on the blood-brain barrier with David Rall in the Cancer Institute. While he was doing that, he was offered a position to work at an NCI experimental program in Baltimore, "an intramural field office in an extramural setting."[7] He would have labs, beds for brain tumor patients, and his own operating rooms – an offer not to be refused by a young neurosurgeon. His talents were recognized and he was soon made Director of the Baltimore Cancer Research Center, where administrative responsibilities became heavier and heavier. Among his charges was a brain tumor cooperative group, which he started and directed.

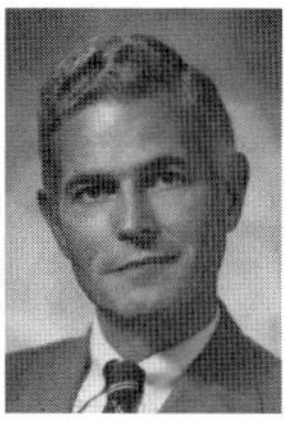

Michael Walker, M.D.

In 1978, Tower asked him to take over the stroke program in NINCDS, which, for a neurosurgeon, seemed a more natural home than the Cancer Institute. When he arrived, there was only one clinical trial in the field of stroke, the third most common cause of death in the United States.

The main obstacle was the defeatist belief that nothing could be done for a patient with a stroke. To find testable drugs, he developed a "Task Order Master Agreement," a contract process in which qualified medical centers were selected in a peer-reviewed process. Qualification depended not only on the talents of the investigators, but their ability to recruit patients. He set conditions for pharmaceutical companies – generic names, uniform package information for treated and placebo patient groups, participation of company scientists but not marketing staff, and provision of placebo preparations. In return, his staff helped the companies obtain FDA data. All results, favorable or not, would be published. The companies did not have a contract and they did not participate in the peer review. Companies and investigators were separate.

Over the course of years, Walker ran dozens of trials, including one evaluating carotid endarterectomy and culminating in the tissue plasminogen activator (TPA) trial that came to a favorable conclusion – but only if patients were treated within three hours of symptom onset. At one point, he supervised 14 trials simultaneously. In the process, the principles and practice of controlled therapeutic trials for cerebrovascular diseases improved continuously.

Another major achievement for Walker was the establishment of centers throughout the country for positron emission tomography (PET), which were used for studies of brain metabolism under different conditions or to evaluate the performance of drug receptors, investigations that are not possible for MRI. The difference is straightforward: MRI shows structure; PET shows function.

The first three PET centers were established at UCLA, Michigan, and Pennsylvania. Others followed in what became a major financial investment by NINDS. At the start, the grants covered installation of the scanners and development of the supporting cyclotrons to make the isotopes for labeled compounds needed for metabolic studies or tags for drug-receptors. This process of preparing the infrastructure took so long that the renewal applications could not report any true research progress, but that soon followed. Many of the scanners became core facilities for multiple research labs in multiple medical centers and grant programs were developed to support individual projects.

After 31 years at NINDS, Walker retired in 2000 and still consults for the institute. John Marler, who had directed the TPA trial and is now in charge of all clinical trials for the institute as associate director for clinical trials, succeeded him in supervising the stroke grants.

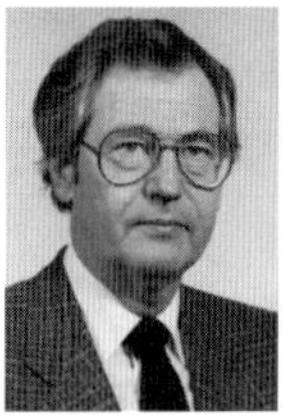

FLOYD JOHN (JACK) BRINLEY, JR., M.D.

Floyd John (Jack) Brinley, Jr., graduated from Oberlin College and went to medical school at the University of Michigan. He interned at the University of California, Los Angeles, and came to NIH in 1957 for neurophysiology training in the joint NINDS-NIMH laboratory of Wade Marshall. Two years later he went to Johns Hopkins and gained a Ph.D. in biophysics in 1961. He remained on the faculty there as an assistant professor and then, in 1966, he was appointed associate professor. He was also a professor of physiology at the University of Maryland until he returned to NINDS in 1979.

At first, Brinley headed the extramural Neurological Disorders Program, guiding research grants, contracts, and fellowships that supported basic research in areas such as developmental disorders, Parkinson disease, Huntington disease, Alzheimer disease, epilepsy, sleep, multiple sclerosis, amyotrophic lateral sclerosis, neuromuscular disorders, infections, neuroendocrine disorders, and neurotoxicology. One of his first achievements was to help set up the Lake Maracaibo study with Nancy Wexler.

Three years after he started, however, it was evident that his responsibilities were excessive and the program was split in two. The neurodegenerative diseases went to Carl Leventhal, and Brinley covered epilepsy, developmental conditions, and neuromuscular disorders. In 1996, another reorganization gave him the convulsive, infectious, and immune disorders, now including neuro-AIDS. In

1999, he became associate director for infection and immunity, emphasizing HIV-1 infection and prion diseases.

From 1981 to 1995, in addition to his NINDS activities, Brinley continued to teach as Professor of Biophysics at the University of Maryland. He won several Public Health Service honors and served on editorial boards of the *Journal of Neurophysiology, Cell Calcium*, and *Cellular and Molecular Neurobiology*. He retired in February 2001, after 23 years of service.

Veterans

Mathilde Solowey, Ph.D.

Dr. Solowey's interview with the author took place when she was 90 years old.[8] She received her bachelor's degree in chemistry from NYU in 1931. She spent several years as a medical student, bacteriologist, and air pollution analyst. In 1942, she earned her Ph.D. in bacteriology with Beatrice Seegal at Columbia University. After working in the Department of Agriculture and private bacteriology laboratories, she came to NINDS in 1961, just when neurological clinical research centers were being established. It was her first assignment from Richard Masland. She nurtured the centers for a decade and set the pattern of relations between the principal investigators and the individual scientists responsible for portions of the total production. In that way she determined the modern format of all program projects.

In 1972, Solowey moved to the Cancer Institute where she worked with Mike Walker on brain tumor projects and then returned to NINDS under Donald Tower to review contracts. She resigned from NINDS in 1974, took a position with Dr. Ruth Kirschstein in the General Medical Sciences Institute, and retired altogether in 1979. She subsequently became a grants consultant to medical schools but her heart was always with neurology because of the friends she made throughout the country and her recognition of the challenge of neurological diseases. She has expressed her appreciation in a tangible way by endowing an annual NIH lecture, which is named after her. She is still working to raise enough money to increase the honorarium.

Levon Parker, B.S.

Levon Parker came to what was then NINCDS in 1962 to work in the Laboratory of Molecular Biology. Parker, who was born in a small town on the eastern shore of Virginia, had received a B.S. in biology and chemistry from the University of Maryland, Eastern Shore.

After 12 years in the lab, conducting research and training other young neuroscientists, Parker was offered the opportunity to head up the institute's first Equal Opportunity Employment division.

Levon Parker (right), Minority and Special Concerns Program Officer, talks to a student at the NIH Summer Research Program Poster Day

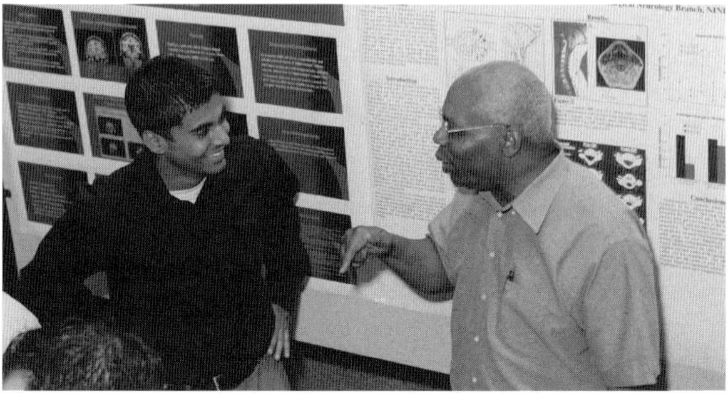

"Ted MacNichol [Edward MacNichol, Jr., M.D., director of the institute from 1968 to 1973] offered me the position, but warned me that it would be a major step away from research," Parker said. "He asked me to think carefully about whether or not I was ready to take the step."

Parker decided he was ready. "I was training people in the lab, but none of them were women or minorities and I was concerned about their lack of representation in the work force. Not enough was being done to bring minorities, women, and people with disabilities into the areas of brain and nervous system research. At that time, there was no office or central program or anything, and we decided that since we had a background in science and had done research, we might be in a better position to work with academic institutions and minority organizations to tell them about the opportunities at NIH."

Parker wrote the first draft of the institute's affirmative action plan and then went to work implementing it. The summer program for students was one of the first programs launched, followed by a lecture series for the students that has since become an NIH-wide event. Minority outreach initiatives were put into place, and had Parker visiting colleges, career fairs, and conferences to recruit potential young neuroscientists to the institute.

In 1975, Parker began to work with the Society for Neuroscience to sponsor a workshop at their annual meeting to pitch neuroscience, and NINDS, to minorities, women, and the disabled. "When Zach Hall came in as director," Parker says, "he encouraged me to broaden the workshops to include all neuroscience research at NIH, and so we also began to work with NIMH and NIA and all the other institutes that fund the neurosciences."

Mentoring is something else that Parker, and the institute, took the lead on within NIH. In the beginning, the summer program for students was focused on job training. But Parker convinced the late Dale McFarlin to use the summer students as researchers – not just lab assistants – and to act as a mentor. Once McFarlin was on board, other intramural researchers followed, supported wholeheartedly by intramural director Story Landis.

Now, when students arrive for the summer program, they have a mentor or preceptor with whom they actually have a chance to do research. Students have the opportunity to become co-authors on scientific papers even before they graduate from college. "That was the difference," says Parker. "We were trying to whet their appetite, to stimulate them to become investigators, to let them know that there is joy, excitement, and challenges when you're involved in biomedical research."

In his current position as the Minority and Special Concerns Program Officer and Director of the Summer Program in the Neurological Sciences at NINDS, Parker continues to build on past successes and broaden the outreach even further. "There aren't enough Native Americans being recruited," he says. "We need to focus more on that, especially because of the health disparities in the Native American community." Parker is also working with Clinical Neuroscience director Henry McFarland to recruit more M.D.s to the clinical training program.

"The program we have at NINDS has become a model for the rest of NIH," says Parker. "When we began, no one else was doing this." Now NIH as a whole continues to build and push forward efforts to increase diversity in training programs and the workforce. "I try to make them feel welcome in biomedical research as an investigator and as a member of the team at the bench. They know that they are here not because of their race or gender, but they are here because of their qualifications."

John Marler, M.D.

John Marler went to Bowdoin College and then to the University of West Virginia School of Medicine. He trained in neurology at the Mayo Clinic, and came to NINDS in 1984 as an assistant to Mike Walker in the extramural stroke program. Walker's extensive experience in brain tumor clinical trials was to be applied to stroke. Together the two scientists developed guidelines where there had been none. He considered one particular trial "a key event in all of neurological research."[9]

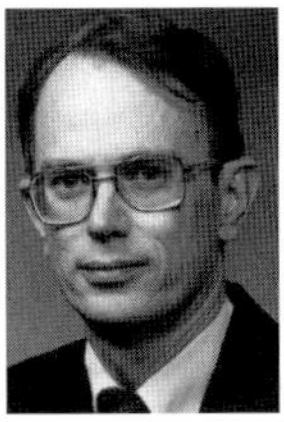

JOHN MARLER, M.D.

This controlled study was set up to determine whether bypass surgery ("extracranial to intracranial" or ECIC) could help ameliorate the effects of a stroke, bringing blood to the part of the brain that had been denied nourishment by the occlusion of a feeding artery. In fact, it did not help, but the trial was a marker of the progress that had been made in the development of clinical trials.

Marler has become increasingly skilled in leading the trials, which are expensive but have never taken more than 8 percent of the total institute budget. The major obstacle to trials is not the cost but enrolling the patients. As Marler has assumed more responsibility he has become convinced that more trials will have favorable results, as in the TPA trial. The NINDS took the lead in announcing the scientific breakthrough – the first-time treatment for stroke – and within a year hosted a symposium to organize all the medical professionals, EMTs, nurses, and others whose practices would change dramatically as a result of the new stroke treatment. The proceedings from this meeting serve as informal guidelines on how to treat stroke on an emergency basis. The NINDS now sponsors a major national campaign to educate people about the symptoms of stroke, and the need to call 911 and get to the hospital in time to get this important treatment.

Extramural Changes for the Millennium: Clusters and Minorities

When Harold Varmus became head of NIH in 1993, he aimed to restore the emphasis on science in the manner of James Shannon. Like Shannon, Varmus himself had been an outstanding scientist before he turned to administration. In fact, Varmus was a Nobel laureate and he insisted on keeping an active research laboratory while he was Director of NIH. He wanted to appoint individual NIH institute directors who had the same values. One of his first opportunities came when Murray Goldstein retired as Director of NINDS in 1993.

There was, of course, a search committee – but it was undoubtedly and properly influenced by Varmus' programmatic views. The committee chose Zach Hall, a molecular biologist who had worked on the neuromuscular synapse. Like Varmus, Hall accepted the position on condition that he could maintain his own laboratory.

As highly respected as Goldstein had been, he was not himself a scientist. The appointment of Hall was a signal that changes were coming. As far as the extramural programs were concerned, change was expedited by the imminent retirements of Leventhal, Streicher, Walker, and Brinley.

In fact, Goldstein himself had instituted a major change himself. In 1992, shortly before he retired, he had appointed Constance Atwell as Associate Director and Director of the Division of Extramural Activities, NINDS.

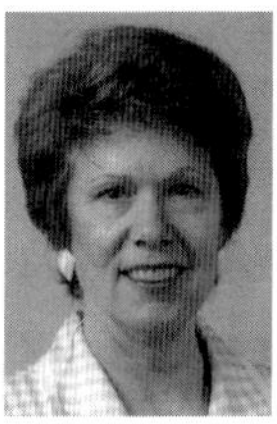

Constance Atwell, Ph.D.

Constance Atwell graduated from Mt. Holyoke College and received a Ph.D. in psychology from the University of California in Los Angeles. Her research combined the physiology and psychology of vision. From 1967 to 1978, she rose through the ranks to become professor of psychology at Pitzer College and Claremont Graduate School in California. For one of those years she taught at the University College of Nairobi in Kenya.

Dr. Atwell came to NIH in 1978 as a grants associate. The next year she became chief of a program on clinical applications of vision research at the National Eye Institute. She was also chief of the branch dealing with strabismus, amblyopia, and central visual processes. In 1992, she moved to NINDS and, for 7 months in 1998, served as Acting Deputy Director.

With the arrival of Hall, investigator-initiated research continued to be primary.[10] But program projects had been more important for clinical investigators than for basic scientists and that aspect was re-evaluated – only to leave it unscathed.

Training was revised to facilitate career development awards. And the administrative structure of the entire institute was revised. The extramural programs were grouped under three rubrics: Fundamental Neuroscience and Developmental Disorders; Convulsive, Infectious, and Immune Diseases; and Stroke, Trauma and Neurodegenerative Diseases.

Hall enthusiastically enlisted NINDS in helping to develop a neuroscience center at the Morehouse School of Medicine. This involved cooperation with the university to develop leadership, scientific and administrative staffs, and infrastructure. NIH leadership was also involved; the National Center for Research Resources and the Office of Research on Minority Health shared funding. Alfred W. Gordon, formerly a scientific review administrator, has led the program for NINDS, which developed so rapidly in several medical centers that it is now a full-time occupation for him.

Al Gordon received his undergraduate degree from Talladega College in Talladega, Alabama, did postgraduate work at the University of South Carolina, and earned his master's of science and doctorate degrees at Atlanta University in Georgia.

Among the goals set for Gordon and his staff is to develop neuroscience in minority institutions and implement strategies for the NINDS to reduce health disparities in populations that are historically at increased risk for disorders of the brain, spinal cord, and peripheral nervous system.

Gordon has said that he hopes "to better promote neuroscience research and research training opportunities for African Americans, Native Americans, Hispanics, and other minority populations nationwide. By doing so, we hope to reduce the burden of stroke and other disease disparities among underserved populations, create partnerships with minority academic and medical schools to attract and train future neuroscience health and research leaders, and promote greater scientific discussion of and minority recruitment in clinical trials. We hope to develop kindergarten through grade 12 educational programs that will bring brain and nervous system science into classrooms, homes, and communities nationwide; increase stroke awareness and treatment options among underserved populations; and encourage minority medical schools to develop programs on stroke and other neurological disorders that have a strong impact on minority populations."

Minority populations are at greater risk for stroke, epilepsy, neurological complications of HIV infection and diabetes, trauma to brain and spinal cord, and developmental disorders. Research programs at minority-led institutions are meant to develop a new group of minority physicians and investigators who will enhance the efforts to combat these conditions.

Under Hall, collaborative programs with other institutes increased. Areas of research emphasis were developed too, but the number of requests for applications increased only slowly. Then, in 1998, when Gerald Fischbach arrived as director of NINDS, there was more active advance planning and more requests for applications emerged. These proposals were developed in consultation with panels of external advisors. Fischbach wanted the program directors to be leading the science, not just responding to grant applications. He made a vigorous attempt to join forces with neuroscientists in other institutes, to collaborate rather than compete.

The balance between the number of individual grants (RO-1s) and program projects is not decided in advance but is determined by the merit of the applications that come in – the results of peer review. Study sections in the Center for Scientific Review consider the RO-1 applications. Program projects, in contrast, are reviewed by an NINDS committee. Clinical trials are RO-1s in NINDS, but are in a special category and are reviewed by the institute.

Under Fischbach, planning became more visible. Leading scientists, patient advocates, and NINDS staff convened in 1998 to determine the "needs, opportunities and priorities."[11] Discussion was continued on the Internet and comments were solicited from 250 advocacy groups. The extramural program directors were then reorganized into seven administrative offices and eight scientific clusters: Channels, synapses and circuits; Clinical trials; Systems and cognitive neuroscience; Neural environment; Neurodegeneration; Neurogenetics; Repair and plasticity; and Minority health and research. The combination should cover almost every aspect of neuroscience and all relevant disorders. A vigorous campaign has been engaged to recruit excellent scientists to fill more of the ranks of the program directors.

In 1999, the success rate for grants rose to 35 percent and NINDS funded 2,200 projects. The process for reviewing and awards is likely to change again when a new director of NINDS arrives and a new era commences. But the priority of investigator-initiated research is not likely to change, and whatever they are called, study sections (now Scientific Review Groups) will play a role. The number of requests for applications is likely to rise and fall in parallel with the overall budget for NIH.

1 Strickland SP. An interview with Dr. Murray Goldstein on the Occasion of the 100th Anniversary in 1987 of the National Institutes of Health and the 150th year of the National Library of Medicine. (June 1986) Transcript in the History Office of the National Institutes of Health, Bethesda, Md.

2 Malakoff D. NIH prays for a soft landing after its doubling ride ends. *Science* 2001;292:1992-1995.

3 Landau W. Recorded Interview with author, March 14, 2000.

4 Turner TB. The medical schools twenty years afterwards: impact of the extramural research support programs of the National Institutes of Health. *J Med Edu* 1967;42:109-118.

5 Streicher E. Recorded Interview with author, February 16, 2001.

6 Leventhal CM. Recorded Interview with author, March 20, 2001.

7 Walker M. Recorded Interview with author, August 10, 2000.

8 Solowey M. Recorded Telephone Interview with author, February 27, 2001.

9 Marler J. Recorded Interview with author, April 25, 2000.

10 Atwell C. Recorded Interview with author, March 28, 2000.

11 *Neuroscience at the New Millennium: Priorities and Plans for the National Institute of Neurological Disorders and Stroke. Fiscal years 2000-2001. Implementation update.* May 2000, NINDS, Bethesda, MD.

CHAPTER EIGHT

TRAINING

Chapter 714. *Be it enacted by the Senate and House of Representatives of the United States of America in Congress Assembled*, That the purpose of this Act is to improve the Health of the people of the United States through the conduct of researches, investigations, experiments, and demonstrations relating to the cause, prevention, and methods of diagnosis and treatment of arthritis and rheumatism, multiple sclerosis, cerebral palsy, epilepsy, poliomyelitis, blindness, leprosy, and other diseases; assist and foster such researches and other activities by public and private agencies, and promote the coordination of all such researches and activities and the useful application of their results; provide training relating to such diseases; and develop, and assist States and other agencies in the use of, the most effective methods of prevention, diagnosis, and treatment of such diseases.

Section 433. In addition, the Surgeon General is authorized to provide training and instruction and establish and maintain traineeships and fellowships, in such institute and elsewhere, in matters relating to the diagnosis, prevention, and treatment of such disease or diseases with such stipends and allowances (including travel and subsistence expenses) for trainees and fellows as he may deem necessary, and, in addition, provide for such training, instruction, and traineeships and for such fellowships through grants to public and other nonprofit institutions.

S. 2591. Public Law 692. August 15, 1950

The directives of the enabling legislation for NINDB included several kinds of training, not only for research, but also for "diagnosis and treatment." The prescription followed the lead of the National Cancer Institute in 1937, which was adopted by the Heart Institute in 1948. At the start, the NINDB training programs therefore included both clinical and scientific training. This was true throughout NIH, but it is a matter of record that the very existence of clinical neurology in the United States was largely a result of these training programs and fellowships. The diffusion of neurology training was aided by the post-World War II shifts of population that expanded the medical schools and universities in the South, Southwest, and West.

Former NINDS director Murray Goldstein[1] has described the goals of the training programs: to train physicians to practice and to do research where there had been none previously and to train basic scientists where there had been few. This required more than support of trainees. It required institutional support to develop teachers, curricula, and facilities.

The programs succeeded in creating clinical neurology as we now know it. Support from NINDS and the Veterans Administration established training centers throughout the country, but it did much more than that. NINDB was established to foster disease-oriented research, which required the training of clinical investigators as well as basic neuroscience research training.[2]

The results are evident in the numbers. In 1948, the American Academy of Neurology was founded with 52 charter members. A year later, there were 710. The membership did not pass 1,000 until 1955, but growth was steady thereafter. In the year 2000, Academy members numbered 17,000. The annual meetings now attract more than 10,000 American and international neurologists.[3]

In 1947 there were only 32 neurology residency positions in American hospitals; by 1971 there were more than 700.

In 1955, there were 15 independent departments of neurology and 61 programs that were part of departments of medicine or psychiatry.[4] By 1970, there were 49 independent departments and 36 programs in the medicine or psychiatry departments.

There have been similar changes in basic neuroscience. In 1950, there was no such field as neurobiology, which emerged by natural selection but was fueled by NINDS training grants (awarded to an institution in which fellows were selected for research training) and fellowships awarded by NIH to individuals. As a result of these training funds from NINDS, the number of young Ph.D. investigators escalated rapidly.

They migrated organizationally from physiology and biochemistry to their own Society for Neuroscience, which was founded in 1969 at the instigation of University of Chicago physiologist Ralph Gerard. Others who played key roles were neurophysiologist Edward Perl, psychologist Neal Miller, and Louise Marshall,[5,6] who was then Director of the Committee on Brain Sciences of the National Research Council and National Academy of Sciences. From the start, behavioral science was prominently represented among the leaders. Within a year, the membership was 1,100; by 1980, 7,100; 1990, 17,500; and, in 2000, there were 28,500 members.[7] The annual meetings now attract 25,000 scientists.[8]

A glance at the Nobel Prizes provides another measure of the advance of neuroscience, which has been the subject of 13 awards in the last half-century.

The results of the clinical training programs have been equally dramatic. From a profound dearth of neurological consultants and investigators, healthcare planners now contend that there may be too many neurologists, a highly contentious issue within the profession. From a field in which research opportunities 50 years ago were essentially limited to EEG and neuropathology, clinical investigation now includes molecular genetics, genomics, transgenic animal models, stem cells, clinical trials, population studies, and outcomes research.

Yet there is concern about the future for M.D.-investigators. This issue is not restricted to neurology and neurosurgery; it affects all other NIH institutes. The reasons are many – rising amounts of debt upon graduation from medical school, the increasing sophistication of biomedical research with longer and longer periods of preparation, and escalating competition from well-trained basic scientists, all combining to make it ever more difficult for one person to succeed in the traditional triad of academic medicine: teaching, patient care, and research. The evolution of medical science would have created these problems under any system, but now medical school faculties must spend more and more time seeing patients to compete for managed care contracts. The time lost and the administrative hassles involved have thwarted clinical research.

The trajectory has not always been upward, and NINDS was always linked to other NIH institutes in the annual congressional allocation for training budgets. But only NINDB and NIMH had full clinical and research training programs.[9] According to Murray Goldstein, NIH Director James Shannon brought pressure on NINDB to cease clinical training. The role of NIH, he said, was research, not clinical practice. NINDB officials responded that clinical investigation required clinical training. Shannon did not back down, even when records showed that the vast majority of trainees made life careers on medical school faculties. The compromise was to restrict NINDB support to a year or two of research training during a residency. Shannon[10] later noted in his review of federal support for biomedical research:

> The training programs in being were again analyzed in the mid-1950s, and it was concluded that medical specialty training could carry on with its own momentum in most areas. However, there was clear evidence of an acute shortage of trained scientists sufficient to impair both the further development of a number of new scientific fields and the provision of an adequate science base for an increasingly complex educational process. In consequence, except in mental health and neurology, the NIH fellowship and training programs were redesigned to emphasize the training of both fundamental and applied scientists.

In a footnote, he amplified the comments about neurology and psychiatry to recognize the "shortage of trained professionals for a combination of practice, education, and advanced training in the associated medical specialties."

Nevertheless, in public, Shannon[10] was a staunch advocate of research training and the issue for neurology continued. In the 1970s, the Nixon administration acted on the remaining clinical training programs. According to Shannon, "These judgments were made by HEW Secretary Caspar Weinberger without public discussion and without providing the basis of his judgment. The economy was said not to have been a factor in the decision." The clinical training programs were ended abruptly on grounds that no other profession received a federal subsidy for training and, more, there should be no such subsidy for people who are likely to have high incomes. By that time, clinical training programs had been established throughout the country. The costs had been transferred to hospitals and were partially supported by Medicare.

What the Nixon administration said and what they really meant were two different things. The heart of the attack on clinical training was about both money and policy.

As Shannon and others noted, officials in the Executive Branch felt they were being criticized because too many approved research grant applications were going unfunded, which could only mean that there were too many researchers seeking support. They thought that by cutting back on the number of investigators – which was most easily done by restricting the number of training positions – they could automatically decrease the demands for more research dollars.

Congress, under the leadership of Senator Edward Kennedy and Representative Paul Rogers, defended the training programs, but in doing so they devised a 1974 law that contained new provisions: training only for areas of health needs, and a payback requirement whereby trainees had to serve in research and teaching or work in areas underserved by medical care. The National Academy of Sciences was to track the program and report to Congress periodically.[11]

The Academy has taken this responsibility seriously, publishing the results of ten studies between 1975 and 1994. The focus has been more on the "areas of health needs" than on the payback provision. By 1994, the committee recommended no increase in training levels. Overall, there has been relative stability in training for Ph.D. scientists, from 14,443 in 1975 to 15,681 in 1999, less than a 10 percent increase in 25 years. During the same interval there was a vast increase in the number of research grants and dollars.[12]

In 1995, however, one analysis[13] concluded that the size of a doctoral program is driven more by the needs of investigators for assistants than by the market for the services of the new Ph.D.s. The result of overproduction was underemployment. Another major concern was the lengthening amount of time it took to obtain a degree and the increase in the number of postdoctoral fellowships required for each young scientist, which led to greater difficulty in finding an independent position and an advance in the ages of researchers applying for their first NIH research grant.[14]

In 2000, the National Research Council report noted an increase in women investigators and an increased number of minority researchers. They concluded that the system was in balance and recommended against any further increase in training positions for "basic (Ph.D.) biomedical scientists." Committee members feared that new Ph.D.s might not find research employment.

Cutting back, however, is not so easy. The number of researchers entering *training* grants can be tracked readily because the information is available in annual reports to NIH from recipient universities. But tracking becomes more complicated because investigators also add predoctoral and postdoctoral fellows to positions on research grants. Another force directs postdoctoral scientists to *research* grants rather than fellowships – foreign nationals are not eligible for individual fellowships, but they can be hired on a grant. It is then difficult to identify which investigators supported by a research grant are fellows and which are junior faculty – because academic titles differ among universities. Whether this arrangement can be controlled remains to be seen. Whether it should be controlled is open to debate.

NIH has responded to the recommendations of the NAS.[15] Among the several considerations, leaders of NIH are uncertain about the need for constraints on the number of Ph.D.s because research opportunities change and may increase. They agree that training time should not be extended unduly and that diversity among trainees is desirable. A tracking system should be designed to follow trainees supported by research grants (as well as those supported by training grants and fellowships).

Training for clinical investigation is another matter because the questions differ from those concerning Ph.D. basic neuroscientists. For more than two decades[16] the number of M.D.-investigators has continued to decline as the number of Ph.D.-investigators has increased. The American Medical Association has noted a fall in the number of physicians identifying research as their primary activity – from almost 23,000 in 1985 to 14,434 in 1997.[17] The percentage of grants awarded to M.D.s has declined each year. Leon E. Rosenberg,[18] former Dean of the Yale School of Medicine, has projected the slope of decline to zero in the year 2015. Again, this problem has affected all of NIH, not only NINDS.[19,20]

NIH as a whole has responded[21] with a series of awards that provide more support for clinical trials and other forms of clinical investigation, including more support for training and for mid-career clinical investigators. Rosenberg's extrapolation to extinction of the clinical investigator may have been merely a drop from a fluctuating peak in one year, a drop more apparent than real.

Training in neurological research presents special problems.[22-24] Advances in disease-oriented research depend on – and flow from – advances in basic science and so one could ask what difference it makes if M D.-investigators disappear. The answer to this question has been provided by several analysts.[12] First, according to Dennis Landis,[25] Chair of Neurology at Case-Western Reserve University in Cleveland, and consultant to the Director of NINDS, M.D.s are more likely to recognize the opportunities of advances in basic sciences for human disease and they are also more likely to cooperate with basic scientists in *disease-oriented* research. M.D.-investigators are needed, as well, for *patient-oriented* research, including controlled clinical trials of new treatments. Many are trained to apply basic neuroscience to human disease in what is called translational research. M.D.-scientists are also invaluable because they tend to communicate well with advocacy groups and participate in the education of practicing physicians.

NIH has responded to these challenges with special research training programs, starting with several that lead to a combined M.D.-Ph.D. degree. Others focus on the post-residency years, providing for five years of mentored research training and experience. There are also grants to support newly independent investigators.

Landis[21] has proposed to the NINDS that programs be put into place to encourage interest in clinical neuroscience among medical students, provide support for participation of medical students in research, initiate a direct educational program for medical students about the attractions of a research career, offer debt relief during periods of training in basic research, and support researchers throughout their career development. The former director of NIH, Harold Varmus, had also urged a similar approach for all of NIH in 1995,[26] but Landis has provided more detail for NINDS specifically.

Richard Johnson[27] has summarized the reasons for optimism. Research opportunities have never been better. Clinical investigation attracts M.D.-Ph.D.s and other skilled young scientists. NIH is moving to promote clinical investigation. And we have broad support from administration, Congress, other legislative bodies, and patient advocacy groups.

As neurobiology attracts more young neuroscientists and as genomic medicine makes therapy available for neurologic disease, these problems should be surmounted for neurology. As technical and molecular progress is seen, research should flourish in neurosurgery, too.

1 Goldstein M. NINCDS manpower recruitment and training programs (1950 to 1975). In Brady RO, ed. *The Basic Neurosciences*. vol. 1 of Tower DB, ed. *The Nervous System: A Three-Volume Work Commemorating the 25th Anniversary of the National Institute of Neurological and Communicative Disorders and Stroke.* New York: Raven Press, 1975:liii-lvii.

2 Goldstein M. The National Institute of Neurological Diseases and Stroke. In Cohen MM, ed. *The American Academy of Neurology: The First 50 Years. 1948-1998.* St. Paul, Minn.: American Academy of Neurology, 1998:174-185.

3 Data from Thomas Cooper and Michael Bisping, American Academy of Neurology, February 21, 2001.

4 Masland RL. National Institute of Neurological Diseases and Blindness: development and growth (1960-1968). In Brady RO, ed. *The Basic Neurosciences*: xxxiii-lii.

5 Perl ER. Society for Neuroscience – a history of beginnings. *Neuroscience Newsletter* 1986;17:1-5.

6 Marshall L. Careful planning created the Society for Neuroscience. *Science* 2000;290:2259.

7 Data from Nancy Beang, Executive Director, Society for Neuroscience, February 20, 2001.

8 Helmuth L. Neuroscience meeting draws crowds, gripes, loyalty. *Science* 2000;290:698-699.

9 Goldstein M. Interview with author, April 19, 2000.

10 Shannon JA. Federal support of biomedical sciences: development and academic impact. *J Med Edu* 1976;51 no. 7, pt. 2:1-98.

11 Walsh J. NIH training grants: the uncertainty factor. *Science* 1975;188:1092-1094.

12 National Research Council. *Addressing the Nation's Changing Needs for Biomedical and Behavioral Scientists*. Washington, DC: National Academy Press, 2000.

13 Massy WF, Goldman CA. The production and utilization of science and engineering doctorates in the United States. Stanford Institute for Higher Education Research Discussion Paper, Stanford University School of Education, Stanford, CA, 1995.

14 Marinacola E, Solomon F. The career structure in biomedical research: implications for training and trainees. *Mol Biol Cell* 1998;9:3003-3006.

15 NIH statement in response to the NAS report: addressing the nation's changing needs for biomedical and behavioral scientists. March 22, 2001 [http://grants.nih.gov/grants/guide/notice-files/NOT-OD-01-027.html].

16 Wyngaarden JB. The clinical investigator as an endangered species. *N Engl J Med* 1979;301:1254-1259.

17 Pasko T, Seidman B. *Physician Characteristics and Distribution in the US, 1999*. Chicago: American Medical Association, 1999.

18 Rosenberg LE. Physician-scientists – endangered and essential. *Science* 1999; 283:3331-3332.

19 Goldstein JL, Brown MS. The clinical investigator: bewitched, bothered, and bewildered. *J Clin Invest* 1997;99:2803-2812.

20 Zemlo TR, Garrison HH, Partridge NC, Ley TJ. The physician-scientist: career issues and challenges at the year 2000. *FASEB Journal* 2000;14:221-230.

21 Nathan DG, Varmus HE. The National Institutes of Health and clinical research: a progress report. *Nature Medicine* 2000;6:1201-1204.

22 Griggs RC, Martin JB, Penn AS, Roses AD, Toole JF. Training clinical neuroscientists. *Ann Neurol* 1987;21:197-201.

23 Rosenberg RN. Where will future neurologists and neuroscientists come from? *Neurology*. 1993;43:1637-1640.

24 Griggs RC. Careers in academic neurology in the Decade of the Brain. *Ann Neurol* 1994;35:753-758.

25 Landis D. Proposal to the National Advisory Council for Neurological Disorders and Stroke: NINDS Research Training Program for Physician Scientists. January 2001.

26 National Institutes of Health Director's Panel on Clinical Research. *Report of the Advisory Committee to the NIH Director*. Bethesda, MD: National Institutes of Health, 1997.

27 Johnson RT, First RD. Adams Lecture: Training Clinical Investigators in Neuroscience. Annual Meeting of the American Neurological Association, Boston, MA, October 15-18, 2000.

CHAPTER NINE

BIG TICKETS: COLLABORATIVE AND FIELD STUDIES

In the first 25 years, NINDB supported research programs far afield. Two of these were resounding successes – the kuru investigations of Carleton Gajdusek and Joe Gibbs, and the Lake Maracaibo project developed by Nancy Wexler. One, an attempt to discover the source of a high incidence of neurological disease on the island of Guam, has been a target of study for almost the life of NINDS, but the source still remains a mystery. Another, the Perinatal Project, had a grand design but its contributions to neuroscience have not been so clear.

Neurological Disease on Guam

"Clusters" they are called, areas of unusually high prevalence of a disease. People in the neighborhood worry about the personal risk of contracting the disease. Epidemiologists and other investigators look for a clue to the cause.

The site may be a football field or an office building, but often these places turn out to be a statistical fluke, a blip in the natural variations of prevalence and clues to nothing. Geographic isolates, however, may be important for genetic diseases – as in Finland or Tunisia, where the rate of cousin marriages is higher than in other places, making it more likely for autosomal recessive diseases to appear.

Some islands harbor isolated populations, too. Iceland is now a favorite place for genetic studies, partly because most current inhabitants can be traced back to a few founders.[1] Oliver Sacks,[2] the famous chronicler of medical oddities that have strong implications, traveled to remote Pacific islands in Micronesia to find out about familial achromatopsia – color blindness. In the resulting book, he related the story of the remarkably high incidence of neurodegenerative diseases in Guam. Also tantalized by the Guamanian phenomenon, Terence Monmaney described it in *The New Yorker* magazine.[3]

The modern story of neurodegenerative diseases on Guam begins with Harry Zimmerman in 1945. He had been an Assistant Professor of Pathology at Yale and, at age 43, had established himself as a new kind of neuropathologist. Instead of merely observing changes in diseased tissue, which was then the custom for many academic neuropathologists, he did experiments to find out the effects of specific infections or dietary deficiencies, or how brain tumors behaved under controlled conditions. His talents, however, were not fully recognized by his departmental chairman; after he returned from service in World War II, Zimmerman never went back to Yale.

Instead, he took a position at the Montefiore Hospital in New York and, later, became the first Dean of the Albert Einstein College of Medicine. He was one of the first to use the electron microscope

(EM) in neuropathology and had a string of outstanding students. Robert Terry was among them; he was the one whose EM photographs established the importance of plaques and tangles in Alzheimer disease. So was Asao Hirano, who was to play an important role in Guam and to follow Zimmerman as chief neuropathologist at Montefiore.

In the Navy, Zimmerman was assigned to a research unit; their mission was to understand the tropical diseases American troops would encounter. Zimmerman landed on Guam in mid-January 1945 and helped in the local hospital by carrying out autopsies. By May, he had examined at least seven cases of amyotrophic lateral sclerosis (ALS or Lou Gehrig's disease); at home, he would not have been surprised if he had seen no cases at all because the disease is rare. He duly recorded and reported this experience to the authorities.[4]

Subsequently, two teams of naval physicians confirmed Zimmerman's observations of the high frequency of ALS and published their results in December 1952 and early 1953. The incidence of ALS was 50 times higher than that in the United States, and it seemed often to be linked in the same family with dementia and parkinsonism. Everywhere else in the world the frequency of ALS was the same – infrequent. Nothing like this had ever been reported; something special was happening on Guam.

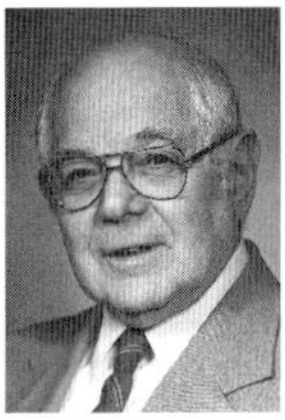

Leonard Kurland, M.D.

Back home, word of this uniquely high prevalence reached Leonard Kurland. Having pioneered epidemiological studies of multiple sclerosis in 1947, he set up the first epidemiology program at NIH. At first, he was assigned to NIMH. However, when Pearce Bailey arrived at NINDS, he wanted Kurland to get training in neurology and suggested that he go to the residency program led by Houston Merritt. Instead, Kurland wanted to go to the Mayo Clinic because of a singular experience:[5]

> Over the Christmas holiday of 1948, I was traveling home to Baltimore when I stopped in New York for a medical meeting at the Roosevelt Hotel. The third paper presented that day was by Alex MacLean and his colleagues, Henry Woltman and Joseph Berkson at the Mayo Clinic. They described multiple sclerosis in the population of a small urban community.

The authors had convincing figures that were quite different from the ones Kurland had found a year earlier in his Master's dissertation. Multiple sclerosis was twice as common in the rural area around Rochester, Minnesota – home of the Mayo Clinic – than it was anywhere else in the world. The duration of symptoms was also remarkable, three times longer than textbooks recorded. Kurland said, "It was obvious to me that they had the data. In effect, my dissertation was torn apart, but it had an electrifying effect on me."

In speaking to MacLean after the lecture, Kurland learned that the secret was the Mayo record system, which had been set up by internist Henry Plummer and then refined by statistician Joseph Berkson. He was determined to go there some day and learn how it was done.

A few weeks later, Kurland visited NIMH. He explained how he discussed his interest in multiple sclerosis:

> Well, I had seen some cases when I was an intern. I was interested in the geographic distribution. When it came time for me to select a topic for my Master's thesis at Harvard School of Public Health, that would have been 1947, I really wasn't that interested in tuberculosis control. I wanted to do the epidemiology of multiple sclerosis as my topic. They thought about it for a while because, in those days, doing chronic disease problems was not the usual thing. But they finally approved it. I went ahead with my dissertation, which had two main parts: a review of the world literature or what was available on the geographic distribution, incidence, prevalence, and survival outcome of multiple sclerosis; the second part was a study to clarify some of the problems, mainly the geographic distribution. So my plan was to carry out the study in five cities in the United States and Canada. That dissertation came to the attention of the head of — there was no Neurology Institute at that time — it came to the attention of the Associate Director of the National Institute of Mental Health, Dale Cameron. He called me in one day and I met him and I also met Larry Kolb whom I hadn't known. In fact, I didn't even catch his name. He later came to Mayo and was on the staff here at Mayo for a while.
>
> When I was introduced to him I hadn't caught his name. He wanted to know what the basis – he said, "We're interested in multiple sclerosis and we'd like to get a study going. What was the basis for your dissertation?" I had available the literature from Scandinavia. And there was one good study in the United States, the one in the Eastern Health District in Baltimore by Kolb and Langworthy. I'm talking to Kolb and he's sitting there with a straight face and I'm telling him what a great study he did! So that went over very well.
>
> The next thing I knew, I got a call from the Mental Health Institute and they wanted me. They said, "We like your project and we'd like you to do it." So we got the funds. They had some grant money from the Public Health Service and they got some money from the Multiple Sclerosis Society, I think, and I was told to go ahead and do the project. So I did the five-city study.

Kolb asked Kurland to direct the study; it may have been on the same day as that interview.[6] "All of sudden, my plan, based on my Master's thesis, became the national plan for the study of multiple sclerosis in the United States and Canada,"[3] said Kurland. In that study he recorded the incidence and prevalence of multiple sclerosis in Winnipeg and New Orleans; the numbers were much higher in the northern city.

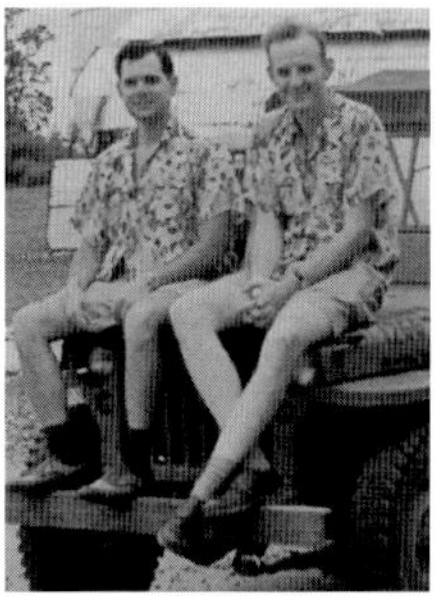

LEONARD KURLAND, M.D. (LEFT) AND DONALD MULDER, M.D. (RIGHT) IN GUAM, 1953

Kurland then went to the Mayo Clinic for training in neurology and instruction in the use of the record system for epidemiology. That is where he was when he heard about ALS on Guam. He recognized the opportunity this afforded and arranged to visit Guam in 1953. A neurologist, Donald Mulder, who had been Kurland's teacher at Mayo, accompanied him. José Torres, a Chamorro who spoke the local language, went with them.

In the Guamanian village of Umatac, where the prevalence was by far the highest, they found that more than a third of adult deaths were attributable to ALS. They immediately confirmed the earlier observations of increased prevalence.

Kurland was to spend the next 50 years thinking about Guamanian ALS, probably longer and harder than anyone else. The secret of ALS – or, at least, a secret of ALS – should have been uncovered, but it is still elusive. Back then, no one knew how elusive it would prove to be, and so it was Kurland who involved NINDB. He served as Chief of the Epidemiology Branch at NINDS from 1955 to 1964, when he returned to the Mayo Clinic and chaired the department of medical statistics, epidemiology, and population genetics from 1964 to 1986. He is now an emeritus professor, widely regarded as the father of neuroepidemiology.

In 1956, under Kurland's direction, NINDB opened the Guam Research Center, which comprised a clinic and a laboratory on the island. In addition to the increased prevalence of ALS, they found a similarly high prevalence of parkinsonism and dementia, which they called the "Parkinson-dementia complex." About a quarter of those patients also had the signs of ALS. It was not clear whether these were three separate diseases, or perhaps more likely, three different manifestations of a condition that had the same cause.

The next advance in the story came from pathology. Asao Hirano started to review the postmortem examinations and found abnormal structures called neurofibrillary tangles in neurons throughout the nervous system of patients dying with any of the three syndromes – ALS, parkinsonism, or dementia. The tangles had been seen in Alzheimer disease, but not ALS. This contribution of Hirano's added to the evidence that the disorders on Guam were related to each other and that Guamanian ALS differed from the disease in America and Europe.

In the next decades, a parade of notable neuroscientists tackled the problem of ALS on Guam: Asao Hirano, the neuropathologist who succeeded Zimmerman at Montefiore; Gajdusek and Gibbs at NINDB; Darab K. Dastur, neurologist and neuropathologist in Bombay; Peter Spencer, neurotoxicologist at Albert Einstein Medical School; Daniel Perl, head of neuropathology at Mt. Sinai Hospital in New York and an expert on aluminum and Alzheimer disease; Jacob Brody, one of the first epidemiologists at NINDS; and John Steele, a Canadian neurologist eponymized in the Steele-Richardson-Olszewski syndrome (progressive supranuclear palsy, another age-related neurodegenerative disease). Steele moved permanently to Umatac in Guam.

Singly or together these outstanding investigators all failed to come up with a satisfactory explanation. Heredity was first suspected, then ruled out because spouses seemed to be affected often. Kurland and Peter Spencer incriminated a local plant, the cycad, but Gajdusek concluded that the fern had nothing to do with the diseases. Oliver Sacks, too, concluded that cycad was not a likely cause, nor were any of the constituents of cycad flour that had been isolated and studied by Spencer. Similar areas of increased prevalence were found in Japan, where cycad did not grow. Also, some experiments showed that the preparation of flour from the cycad leaves involved so many steps that almost none of the original material persisted. Animal experiments did not show any consistent toxin. Gibbs and Gajdusek failed to transmit ALS – Guamanian or American – to primates, thus excluding a slow virus. They and others in their group advanced the thought that a mineral imbalance in the local drinking water might be responsible – another idea that fizzled.

In 1982, after 30 years of frustration and millions of dollars, NINDS closed the Guam Center with the approval of Carleton Gajdusek, who said "all that can be done scientifically can be done without the lab."[2] Kurland continued, and in 1990 he led another program project on Guam, this one sponsored by the Aging Institute.

In 2001, Kurland still favored the cycad theory:[6]

> The epidemiology of ALS conforms quite well to the use of cycads in Guam. Cycad, before World War II, was essentially a famine food. But they had a 7-day ritual washing in which they would leach out the water-soluble toxins. That worked pretty well. But during the war, during the Japanese occupation, many of the Chamorros were in the equivalent of concentration camps. They had to eat what was available. The Japanese would not eat the cycad; they left that to the natives. But if they were in a concentration camp situation, could they soak the seeds for 7 days? If they were starving they might consume them before the toxin washed out. At least, that was my thought on this.

Wigbert Wiederholt was another intrepid investigator of the Guamanian diseases. He had been chair of neurology at the University of California, San Diego, from 1978 to 1983. He then became an epidemiologist and worked at the Mayo Clinic, first on the vexing question of whether the Guillain-Barré syndrome could be caused by swine flu vaccination (the answer turned out to be negative). When that project was completed he turned to Guam, where he spent much of the last 10 years of his life before he died in March 2000 at age 68.[7]

In 1997, Wiederholt organized another program project to confront the Guamanian diseases. This one involved six American universities and also the University of Guam.[8] In the year 2001, they reported their new findings at a neurological meeting in a poster hung immediately adjacent to one by Kurland's team.[9,10] Their findings were similar. The incidence of both ALS and parkinsonism-dementia has declined notably on Guam. (Incidence is defined as the number of new cases each year.) The age at onset of symptoms has increased from 40 to 58 for ALS and from 50 to 65 for parkinsonism-dementia. But neither has disappeared.

In favor of a genetic cause is the evident occurrence in families, and relatives of affected people have high risks for both ALS and the parkinsonism-dementia complex. However, the pattern does not fit any Mendelian pattern of inheritance and the distribution of the disorders in a community would be consistent with an environmental agent, a genetic cause, or – more likely – both.

In favor of an environmental cause is the declining incidence between 1960 and 2000 as diets changed and Guam became modernized. But the years of intense scrutiny have failed to come up with a single cause more likely than the cycad.

Neurologist Oliver Sacks thinks the disorders may disappear because of the very characteristics that led to the anomalously high incidence in the first place, including the island location. He found that congenital deafness had disappeared from the island of Martha's Vineyard off Cape Cod. "So it was with Fuur, the little Danish island of the colorblind; so, most probably, it will be with Pingelap (another site of colorblindness) and so, perhaps it will be with Guam – odd genetic anomalies, swirls, transients, given a brief possibility, existence, by the nature of islands and isolation. But islands open up, people die or intermarry; genetic attenuation sets in, and the condition disappears. The life of such a genetic disease in an isolate tends to be six or eight generations, 200 years perhaps, and then it vanishes, as do its memories and traces, lost in the ongoing stream of time."

The Collaborative Perinatal Study

It must have been an exciting time for Pearce Bailey when he first had authority to set up the programs for NINDB. How did he set his priorities? He left no diary, and his public writings do not describe why or how one of his first acts was to set up a "Collaborative Perinatal Study." (Perinatal included fetal events, delivery, and the early months of life.)

From the beginning Bailey appreciated the magnitude of the problem and the need to do something. NINDB had its first budget in 1951. The very next year, he mentioned perinatal disorders in his appearances at the House and Senate Appropriations Committees. He planned to carry out a national study of mothers and their newborns to uncover causes of mental retardation, cerebral palsy, and other congenital abnormalities of the brain.

Statistics from 1950 provide a glimpse of the huge national burden of perinatally related health conditions. The number of births that year was 3.6 million. Perinatal mortality was 743,342 or 21 percent of all births. Brain damage was found in 57,273 or 2 percent of all live births.[11] The numbers barely hinted at the costs in money and misery. Among adolescents with long-term disability, 75 percent had problems that had originated before birth, and 94 percent of these teenagers had neurological problems.[12]

The numbers could be expressed in other specifics found in 1960, when 5 million Americans were found to be mentally retarded. Epilepsy affected 1.5 million, 555,000 had cerebral palsy, and more than 1.1 million were legally blind or legally deaf.[13]

The perinatal program did not actually begin until the mid-50s and the first summary of activities described what happened.[14] The first two centers were funded in 1956 at Yale and Brown universities. The summary continued:

> An ad hoc advisory committee composed of 15 scientists under the chairmanship of H. Houston Merritt had been convened to begin the preparation of a special protocol for the collection of clinical and postmortem data. During the same year (1956), a 3-day conference was held in San Juan, Puerto Rico, to review the present state of research on perinatal influences which may lead to brain damage and impairment of learning, including a review of work of the NINDB Perinatal Laboratory of Physiology . . . . It was sponsored jointly by NINDB, the National Science Foundation, and several voluntary health agencies: United Cerebral Palsy, Association for the Aid to Crippled Children, and the National Multiple Sclerosis Society. Also represented were the National Society for Retarded Children and the Muscular Dystrophy Associations of America.

By 1958, 12 institutions had enrolled at a cost of $1,389,527. Richard Masland arrived as NINDB Assistant Director that year; his assignment was to lead the Perinatal Project. Masland had established his credentials earlier in his career when he was induced by Grover Powers, Professor of Pediatrics at Yale, to take a year off from his professorial position at Bowman Gray School of Medicine to do a survey for the National Association for Retarded Children. In that capacity he had visited all the centers where research was being done and had written a monograph on "mental subnormality."[15] This experience gave him valuable information about the current state of the field.

Masland recalled that important figures in the perinatal program were Nicholas Eastman, Chair of Obstetrics at Johns Hopkins, and

Stewart H. Clifford, a pediatrician who gave up his practice to supervise the program in Boston.

The extent of the activities of the project may now seem beyond comprehension, especially considering the limitations of the time. When the program started, the number of pediatric neurologists was "shockingly small" and there were virtually none in the United States "who had ever studied the newborn."[3] Also, computers were as infantile as their subjects, so record keeping was relegated to punch cards and tapes.

The logistics of gathering data were horrendous. The planners recognized the problems of earlier studies. For example, if mental retardation or some other disorder were first recognized when a child was 5 years old, it would be impossible to ascertain which problems at birth had been responsible. Memories would be fallible. Requisite specimens would not have been taken, nor would the record keeping have been relevant. The study had to be prospective, planned in advance.[16] The general outline for the program, therefore, included registration of 50,000 consecutive pregnancies in the 14 participating institutions, keeping data on each pregnancy and delivery, examining the placenta according to a standard procedure, and taking and storing specimens from the time of birth. Each child would then have to be examined periodically, according to standard protocols of examination and record keeping, noting intelligence and any neurological, hearing, or language disorders. The children were to be followed until they were 8 years old. If there were any deaths, autopsies would be done, also in a standardized manner.

There would also be a prenatal research laboratory under the direction of William Windle, a noted neuroanatomist and developmental neurobiologist. This would allow experiments to be carried out in monkeys as a way to validate observations made in the perinatal human studies. The laboratory was set up at the University of Puerto Rico, where a colony of free-ranging monkeys was established. Windle experimentally studied the effects of several threatening circumstances: premature separation of the placenta, asphyxia at birth, exposure to breakdown products of hemoglobin in kernicterus (the autoimmune condition that results from Rh blood group incompatibilities in the parents), and postnatal exposure to lead.[17] For his work, Windle was awarded a Lasker Prize in 1968.

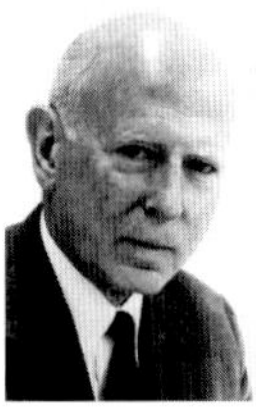

William F. Windle, Ph.D., Sc.D., head of the primate lab in Puerto Rico, and winner of a 1968 Lasker Award in Basic Science

There were problems of coordination and conflicts about authorship. Some sites had difficulty following the children and gave up with the seventh birthday instead of the eighth. At a Congressional hearing in 1963, James Shannon complained that federal restrictions on salaries impeded full staffing of the project in the medical schools.[18] But in the end, the investigators published hundreds of scientific papers and dozens of books.[19,20] The program did not end until 1981; it lasted more than 25 years and cost more than $100 million dollars.

What did it achieve?

Paul Nichols answered succinctly:[7] "There weren't any major breakthroughs. They did not find out exactly what causes cerebral palsy, mental retardation, epilepsy, or other disorders of infancy and childhood. But a lot of things were done," as documented in all the books and papers. He also noted that investigators are still putting in requests to use the stored data.

Nichols was in a position to know. He had a Ph.D. in genetics from the University of Minnesota. His faculty sponsor, Elving Andersen, had spent time devising forms for the perinatal project and suggested that Nichols use the NINDB data, which he did. Comparing psychological test scores among twins and siblings, Nichols found evidence of a genetic trend. Andersen then recommended Nichols for a position at NINDB, which he accepted in 1971. His first assignment was the Perinatal Collaborative Project. He was an author of two of the project's monographs – one on minimal brain dysfunction was published with Sally Broman and another concerned preschool IQ. (Thirty years after he started, Nichols is still a program director at NINDS.)

Some of the achievements were listed as early as 1968, providing data to ascertain long-held beliefs:[21] Risk factors for neurological or psychological abnormalities included mother's age over 50 or under 15, incompetent cervix, and prematurity. Thirty percent of 1-year-old babies with neurological problems were born prematurely.

Banked blood samples from the Perinatal Project were still being used in 2001; using serum from the Project, Matthew Longnecker and his associates found that exposure to the anti-malarial insecticide DDT increased the risk of pre-term births, a contributor to infant mortality.[22]

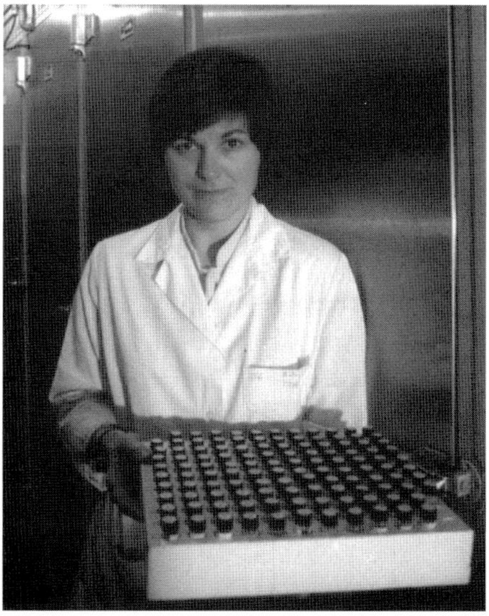

Lab technician holds vials of blood collected during Perinatal Project

There were indirect effects, too: improved prenatal care and hospital practices for newborn infants; new interdepartmental research in medical schools; training of medical students and residents; and the importance of documentation for later studies. The whole field of perinatal research was stimulated and neonatal intensive care units soon became a dominant force. The methods for data collection, test-and-retest validations, became staples of epidemiologic studies and therapeutic trials. Longnecker has compiled a bibliography of more than 400 titles that emanated from the project.[23]

Joseph S. Drage, M.D.

Sam Drage is another veteran of the Perinatal Project. He graduated from medical school at the University of Minnesota and was trained in pediatric endocrinology there. Faced with the physician draft, he was concerned about being sent to some remote area where his wife, also a physician, would not be able to find work. Heinz Berendes, one of his teachers in Minnesota, had come to NINDB as Chief of the Perinatal Research Branch at NINDS, the central coordinating unit of the entire project. Drage asked Berendes if a position were available and, in 1962 – shortly after the start of the program – found himself assigned to the Perinatal Branch. He was primarily involved in developing the examinations for 7-year-old children.[12]

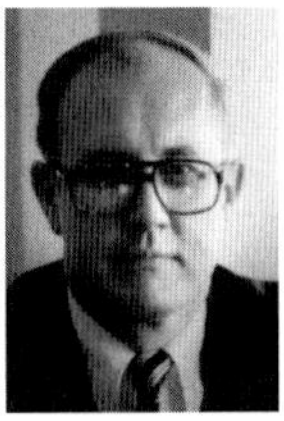

JOSEPH S. "SAM" DRAGE, M.D.

In 1968, the nature of the project changed from grants to contracts. Instead of the Project Directors at each institution setting policies, the NINDS Committee now largely determined and coordinated activities. In 1971, Berendes went for a Master's degree at Hopkins and Drage became acting chief of the branch. He had two major tasks: prepare a comprehensive plan for analyzing the data and complete the process of collecting data. With Janet Hardy he published a monograph on the first year of life. The last children in the project were born in 1966; they would finish their 8-year examinations in 1974. There was no formal attempt to keep the study going after that, but data analysis continued.

Drage credits the Perinatal Project with changing concepts about the origins of cerebral palsy from birth injuries to earlier events when the fetus was still developing in the uterus. He also credits the project for validating the scoring system developed by Virginia Apgar, Professor of Anesthesiology at Columbia University. As he put it:

> The anesthesiologists and obstetricians were paying all the attention to the mother and the poor little baby was just plunked aside. But there was no one really paying attention to the baby. Apgar's scoring system was still very controversial at the time. The study included Apgar scoring in the nursery. We had trained observers to do it.

It is now recognized that an infant's behavior in the Apgar score is a reliable, if not infallible, predictor of later cerebral function. The controversies had to do with variability in scores at different sites; the collaborative project brought a standard of consistency from place to place.

In the mid-80s, when the monographs had all been published, Drage became Chief of the Developmental Neurology Branch, in charge of both basic and clinical research programs. In that capacity he became the NINDS representative to the task force that sponsored the studies linking aspirin to Reye syndrome. He also participated in the studies linking folic acid deficiency to neural tube defects.

Drage never had formal training in neurology, but he was so completely immersed in the diseases of pediatric neurology and the training of pediatric neurologists that he was elected to membership in the Child Neurology Society. He retired from NINDS in 1999, 28 years after he started with the Collaborative Perinatal Study.

Karin B. Nelson, M.D.

Karin Nelson is an investigator whose professional life was shaped by the Collaborative Perinatal Project. She is now Acting Chief of the Epidemiology Branch of NINDS.

Nelson grew up in a suburb of Minneapolis, did her undergraduate work at the University of Minnesota, and went to medical school at the University of Chicago. When she completed her internship, her husband – the noted neurophysiologist Phillip G. Nelson – came to NIH and Karin sought neurology training in the area. She started at the University of Maryland, found the commuting awkward, and finished at George Washington University. She did electromyograms for Milton Shy. Then the Nelsons made another career move together. Phil had a postdoctoral fellowship with Sir Bernard Katz in London. Karin spent the year at the National Hospital Queen Square, a shrine of clinical neurology.

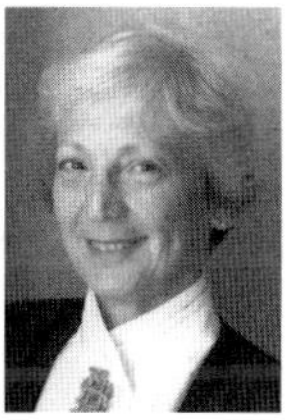

Karin B. Nelson, M.D., currently Chief of the Epidemiology Branch

When they returned to Washington, Richmond Payne offered Karin a position at the Children's Hospital. Assuming her duties there required some reorienting because she had had no training in pediatrics. At that time, there were few training programs in child neurology and it was not uncommon for adult neurologists to take responsibility for children. There she became interested in the most common form of epilepsy, febrile seizures. There was a paucity of knowledge and, therefore, much controversy about management. She was questioned about this so often that, when she was offered a position at NINDB's Perinatal Project, she quickly accepted it.

As she practiced child neurology without formal training, so she became an epidemiologist without formal training – by working with statisticians and epidemiologists with the perinatal data. With them she turned to the question of febrile seizures. Some leading figures advocated chronic treatment with barbiturates to prevent later recurrence of seizures. But that method was questioned from the start and became more of a problem when impaired school performance was blamed on the drug treatment.

Nelson's approach was influenced by the primitive card-sorting approach to data analysis from the days before computers were so well developed. Her views were clearly articulated:[24]

> I came to do the febrile seizures, but it was also easier to do that with a subset than it was to attack the whole data set. So the febrile seizures were first. That was the first study of natural history with an epidemiologically sensible basis that was ever done on febrile seizures. It has been confirmed by several national studies since. It changed the management of the most common seizure disorder in childhood. There was a consensus conference about management, and then there was a randomized trial of treatment. It was a succession of steps from . . . you cannot figure out what is a sensible course of action until you know the natural history of a disorder. The outcomes had been studied in samples that were just ridiculous. They went to clinics for the mentally retarded and asked who had had a febrile seizure and said, "Ah-ha, it causes mental retardation." That is just not a sane way to do it. So this was the first. Here is something as common as grass, 3-4 percent of all kids have them. Why do you have to be as ignorant as we were? And the answer was that there wasn't a dataset to take the questions in an A-B-C set of steps – natural history and then randomized trials changed the management of a major neurological disorder.[25]

Karin Nelson has made numerous contributions to the issues considered in the collaborative project. One of her favorites was evidence that the cause of cerebral palsy is more often associated with intrauterine events than with difficult births. In recent years she has moved from analytic epidemiology to molecular epidemiology, which she explains as follows:

> Epidemiology is the **distribution** of the determinants of a disease. Distribution is the nose-counting aspect, but to my point of view that is interesting only in so far as it takes you to the next step about why. The study of etiology within epidemiology isn't so different from what a clinician might undertake, except that, instead of dealing with a patient as the denominator, it deals with populations, and that makes a more generalizable result . . . . The distribution of disease is a very important description. If you are going to make public health decisions, you have to know who's got it, where is it, and how it is distributed according to demographics.
>
> My interest, in fact, is the next stage, which is "why"? That is also appropriately a topic of epidemiology, but it is approached

a little differently. The question is: what determines the disease distribution in populations? And where does that get you in understanding what is really going on? There is **descriptive** epidemiology, to say "who's got what," and there's **analytic** to say, "and how far can that take you in understanding mechanisms of disease and what are the etiologies." The latest finesse added to analytic epidemiology is **molecular** epidemiology, which means biologic sampling and integrating that with the analytic epidemiology. That is what we are into at the moment. Then you come head-on into the question of, say you do biologic sampling. You are going to measure something. What is it going to be and how are you going to interpret it when you get it? Directly back in the ballpark of the basic scientists from whom many of the important hypotheses come, but the opposite is also happening. Observations in humans can generate the hypotheses, which are then tested, even in the basic science labs. And that is what's happening here. Observations in humans, testing of biochemical differences between cases and non-cases, and then taking that back to the basic scientists and asking, "how do we understand what's going on here?"

Nelson has applied this theoretical approach to the question of autism. In her studies, archived neonatal blood samples were assayed for "biological regulators of cerebral development," that is they measured the blood content of nerve growth factors and related peptide substances. Nelson and her colleagues found that several of these regulators were present in higher concentration in children who later showed signs of autism, or were mentally retarded without signs of autism, than in children who had cerebral palsy or were asymptomatic.[26] The data would implicate impaired development of the brain in the etiology of autism, which has been a challenge to neuroscientists seeking an explanation.

From the Collaborative Perinatal Project to molecular epidemiology was a straight line for Karin Nelson, another indirect contribution of the project.

1 Sveinbjörnsdóttir S, Hicks AA, Johnsson T, et al. Familial aggregation of Parkinson's disease in Iceland. *N Engl J Med* 2001;343:1765-1770.

2 Sacks O. *The Island of the Colorblind.* New York:Vintage Books/Random House, 1997.

3 Monmaney T. Annals of Science. This obscure malady. *The New Yorker*. October 29, 1990:85-113.

4 Zimmerman HM. Monthly report to medical officer in command. U.S. Naval Medical Research Unit No. 2, June 1, 1945.

5 Heussner R. At the epicenter. *Minnesota Med* 1998;81:6-9.

6 Kurland LT. Recorded Telephone Interview with author, March 27, 2001.

7 Trautner DA, Thal L. In memoriam. Wigbert C. Wiederholt M.D. (1932-2000). *Neurology* 2001;56:1444.

8 Wiederholt WC. Neuroepidemiologic research initiatives on Guam: past and present. *Neuroepidemiology* 1999;18:279-91.

9 Galasko DR, Plato CC, Garruto PM, Gamst A, Craig UK, Torres J, Wiederholt WC. ALS and Parkinson-dementia complex of Guam: a 40-year follow-up of a prospective case-control study. *Neurology* 2001:56 (suppl. 3): A115-6 (P02.072).

10 Waring SC, Reed DM, Petersen RC, Craig LK, Kurland LT. Parkinson-Dementia Complex of Guam 1950-1989. *Neurology* 2001; (suppl 3): A116 (P02.073).

11 U.S. Congress. House. Committee on Appropriations. *Departments of Labor and Health, Education, and Welfare Appropriations for 1957: Hearings before the Subcommittee on Departments of Labor and Health, Education and Welfare and Related Agencies Appropriations.* 84th Cong., 2nd sess., January 30-31, February 2-3, 6, 8, 9, 13, 19-20, 1956, p. 776.

12 Masland RL. Forword to Niswander KR, Gordon M, Berendez HW, et al. *The Women and Their Pregnancies; The Collaborative Perinatal Study of the National Institute of Neurological Diseases and Stroke.* [Washington]: National Institutes of Health, 1972:73-379.

13 Niswander, et al. *The Women and Their Pregnancies*: 2.

14 U.S. Congress. House. Committee on Appropriations. *Departments of Labor, Health, Education and Welfare Appropriations for 1964. Part 3, National Institutes of Health: Hearings before the Subcommittee on Departments of Labor and Health, Education and Welfare and Related Agencies Appropriations.* 88th Cong., 1st sess., May 7-8, 12-14, 1963, p. 798.

15 Masland RL. Recorded Interview with author, September 13, 2000.

16 Barden FO. *History – Perinatal Research Project, Chronological Statement of Volume XVI. Planning, Organization, Direction, Administration.* National Institute of Neurological Diseases and Stroke, National Institutes of Health, Bethesda, MD, 1969.

17 U.S. Congress. House. Committee on Appropriations. *Departments of Labor, Health, Education and Welfare Appropriations for 1968. Part 5, National Institutes of Health, National Institute of Mental Health: Hearings before the Subcommittee on Departments of Labor and Health, Education, and Welfare and Related Agencies Appropriations.* 90th Cong., 1st sess., April 6-7, 11-13, 17, 1967, pp. 480-481.

18 U.S. Congress. House. Committee on Appropriations. *Departments of Labor and Health, Education and Welfare Appropriations for 1963. Part 3, National Institutes of Health: Hearings before the Subcommittee on Departments of Labor and Health, Education and Welfare and Related Agencies Appropriations.* 87th Cong., 1st sess., February 7-9, 19, 1962, p. 1505.

19 U.S. Congress. House. Committee on Appropriations. *Departments of Labor, Education and Welfare, and related Agencies Appropriations for 1981. Part 4, National Institutes of Health: Continuation of Hearings before the Subcommittee on Labor and Health, Education and Welfare Appropriations.* 96th Cong., 2nd sess., February 25, 28, 29, March 3-6, 1980, p. 857.

20 Drage JS. Recorded interview with author, January 18, 2001.

21 U.S. Congress. House. Committee on Appropriations. *Departments of Labor, Health, Education and Welfare Appropriations for 1968. Part 5, National Institutes of Health, National Institute of Mental Health: Hearings before the Subcommittee on Departments of Labor and Health, Education, and Welfare and Related Agencies.* 90th Cong., 1st sess., April 6-7, 11-13, 17, 1967, pp. 480-481.

22 Longnecker MP, Klebanoff MA, Zhou H, Brock JW. Association between maternal serum concentration of the DDT metabolite DDE and preterm and small-for-gestational-age babies at birth. *Lancet* 2001;358:110-114.

23 Longnecker W. Bibliography for Collaborative Perinatal Project, 2001.

24 Nelson KB. Recorded Interview with author, September 27, 2000.

25 Nelson KB, Ellenberg JH. Prognosis in children with febrile seizures. *Pediatrics* 1978;61:720-727.

26 Nelson KB, Grether JK, Croen LA, et al. Neuropeptides and neurotrophins in neonatal blood of children with autism or mental retardation. *Ann Neurol* 2001;49:597-606.

CHAPTER TEN

DECADE OF THE BRAIN: DAVID MAHONEY AND THE DANA ALLIANCE FOR BRAIN INITIATIVES

On March 8, 1989, the United States Congress passed a joint resolution that designated the "Decade of the Brain" to commence on January 1, 1990. On July 18, 1990, President George H.W. Bush issued the formal proclamation.[1] In doing so, he recognized the advances in neuroscience and he noted that these advances gave hope for more effective treatment for Alzheimer disease, Parkinson disease, cerebral palsy, spinal cord injury, schizophrenia, depression, stroke, and AIDS.

The President did not originate the idea of designating a decade to support neuroscience and disorders of the brain. Murray Goldstein, former Director of NINDS, claims that it started in NINDS.[2]

> In the late 1980s a few of us were sitting around and trying to say what can we sell that takes neurology to public attention? We keep talking about stroke and head injury but neither has the catch. In a small meeting we came up with the idea. We didn't want a war on something again; that had been played to the death. We came up with the idea of the Decade of the Brain. Here, neuroscience was exploding. For the first time we were having clinical interventions for neurological disorders, not only being expert diagnosticians, but we had something to do. The future was all there.
>
> It was done in my office. I would be talking in my weekly staff meetings about this. Getting ideas from Carl Leventhal and Mike Walker and Gene Streicher and others. That was my inside group. I don't know if one of them said, "Hey, why don't we call it the Decade of the Brain?" or whether I said it. All I can tell you is one day I said, "We're going to have a Decade of the Brain." I tested it out with two Congressmen. By this time, I had become reasonably informally acquainted with a couple of key Congressmen, where I could invite them to lunch privately, or I'd go to their office and have a cup of coffee and we'd talk off the record. And I tried it. Both of them said it was a good idea.

One of the two was Silvio O. Conte, a Republican from Massachusetts, who became a vigorous and influential supporter of the program in Congress, thanks to the efforts of Lawrence Hoffheimer, executive director of the NINDS-linked National Committee for Research in Neurological Disorders. But it was not to be all smooth sailing. Goldstein went to Lewis Judd, Director of NIMH, to propose a joint effort. That proved to be impossible – several NIMH officials claimed priority for the idea. Even with the aid of skilled mediators – Roger Porter (Deputy Director of NINDS from 1987 to 1992) and Alan Leshner (then with NIMH, now

Director of the National Institute on Drug Abuse) – the two institutes could not fully join forces.

Soon, however, all the other NIH institutes with neuroscience programs had their own variations of the Decade of the Brain. Professional organizations came on board with supporting efforts; they put the Decade of the Brain logo on journals, meeting announcements, and letterheads. Decade of the Brain lectures and symposia featuring scientific leaders became prominent in the annual meetings of clinical and scientific societies. Nevertheless, during the first years of the Decade, the multiplicity of organizations blurred its focus and there was a background doubt that all the effort would ever result in a surge in neuroscience funding – which was one of the key goals of the initiative.

PROCLAMATION 6158
DECADE OF THE BRAIN

DECADE OF THE BRAIN, 1990 – 1999

By the President of the United States of America

A Proclamation

The human brain, a 3-pound mass of interwoven nerve cells that controls our activity, is one of the most magnificent – and mysterious – wonders of creation. The seat of human intelligence, interpreter of senses, and controller of movement, this incredible organ continues to intrigue scientist and layman alike.

Over the years, our understanding of the brain – how it works, what goes wrong when it is injured or diseased – has increased dramatically. However, we still have much more to learn. The need for continued study of the brain is compelling: millions of Americans are affected each year by disorders of the brain ranging from neurogenetic diseases to degenerative disorders such as Alzheimer's, as well as stroke, schizophrenia, autism, and impairments of speech, language, and hearing.

Today, these individuals and their families are justifiably hopeful, for a new era of discovery is dawning in brain research. Powerful microscopes, major strides in the study of genetics, and advanced brain imaging devices are giving physicians and scientists ever greater insight into the brain. Neuroscientists are mapping the brain's biochemical circuitry, which may help produce more effective drugs for alleviating the suffering of those who have Alzheimer's or Parkinson's disease. By studying how the brain's cells and chemicals develop, interact, and communicate with the rest of the body, investigators are also developing improved treatments for people incapacitated by spinal cord injuries, depressive disorders, and epileptic seizures. Breakthroughs in molecular genetics show great promise of yielding methods to treat and prevent Huntington's disease, the muscular dystrophies, and other life-threatening disorders.

Research may also prove valuable in our war on drugs, as studies provide greater insight into how people become addicted to drugs and how drugs affect the brain. These studies may also help produce effective treatments for chemical dependency and help us to understand and prevent the harm done to the preborn children of pregnant women who abuse drugs and alcohol. Because there is a connection between the body's nervous and immune systems, studies of the brain may also help enhance our understanding of Acquired Immune Deficiency Syndrome.

Many studies regarding the human brain have been planned and conducted by scientists at the National Institutes of Health, the National Institute of Mental Health, and other Federal research agencies. Augmenting Federal efforts are programs supported by private foundations and industry. The cooperation between these agencies and the multidisciplinary efforts of thousands of scientists and health care professionals provide powerful evidence of our Nation's determination to conquer brain disease.

To enhance public awareness of the benefits to be derived from brain research, the Congress, by House Joint Resolution 174, has designated the decade beginning January 1, 1990, as the "Decade of the Brain" and has authorized and requested the President to issue a proclamation in observance of this occasion.

NOW, THEREFORE, I, GEORGE BUSH, President of the United States of America, do hereby proclaim the decade beginning January 1, 1990, as the Decade of the Brain. I call upon all public officials and the people of the United States to observe that decade with appropriate programs, ceremonies, and activities.

IN WITNESS WHEREOF, I have hereunto set my hand this seventeenth day of July, in the year of our Lord nineteen hundred and ninety, and of the Independence of the United States of America the two hundred and fifteenth.

G Bush

The mood changed to one of optimism a few years later when The Charles A. Dana Foundation's David Mahoney entered the scene and showed how the power of a forceful and committed individual could energize and focus an effort.[3]

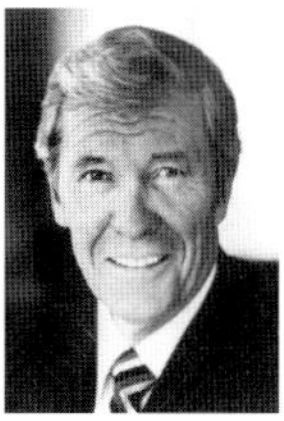

David Mahoney, former chairman of The Dana Foundation

David Mahoney was born in the Throggs Neck section of the Bronx in New York City. One of his childhood companions in playing stickball on the streets was John O'Connor, who later became Cardinal of the New York City Diocese. Mahoney graduated from La Salle Military Academy and during World War II served as a Captain in the infantry. After the war, he applied to the Wharton School of Business at the University of Pennsylvania. While awaiting the admissions decision, he worked for an advertising agency in New York. After he was accepted, his father was ill and money was tight. He therefore continued to work for the agency in New York and commuted to Philadelphia for night classes.

After Mahoney graduated, he became Vice President of the agency – at age 25. Three years later he started his own advertising company, which he sold 5 years later to run the Good Humor Company. Another 5 years later he joined Colgate Palmolive as executive vice president, and became president of the Canada Dry soft drink company in 1966. In 1968, Canada Dry consolidated with several other large corporations to form Norton Simon, Inc. Two years after that, Simon retired and Mahoney became CEO and Chairman of the Board.

In 1983, Mahoney tried to take Norton Simon private but was outbid. He was given a lucrative buyout package and was now richer than ever – but without a job. A long article about his plight appeared in *The New York Times*. His restlessness and depression did not last long because, over the years, he had developed an interest in neuroscience. He now expressed that interest through The Charles A. Dana Foundation, of which he had been Chairman since 1977.

Under Mahoney's leadership, The Dana Foundation changed its focus from that of a philanthropic foundation primarily involved in

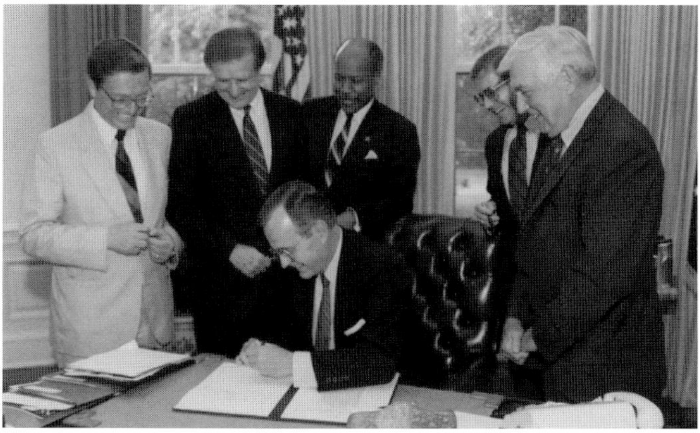

President Bush signing Proclamation of the Decade of the Brain

the erection of buildings for hospitals and universities, to one fully devoted to brain science and education.

Mahoney's interest in neuroscience arose at a meeting James Watson had arranged for business leaders at Cold Spring Harbor. Maxwell Cowan, a leading developmental neurobiologist, was also Vice-President and Chief Scientific Officer of the Howard Hughes Medical Institute. Cowan, wrote[4] that he was one of six neuroscientists

> who were invited and, as it happened, I was asked to give the first talk on the structure of the brain. It occurred to me that most of the participants had probably never seen a normal brain, so I brought a formalin-fixed human brain with me and . . . proceeded to demonstrate and dissect it. Unlike most of the students, who seemed rather blasé about seeing and even handling the brain, this group of distinguished businessmen was completely fascinated to learn about it and, at one point, to actually touch the brain.

Two years later, Mahoney told Cowan:

> I can still remember vividly your dissecting a brain for us. That weekend had a profound effect on me. I went home afterwards and said to my wife, "Hillie, I think I should give up working and spend the rest of my life trying to do something to promote research on the brain and its disorders."

Under Mahoney's initiative, in 1992 The Dana Foundation funded and organized a meeting at Cold Spring Harbor, gathering together a group of the country's top neuroscientists to explore ways to invigorate the Decade of the Brain. Mahoney confronted them, warning that the public would not respond to their announced goal of "understanding the brain." People, he said, wanted more direct help from research and they wanted the science explained in plain English.[5]

By the end of the meeting, 60 scientists has signed a Declaration that set ten research goals[6] to be achieved by the end of the decade. Each goal was created to be meaningful to the public, and each scientist made a personal commitment to go forth and talk to the public in layman's language. Mahoney convinced Nobelist James Watson and Max Cowan to lead a group of elite neuroscientists under the aegis of The Dana Alliance for Brain Initiatives. By 2001, the Alliance included more than 200 neuroscientists and nine Nobel laureates. A similar organization was formed in Europe.

Mahoney became evangelical in bringing the power of brain science to public attention. He used all his marketing skills to charm, cajole, and coax – all based on the facts. He used every arrow in his quiver of public relations experiences – an annual progress report on brain science; a biweekly newspaper (*The Brain in the News*); a bimonthly newsletter (*BrainWork*); a quarterly journal with in-depth articles by authorities (*Cerebrum*); a guide to organizations concerned with the brain and brain disorders; a press office to field and direct inquiries from journalists interested in neuroscience; as well as a web site, advertisements, videos, and course material for children and young adults.

The Foundation also gave out $34 million in grants for brain research, including some for projects that enhanced technology, especially novel approaches to brain imaging. The Dana Foundation awarded coveted prizes to brain scientists and education leaders. Mahoney and the Alliance leaders did not separate psychiatric and neurologic research, and they became a strong force in the unification of clinical and basic neurosciences.

Undoubtedly the most influential of these approaches was Brain Awareness Week, which started in 1996 and is now celebrated by more than 1,300 partner organizations in 46 countries. During the last 5 years of the Decade of the Brain, a major focus of Brain Awareness Week was the presentation of an annual report on the progress of brain research to an assembly of prominent neuroscientists, patient advocacy groups, and policy makers in Washington, D.C. The education program gave visibility to advances in neuroscience, and by the end of the Decade of the Brain, the combined efforts of the Dana programs had reached 15 million people in the United States and Europe. Now the impact is worldwide. The momentum did not end when the Decade ended and David Mahoney died in 2000 at age 76.

Mahoney did not work solely through The Dana Foundation. He had a personal impact, too. He made a donation to the University of Pennsylvania in 1983 to create the David Mahoney Institute for Neurological Sciences. In 1990, he founded the Harvard Mahoney Neuroscience Institute and, in 1999, Columbia University honored him by naming a neuroscience center for him. In addition, he

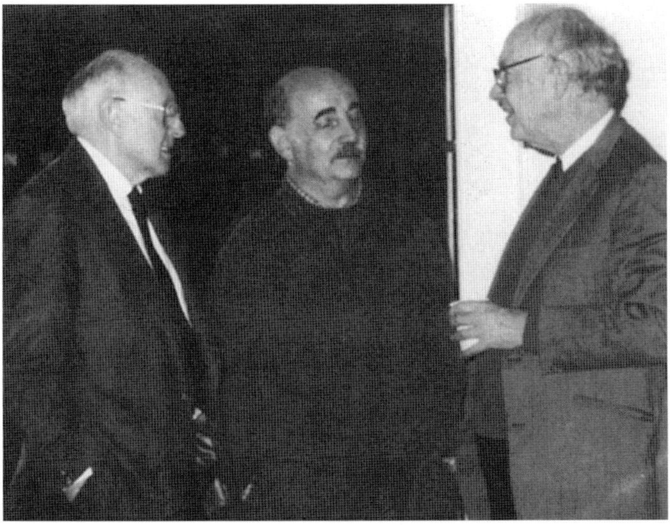

(FROM LEFT) NEUROSCIENTISTS MAXWELL COWAN, M.D., ALBERT AGUAYO, M.D., AND JAMES WATSON, M.D., AT THE 1992 COLD SPRING HARBOR MEETING

wrote a book, *The Longevity Strategy*, with neurologist-author Richard Restak.[7]

For all of this, Mahoney was recognized with awards from the Lasker Foundation, the American Academy of Neurology, and the Society for Neuroscience. His gracious wife Hillie was involved in it all.

In the year 2000, Joseph B. Martin, M.D.-Ph.D., neurologist, neuroscientist, and Dean of the Harvard Medical School, evaluated achievements on the goals set in that 1992 Cold Spring Harbor meeting.[8] He concluded, "the report card reflects great accomplishments in defining the underlying mechanisms of neurological and psychiatric disorders. New and more effective treatments for many of these are certain to appear in the first decade of the twenty-first century.

Yet even the goals with high marks are still in need of attention. It is impressive that present-day favorites were not on the 1992 list, which did not mention, for instance, stem cells or the Human Genome Project. There are more opportunities now than ever before.

Looking back, it is difficult to evaluate the Decade of the Brain. The goal was to enhance NIH funding for neuroscience, which largely did not materialize. In fact, some members of the NINDS Advisory Council had doubts from the start, and thought the inter-institutional conflicts were pointless because they were directed towards a pot of money that would never be seen.[9] In interviews at the end of the decade, some NINDS officials concurred.[10]

Ruth Kirschstein,[11] now Acting Director of NIH, put the matter in perspective. "I think it would be more important right now," she said, "because the institutes are working together. I think everybody paid lip service to it, but nothing happened. It was also a period in which our budget was not in very good shape. Maybe it was just too early, because now the neurosciences are the most actively flourishing."

Richard Hodes,[12] Director of the National Institute on Aging, posed a different question – "whether the same progress would have occurred had there not been that banner? Well, I don't know."

Brain Awareness Week Logo

Evaluation of Decade of the Brain Goals

By Joseph H. Martin, M.D., Ph.D.[4]

Goal	Grade
1. Identify genes for familial Alzheimer disease, Huntington disease	A+
2. Identify genes for manic-depressive illness	C+
3. New medications and therapies to reduce nerve cell death and enhance recovery after stroke or other forms of brain damage	B+
4. New drugs or other treatment to alleviate multiple sclerosis, Alzheimer disease, Parkinson disease, and epilepsy	A
5. New treatments to promote nerve regeneration after spinal cord or peripheral nerve injury	C
6. New, more effective treatments of manic-depressive illness, anxiety disorders, and forms of schizophrenia that now resist treatment	B
7. Develop agents to block action of cocaine and other addictive substances	B
8. New treatments for pain of cancer, arthritis, migraine, and other debilitating diseases	B+
9. Identify genes for hereditary deafness and blindness	A+
10. Elucidate neuronal mechanisms of learning and memory	A

And Steven Hyman,[13] Director of NIMH, was even a bit optimistic:

> Well certainly if you look at funding it didn't give the brain sciences any edge over other disciplines, which also grew and deserved to grow, frankly. But it created a wonderful esprit and I think that we shouldn't let it drop. In some sense it was (for much of neuroscience and clinical neuroscience) rather unifying, which is a very good thing. I think a certain number of the behavioral scientists felt left out. We can't afford to leave them out. Ultimately we need to incorporate them and make sure that behavioral science is not separated from the brain, I think that is very, very important. But I think on balance it was a very good thing for the spirit of the enterprise – it made neuroscience feel special. One could really sense that.

Quite independently, Gerald Fischbach, former Director of NINDS, agreed:[14]

> You know it certainly raised a public awareness of brain research. Were important advances made that wouldn't be made anyhow? I don't know, actually. I think it's hard to make a specific claim about that. If I were pressed, I would say that it certainly added to the public awareness of brain research, it raised expectations on the part of patients and the public, and also some of the scientists made people feel more hopeful. But I don't think it's been the cause of discovery. I think that was on its own trajectory.

There was a very real way in which it had an effect and that was public perceptions that get translated into Congressional actions. I think it contributed to this rather remarkable period of budget doubling. It contributed in a very important way, from a variety of different sources.

As a public relations gambit, the Decade was a success. As a way of engaging scientists, legislators, and leaders of voluntary agencies, it was a success. As an education program it successfully mirrored the wonderful scientific and technological advances. As part of the preparation for the bipartisan doubling of the neuroscience budget, the Decade was a clear success.

We cannot be certain the Decade had anything to do with these advances, which might well have come without the public hue, but the advances and the education marched together. Murray Goldstein got it up and running, and David Mahoney energized and pushed it forward, but they did not do it alone. Directors in all the institutes played their roles. So did the professional organizations and the voluntaries. So did the legislators who have set upon a course of doubling the NIH budget, a bipartisan policy supported by President George W. Bush. Many wish we could be clever enough to keep it going in the next millennium.

1 Bush GH. Presidential proclamation 6158. In Decade of the Brain, July 18, 1990.

2 Goldstein M. Interview with author, April 19, 2000.

3 Mahoney D. Conversation with author, 1996; recalled by the author and facts confirmed by Barbara Gill, Director of The Dana Alliance, and Mrs. David Mahoney, April 18, 2001.

4 Cowan M. Remembering David. *Dana Alliance Member News*. Vol. 4, no. 2, (April/May 2000).

5 Nevins J. Philanthropist David J. Mahoney: an appreciation. *Cerebrum* 2000; 2:93-94.

6 How Brain Scientists Broke the Mold. *The Dana Alliance for Brain Initiatives*. New York: The Dana Press, 1999, p. 9.

7 Mahoney DJ, Restak R. *The Longevity Strategy: How to Live to 100 Using the Brain-Body Connection*. New York: The Dana Press/John Wiley & Sons, 1998.

8 Martin JH. On Average, The Decade of the Brain Scores a B+. In *Delivering Results, A Progress Report on Brain Research, Update 2000: Brain Research in the New Millennium*, Washington, DC: A Publication of The Dana Alliance for Brain Initiatives produced and distributed by the Dana Press, 2000, pp. 6-9.

9 Author's personal recollections of the NINDS Advisory Council and its Committees in 1989.

10 Leventhal C. Interview with author, March 20, 2001.

11 Kirschstein R. Interview with author, March 6, 2001.

12 Hodes R. Interview with author, March 23, 2001.

13 Hyman S. Interview with author, February 27, 2001.

14 Fischbach G. Interview with author, April 21, 2001.

CHAPTER ELEVEN

THE VOLUNTARIES

At the 1949 hearings on the bill to establish NINDB, only three neurological diseases were represented by advocates – multiple sclerosis, epilepsy, and cerebral palsy. Of the three, only multiple sclerosis had its own national organization and that one was only 2 years old.

In the year 2001, the Office of Communications and Public Liaison had a list of more than 325 different voluntary organizations that were concerned with the institute's research. Their origins, motives, and operations differ, but many arise from personal interests: particular families affected by particular diseases. They want to foster research, often in search of effective treatments for conditions that lack any treatment at all.

These groups correctly see NIH as the main source of biomedical research, but they raise additional funds. Fund-raising is achieved by actions as different as bake sales or annual telethons. If funds suffice, many voluntaries provide money for their own research grants and research training fellowships. They do not compete with NINDS but rather complement its efforts. Many of these private organizations help in providing patient care or guidance, which NINDS does not do directly, and many organizations, like NIH institutes, serve as a source of educational material.

Other potent forces are the professional organizations – the American Academy of Neurology, the American Neurological Association, the Child Neurology Society, and similar organizations for neurosurgery, neuroradiology, and neurorehabilitation. They all have strong interests in promoting research in the neurosciences and, come budget time, they all want NINDS to be strongly supported by the Congress. The benefits of this relationship between NIH and the voluntaries are reciprocal. The voluntaries are now a powerful force in the daily life of NINDS officials.

One of the earliest organizations was the March of Dimes, which emerged from an anti-polio campaign begun during the Roosevelt administration in 1938. The March of Dimes funded the trials that led to the development of an effective vaccine that was widely distributed after World War II and which, by 1953, had eradicated poliomyelitis in the United States. It is noteworthy that this historic achievement of a private organization preceded the creation of NINDB.

For NINDS, the impact of voluntary agencies started with the National Multiple Sclerosis Society and, once again, with a single determined person – Sylvia Lawry.

Sylvia Lawry was born in 1915. She was a pre-law student at Hunter College in New York City when her brother began to have symptoms of the disease. After a few years of fruitless search for effective treatment, Ms. Lawry placed a small classified notice in *The New York Times* in 1945:

> *Multiple Sclerosis. Will anyone recovered from it please communicate with patient.*

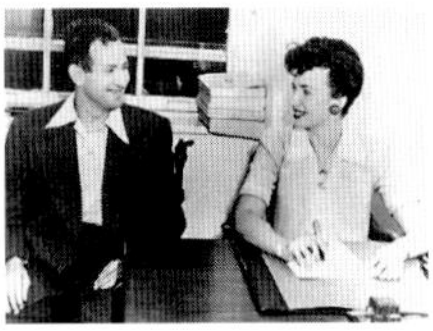

SYLVIA LAWRY, FOUNDER OF THE NATIONAL MULTIPLE SCLEROSIS SOCIETY, AND HER BROTHER, BERNARD LAWRY

More than 50 people responded, all of them involved in the same search for effective treatment and all of them frustrated by the absence of experts on the disease or any kind of research to improve the situation. At about that time, former NINDB Director Richard Masland said to a group of neurologists, "For all the good we do for MS patients, we might as well be asking nuns to take care of them."[1]

Masland, a perceptive, kind, and gentle man, was not being callous. He was bemoaning the total lack of effective treatment for a disease that affects primarily young adults, more often young mothers than fathers. He was emphasizing the need for research as the only way to find and develop treatment. Later events proved his prescience. (But more research does not eliminate the need for comforting caregivers, including clerics.)

Sylvia Lawry recognized the need for an organized movement to stimulate and finance research into the cure, treatment, and cause of multiple sclerosis. In 1946, she took up the challenge and, at age 21, she convened a meeting of scientists and founded the new society.

At first the organization had a different name. The National Multiple Sclerosis Society (NMSS) became the official name in 1947 and the first two chapters were chartered in Connecticut and California. Now, there are chapters in all 50 states, and the Society as a whole budgeted about $30 million to support research in 2001. NMSS has been a forceful advocate on behalf of an increasing budget for MS research, which in 2000, it estimated at about $100 million annually.

Under Lawry's singular leadership, NMSS did more than advocate. Their members raised money for research and for research fellowships. They actively promoted better care through educational programs for health professionals and for public education. Their mission included the goals of NINDS itself – research, training, and education – all aimed at improving patient care. In time, Ms. Lawry became an active adviser in the creation of similar organizations in other countries, and she personally led the way to the creation of an international federation of MS societies. After a lifetime devoted to advocating for MS research and treatment, she died in 2001 at the age of 85.

Other national advocacy organizations were created because of the success of the NMSS. Several local organizations coalesced to form United Cerebral Palsy. Ultimately, several of the epilepsy organizations also combined, but there are still more than one. In time, organizations appeared for Alzheimer disease, Parkinson disease, stroke, and muscular dystrophy and related diseases. All of these organizations have added to the efforts of NINDS by raising money for research, training, and education. Often the voluntaries have cooperated with NINDS officials in funding the same project. That is, a voluntary organization may fund a fellowship for a young investigator working with a senior grantee supported by NINDS. Or vice versa. Or NINDS and a voluntary may share the support of an expensive project of mutual interest.

Increasingly, celebrities have aided the effort. President Franklin Roosevelt himself had had paralytic poliomyelitis and that fact undoubtedly helped the cause of the March of Dimes. For NINDS, the first well-known promoter was Eleanor Gehrig, widow of the famous baseball player who is now immortalized in the eponym for amyotrophic lateral sclerosis or Lou Gehrig's disease. Senator Charles Tobey of Maine had a daughter with MS and testified in the hearings that led to the formation of NINDB.

One of the most effective celebrities is Jerry Lewis, the comedian, actor, and all-round entertainer. He has been National Chairman of the Muscular Dystrophy Association (MDA) for five decades and serves as host of the annual Jerry Lewis MDA Telethon. Since its inauguration on Labor Day Weekend in 1966, the Telethon has raised over a billion dollars for research and patient care. Lewis's tireless efforts have transformed an official national holiday into one that also recognizes the need for biomedical research.[2]

Other celebrities have become advocates for research on and treatment for particular conditions: Mohammed Ali, Michael J. Fox, and Janet Reno for Parkinson disease; Nancy Reagan and the Princess Aga Khan for Alzheimer disease; Catfish Hunter and other baseball players for ALS; and Christopher Reeve for spinal cord injury.

These individuals and their organizations have sometimes done more than raise money and distribute funds to support investigator-initiated research projects. Nancy Wexler and her father gathered scientists who together devised a planned campaign to map the gene for Huntington disease in 1983 (discussed in Chapter 15). In that effort, a voluntary organization – the Hereditary Disease Foundation – combined efforts with NINDS to create and support research of historic import. It was the first research to prove the theory of what is now called "positional cloning," the ability to map the position of disease genes without knowing in advance the nature of the gene product.

Influenced by the Huntington story, the MDA followed with its own drive to find the gene for the most devastating of the dystrophies, the Duchenne type. This condition is symptomatic as soon as affected boys begin to walk and is evident to parents by the time the child is 5 years old. The children are unable to walk by age 12 and most die by age 30. There is still no effective treatment.

In the 1980s, the Scientific Director of MDA was Donald Wood. Supported by Robert Ross, Vice-President of MDA, and scientific advisors, Wood organized a meeting with James Watson, the Nobel laureate and molecular biologist.[3] If they wanted to find the gene for Duchenne dystrophy, Watson advised them to forget the usual and average $50,000 research grant that MDA customarily awarded and consider giving much larger sums to only a few centers. They followed his advice and by 1987 the gene had been mapped and the gene product was identified as *dystrophin*, an essential protein of the muscle surface membranes. This was the first time in history that a previously unknown protein was identified as the problematic target of a human mutation. Credit for this is given to Louis Kunkel and his associates at Harvard, Eric Hoffman, Marcel Koenig, and Anthony Monaco. But others also played key roles: Ute Franck, Kay Davies, Ronald Whorton, and Thomas Caskey among them.

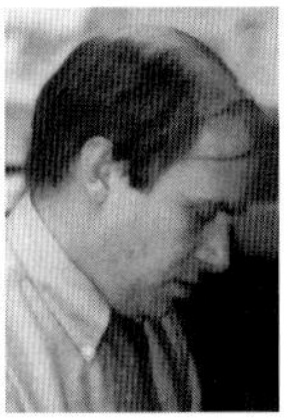

LOUIS KUNKEL, PH.D., WHOSE TEAM AT HARVARD DISCOVERED THE GENE FOR DUCHENNE MUSCULAR DYSTROPHY IN 1986

The Duchenne campaign had another unexpected result. Once the Duchenne gene had been found, it was discovered that some children with a clinically similar disorder did not show the usual mutation. Ultimately these syndromes were found, by Kevin Campbell and his associates at the University of Iowa, to be associated with another set of previously unknown proteins of the muscle surface membrane. Naturally, NINDS also supported these investigators, but the concept of a multi-institutional effort for muscular dystrophies started with MDA.

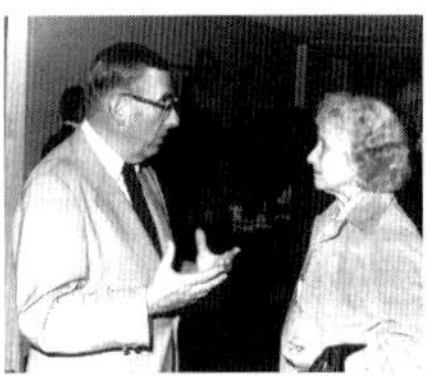

MARJORIE GUTHRIE, FOUNDER OF THE HUNTINGTON'S DISEASE SOCIETY, TALKING TO DONALD TOWER, M.D.

Another initiative at NINDS, initially broached by a voluntary organization, was the development of special research and patient care centers. Marjorie Guthrie, widow of folk singer Woody Guthrie and founder of the Huntington's Disease Society, advocated for the "Centers Without Walls," for which NINDS grants were awarded in 1980, including one to Harvard Medical School to create a center. There, James Gusella and Joseph Martin found the Huntington disease gene.

Similar centers that combine research and patient care have been promoted successfully for Alzheimer disease and stroke. Centers for Parkinson disease have been named in honor of the late Senator Morris Udall of Arizona. These centers focus on research but draw patients with particular diseases in numbers sufficient to carry out therapeutic trials of new drugs. In the process, patient care improves and young investigators are trained.

The Udall Centers, like so much of NINDS activity, again show the impact of dedicated partisans. In this case, leaders of the movement to increase Parkinson research were Joan Samuelson, a young lawyer who is herself affected by parkinsonism, and Morton

Kondracke, publisher of a Washington newsletter about Congress and a recent novel, "*Saving Millie*,"[4] whose wife has Parkinson disease. The five separate Parkinson advocacy groups supported them in that effort.

The voluntary organizations have played an active role in the life of NINDS from the beginning. Representatives of advocacy groups supporting research in head injury, Lou Gehrig's disease, Rett syndrome, epilepsy, spinal cord injury, and Alzheimer disease have sat on the institute's Advisory Council over the years and have added their valuable points of view to the discussion. The influence of the voluntary health agencies has been even further broadened by the advent of television and computers, access to the world wide web, consumerism, political activism, and enhanced patient education.

Input from these organizations has become invaluable for NINDS officials in a mutually beneficial arrangement. Yet NINDS officials must maintain a delicate balance between the demands of the numerous competing organizations. Even more of a concern is the potential conflict between earmarked (or "line item") research funds from Congress and the ability to provide money for investigator-initiated research – yet one more challenge for NINDS administrators.

1 Obituary for Sylvia Lawry. *The New York Times*, February 28, 2001.

2 Schenkenberger R. E-mail Communication to author, May 31, 2001.

3 Rowland LP. Duchenne Dystrophy: behind the discoveries. *MDA Newsmagazine* 1989;6:16-20.

4 Kondracke M. *Saving Millie: Love, Politics, and Parkinson's Disease.* New York: Public Affairs, 2001.

CELEBRATING 50 YEARS OF BRAIN RESEARCH

50th

ANNIVERSARY

SECTION 3

IVE LASKER AWARDS AND SIX NOBELS

Investigators pay attention to prizes. Some occasionally complain about the validity of an award to a particular recipient, and sometimes an award is given for work that later proves to have been erroneous. But for the great majority, there is more concern about scientists who are omitted than about those included. Venerating the awardees is therefore not intended to demean the achievements of others.

Breakthroughs may lead to prizes, but luminous achievements come after "ordinary" scientists have done the spadework. Prize winners usually lead teams of other scientists.

Among the most respected awards for biomedical research are the Albert and Mary Lasker Awards in Medicine, and the pinnacle of awards, the Nobel Prize. Researchers pay attention to the Lasker Awards since they are one of the awards that often prefigure a forthcoming Nobel.

Five investigators from the intramural research program of NINDS or NIMH have won Lasker Awards: Roscoe Brady, Seymour Kety, Louis Sokoloff, Nancy Wexler, and William Windle. Windle, an early developmental neurobiologist and neuroanatomist, received his Lasker in 1968 for his basic discoveries in the field of developmental biology. (His work is described in Chapter 9.)

One intramural NINDS investigator has won a Nobel Prize, D. Carleton Gajdusek. His work, in turn, has been inextricably linked to that of an extramural investigator supported by NINDS and other NIH institutes – Stanley Prusiner – who took both the Lasker and Nobel for discovering the *prion*.

The millennial Nobel Prize was given to three extramural scientists: Arvid Carlsson, Paul Greengard, and Eric Kandel. Each of them was connected to NINDS or NIMH at some point in their careers, and their discoveries were linked, in essence, to those of the intramural Nobelist, Julius Axelrod, who had been recognized three decades earlier. The millennial laureates each exemplify the modern neuroscientist, adroitly adapting new techniques and new approaches through the years. Seymour Kety recruited several of these investigators to the unified research program he headed that included both NIMH and NINDB in the years 1950-1960.

The work of these researchers illuminates the unifying nature of neuroscience. The relationship between Seymour Kety and Louis Sokoloff is a good example. Teacher and student, they were intimate friends for 50 years. Their research, too, was cognate, one leading logically to the other. Yet Kety always made it absolutely clear that Sokoloff's work was a totally independent achievement.[1,2]

Their work also illuminates how investigators can change directions and still make historically important contributions. Kety, in Sokoloff's words, started as a "hard-nosed physiologist" with no particular interest in psychosis, yet he became a hero of modern psychiatry. Sokoloff, in contrast, began his career by practicing psychiatry, with meager training, in the Army during World War II. It was his curiosity about what happened in the brain to cause changes in behavior that led him to studies of cerebral blood flow. In the end, Sokoloff's research became the basis for a modern neuroanatomy of the brain and for imaging methods of wide application, including clinical neurological diagnosis.

When asked for the secret of his success in research administration, Kety[3] said:

> I had confidence that the best way to direct people's interest toward mental illness was by having it directed by themselves. One could hope that this could be accomplished in a consortium of scientists working on their own field but getting together once in a while at lunch, at conferences, and learning a little bit about mental illness and perhaps finding how something they were interested in might fit into the picture.

Seymour Kaufman, a biochemist, provided an example of the value of that approach. When he was first recruited to Kety's team, Kaufman warned that he had no intention of working on mental disease; instead he was interested in the fundamental biochemistry of hydroxylated aromatic amino acids. Kety said that did not matter. A few years later, Kaufman elucidated the molecular basis of a major form of mental retardation, phenylketonuria. He found that the process of converting phenylalanine to tyrosine involved a new co-factor, biopterin.

Ironically, after that, Kety described an incident involving another biochemist, Giulio Cantoni:

> A young man came to Cantoni's laboratory for an appointment as a postdoctoral fellow and Cantoni talked to him for a while and said: "Yes, I think the person you should work with is Seymour Kaufman." And this young man said, "I would rather not because Dr. Kaufman is too clinical."

Gajdusek and Prusiner provide another view of the interface between clinical and basic research. They worked on the same problem but came from totally different backgrounds. Gajdusek was trained as a pediatrician first and then as a virologist. He was led to what he called "spongiform encephalopathies" by his interest in anthropology. Traveling in remote New Guinea, he encountered kuru, a chronic neurological disorder among the indigenous people living there. Ultimately he found that the condition was transmissible, that is, the disease could be induced in monkeys by injecting them with tissue from the brain of a person who had died of it. This was the first time in history that a chronic neurodegenerative disease seemed to be caused by a virus or similar agent. Gajdusek and his colleagues later found another disease with the same characteristics, Creutzfeldt-Jakob disease (CJD).

Prusiner, in contrast, was fully trained in biochemistry before he encountered a person with CJD when he was a resident in neurology. He knew about Gajdusek's work and therefore collaborated with virologists. Ultimately, he worked out the molecular basis of CJD and related diseases. In the process, he discovered a new form of life, a self-replicating protein that he named the *prion*.

The other two prize winners came to neuroscience by other routes. Brady was a lipid chemist, drawn to human diseases with abnormal metabolism of the fatty substances that are major components of nerve fibers in the brain. Nancy Wexler is a psychologist who became a leader in both the ethical and scientific problems generated by Huntington disease, a familial disease with both neurologic and psychiatric manifestations, one that she encountered in her own family.

The work of all these investigators illustrates the unity of clinical neurosciences. The several NIH institutes involved may have different administrations but brain science is brain science.

1 Kety S. Transcript of Oral Interview with Philip S. Holtzman, April 6, 1992, Countway Library of Medicine, Rare Books and Special Collections, Harvard University, Cambridge, MA, pp. 192-193.

2 Kety S. Interview with Eric Kandel, 1999. Living Library. Albert & Mary Lasker Foundation [www.laskerfoundation.com/library/Kety/interview.html].

3 Kety S. Transcript of Oral Interview with Philip S. Holtzman.

CHAPTER THIRTEEN

SEYMOUR S. KETY, M.D.
1915 – 2000

Lasker Award for Special Achievement, 1999

For a lifetime of contributions to neuroscience – including discovery of a method for measuring cerebral blood flow that led to current brain imaging techniques, adoptive studies in schizophrenia that established its genetic origin, and visionary leadership in mental health that ushered psychiatry into the molecular era.

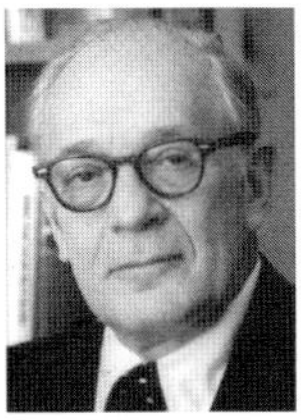

SEYMOUR S. KETY, M.D.

In 1999, Seymour Kety won the Lasker Award for special achievement in medical science. The award was surely well deserved, but it was also a long time coming. Kety was then 84 years old, but the research that gained him his recognition was established even before he came to NIH in 1951 at age 35.

Kety's discoveries of noninvasive methods for measuring cerebral blood flow and local cerebral metabolism were amplified by his student and colleague, Louis Sokoloff, and became the basis for positron emission tomography (PET) and functional magnetic resonance imaging (fMRI), the imaging techniques that have made it possible to relate brain activity to neuropsychological changes.

But Kety's fame does not rest on those accomplishments alone. He was also one of the first investigators to establish the role of heredity in mental disorders – especially schizophrenia. He did that by devising a study of the family histories of the biological and adoptive parents of schizophrenic patients adopted at birth. At the NIH, he directed the intramural programs for both NIMH and NINDB, attracting a group of investigators of unusual talent. He assembled another team later at the McLean Hospital of Harvard Medical School. Because of Kety's own scientific contributions and his ability to select and lead young researchers, he is revered as a founder of biological psychiatry.

Kety was born in Philadelphia in 1915. In childhood[1] he built a chemistry laboratory at home. He cherished his education at Central High School and then attended the University of Pennsylvania for college and medical school.

In college, Kety worked in a commercial toxicology laboratory, measuring urinary lead levels.[1] The method involved precipitation of lead as an insoluble salt, then redissolving it by complexing it with sodium citrate. In medical school, he took a research elective in which he added lead to the diet of rats and found that feeding them citrate increased the urinary excretion of lead. He considered this his first personal "scientific discovery," in contrast to merely repeating the observations of others.

In medical school he made another personal discovery and, immediately on graduation in 1940, married Josephine Gross, who became a pediatrician and a steadfast partner.

Kety interned at the Philadelphia General Hospital. Despite the clinical demands, he managed to spend time in a laboratory studying the kinetics of lead citrate. This led to his first publication, which appeared in the *Journal of Biological Chemistry*. That research also led to an application for a fellowship with Joseph Aub, who was noted for his lead poisoning studies at Massachusetts General Hospital. Because of a childhood leg fracture that left a permanent disability, Kety was ineligible for military service and free to continue doing research.

By the time Kety arrived in Boston, however, Aub had given up the lead project. Instead, as part of wartime research, he was studying shock. In these experiments, Kety and Alfred Pope (later a distinguished neurochemist) were junior members of the team and therefore the ones who stayed up all night to make measurements from animals in shock. Kety and Pope remained close friends their entire lives, sharing a mutual interest in the brain spurred by the experiments in ischemic shock, which showed that adaptive reflexes maintained circulation to the heart and brain while blood flow to other organs shut down.

At the same time, Carl Schmidt, at the University of Pennsylvania, published a paper on measurements of cerebral circulation, so Kety returned to Pennsylvania. Schmidt's experiments on blood flow in the monkey led to some interesting observations about convulsions and anesthesia, but the method was invasive and Kety was increasingly interested in the human brain, which would require noninvasive techniques.

Kety began to think about applications of the Fick principle, which states that blood flow can be measured by assessing the concentrations of a substance within the blood as it enters and leaves the organ being studied. The Fick principle had been used successfully to study the heart and liver, but Kety decided to apply the principle to the brain using a novel method based on an inert gas, nitrous oxide. This involved some fancy mathematics, which proved no obstacle to Kety. One of his later co-workers, Reuben Copperman, a physicist, once said:[2] "Seymour Kety knows just a little bit of mathematics, but what he can do with that little bit is phenomenal!"

Kety carried out preliminary monkey experiments with Schmidt, comparing the two methods to validate the method, and then applied it to humans. He established normal values for the human brain and then evaluated abnormal states, finding decreased brain oxygen consumption in coma, increased consumption in epileptic seizures, and no change in sleep.

These were productive years for Kety. He published 40 papers on cerebral blood flow between 1945 and 1951, culminating in the classic paper on the theory underlying the use of nitrous oxide for measuring cerebral blood flow in humans (including the mathematics).[3] Kety's fame was established by the time he arrived at NIH in 1951.

To his disappointment, however, Kety had found no abnormality of blood flow or oxygen consumption in the brains of patients with schizophrenia. But because he was convinced that there had to be a chemical abnormality in schizophrenia, he concluded that his method must be too coarse to find the changes that might affect particular parts of the brain. Kety realized he needed a method to measure metabolism locally, specifically in small brain structures.

That opportunity came in 1953, when William Landau had an appointment in Wade Marshall's NIMH Laboratory of Cerebral Physiology. Landau had just finished a neurology residency and was already a skilled neurophysiologist. He later became Chair of Neurology at Washington University, St. Louis. At NIH, he visited Kety one day and asked if he could work on local cerebral blood flow.

Soon enough, Kety put together a team comprising Landau, Louis Sokoloff, Walter Freygang, and Lewis Rowland. Kety conceived and developed the method for measuring local blood flow and metabolism by using a radioactively labeled inert gas and analyzing concentrations of the gas with a method called "autoradiography."

Kety was involved in every aspect of every experiment, even synthesizing the gas himself. Sokoloff, recently arrived from Penn, was the first lieutenant and consultant. Landau applied the practical experience he had gained in monitoring circulation, blood pressure, and EEG in experiments with cats. When they needed brain slices for radioautography and wondered how they would do that, Kety later credited Freygang with the idea of using a band saw. Rowland, the totally urban and most junior member, who had never seen a band saw, was sent to Sears to purchase one. It was his job to make the slices and put increasing concentrations of the radioactive gas marker into gelatin cores, which were then incorporated into the slices for later measurement.

Together, this team found that visual stimuli increased the blood flow in the anatomic structures involved in vision and that noises increased blood flow in parts of the brain involved in hearing. Their studies were recorded only in an abstract[4] but were another triumph for Kety and proved to be the basis for later brain imaging. However, the method had one severe limitation: it required decapitation of the subject and hence was not suitable for human use. Sokoloff resolved that obstacle later in a related but independent set of experiments.

Kety's service at NIMH fostered his growing interest in the biologic basis of psychosis. He obtained radioactive adrenaline for studies of schizophrenia and gave some of the labeled compound to his colleague Julius Axelrod for studies that eventually led to the Nobel Prize.

In 1961, Kety was invited to give a special lecture at NIH. The title was "The Brain and Behavior," and it not only solidified his own biological views, but it was globally influential. That same year he became Chair of the Department of Psychiatry at Johns Hopkins University Medical School. This move proved to be an error, largely because he was neither equipped for, nor interested in, the administration of a large clinical department. Kety never moved to Baltimore. Instead, he commuted daily, using the long automobile rides to ruminate. One of the ideas he developed while in transit between his home in Bethesda and his job in Baltimore was a project to evaluate the contribution of genetic factors to schizophrenia.

This was the beginning of Kety's second revolutionary contribution to neuroscience. In 1959 he had reviewed the published papers on the biology of schizophrenia. He could exclude all of the presumed evidence of a biological basis for schizophrenia except for genetics since there was a higher concordance in monozygotic (identical) twins than in dizygotic (fraternal) twins. (That is, the more similar the genetic makeup of twins, the more likely that both would be affected by schizophrenia.) That, however, did not exclude environmental influences, which could differ in the two categories of twins. Kety realized that adoption studies might resolve the problem, since "an adoptee shares his genetic endowment with his biological family but his environment with another family."[5]

Returning to NIH in 1962, Kety joined with David Rosenthal, then chief of the psychology laboratory at NIMH, and Fini Schulsinger, head of psychiatry at the Kommunhospitalet in Copenhagen, who had access to complete records of adoptions. Kety and his team studied hospital records and carried out comprehensive psychiatric interviews with relatives. They discovered that the prevalence of schizophrenia was ten times more common in biological relatives than among relatives of the adoptees.[6] The rigorous design of the project provided powerful evidence of a genetic component in schizophrenia at a time when most psychiatrists believed that the condition was "a way of thinking that one learned from one's parents, which could be treated by education and by psychological and social manipulation."[7]

In 1967, Kety moved to Harvard for yet another chapter in his career. He continued to study adoptees and built yet another group of outstanding psychiatric investigators.

Kety retired from Harvard in 1981 and returned to NIMH as an emeritus scientist. He died in 2000 at the age of 84. Adoring obituaries documented his personal qualities.[8-12]

Sokoloff expressed the feelings of all the memorials for Kety:

> He graced every field in which he worked and those with whom he worked, and I know of no scientist who was so universally respected, admired, and even loved.[13]

1 Kety SS. In Squire LR, ed. *The History of Neuroscience in Autobiography*, vol. 1. Washington, DC: Society for Neuroscience, 1996:382-413.
2 Sokoloff L. Interview with author, March 17, 2000.
3 Kety SS. The theory and applications of the exchange of inert gas at the lungs and tissues. *Pharmacol Rev* 1951;3:1-41.
4 Landau WM, Freygang WH,Jr, Rowland LP, Sokoloff L, Kety SS. The local circulation of the living brain: values in the unanesthetized and anesthetized cat. *Trans Am Neurol Assoc* 1955;80:125-129.
5 *Autobiography: Seymour S. Kety,* Living Library. Albert and Mary Lasker Foundation [www.laskerfoundation.com/library/Kety/autobiography-Kety-html].
6 Kety SS, Rosenthal D, Wender PH, Schulsinger F. Mental illness in the biological and adoptive families of adopted schizophrenics. *Am J Psychiat* 1971;128:302-306.
7 Kety SS. Transcripts of Oral Interview with Philip S. Holtzman, April 6, 1992, Countway Library of Medicine, Rare Books and Special Collections, Harvard University, Cambridge, MA, p. 402.
8 Snyder SH. Seymour Kety: the NIH years. *Clin Neurosci Res* 2001;1:6-7.
9 Butler RN. Seymour Kety: in memory of the father of neuroscience and biological psychiatry. *Geriatrics* 2000;55:3-4.
10 Eisenberg L. Seymour S. Kety (1915-2000). *Nature* 2000;406:472.
11 Holzman PS. Seymour S. Kety, 1915-2000. *Nat Med* 2000;6:727; and *Am J Psychiatry* 2000; 157:1057.
12 DeLisi LE. Seymour S. Kety, MD: the man and his accomplishments. Summary of a symposium in his honor at the VIIIth World Congress of Psychiatric Genetics, Versailles, France, August 30, 2000. *Psychiatr Genet* 2000:10:153-158.
13 Sokoloff L. In Memoriam: Seymour S. Kety, M.D., 1915-2000. *Am J Med Genet* 2000;96:585-9; *J Cereb Blood Flow Metab* 2000;20:1271-1275; and *Clin Neurosci Res* 2001;1:2-5.

CHAPTER FOURTEEN

LOUIS SOKOLOFF, M.D.

Lasker Award for Clinical Research, 1981

For developing a pioneering method of mapping and measuring brain function, both as a whole and in localized areas – a monumental breakthrough in the understanding and diagnosis of brain diseases.

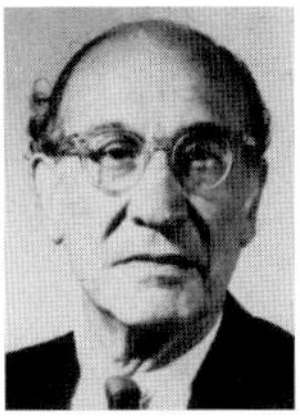

LOUIS SOKOLOFF, M.D.

Louis Sokoloff has spent almost all of his professional life at NIMH, not NINDS, but his groundbreaking work could have been done in either institute. When Seymour Kety headed the scientific programs of both institutes, he recruited a remarkable group of scientists, Sokoloff among them. Why some of them were assigned to NIMH and others to NINDB is not clear, but during the decade when NINDS and NIMH shared laboratory space (until the split in 1960) institutional labels meant little. The labs were close enough to invite collaborations and they were scattered throughout the floor in a way that had nothing to do with institutional affiliation. Both institutes benefited from the collaborative atmosphere, and so did the science.

Like Kety, Sokoloff grew up in Philadelphia.[1] In childhood, his brother set up an aquarium, which fascinated him and set him to read about biology. Like so many other aspiring scientists, he lists Paul de Kruif's *Microbe Hunters* as a major influence.[2]

Sokoloff's family was poor and he could not attend the elite public Central High School because he could not afford the bus fare. Instead, Sokoloff attended South Philadelphia High School, where he nonetheless had an excellent education and qualified for a scholarship to the University of Pennsylvania. As an undergraduate, his interests in research were kindled by Lewis Heilbrunn, the cell biologist who emphasized the role of calcium in cell biology.

Sokoloff went to medical school at Penn and became interested in biochemistry under the influence of outstanding scientists – Henry Bazett, David Drabkin, and the great German immigrant Otto Meyerhof. There he also met Seymour Kety, Julius Comroe, and Carl Schmidt. Sokoloff graduated in 1946 and had a general internship at the Philadelphia General Hospital. His first 6-week rotation was in psychiatry. In the second year, he was assigned again to psychiatry for 6 months.

In 1947, Sokoloff entered the Army and, on the basis of his meager training, found himself ordained as a neuropsychiatrist. At that time, therapy for psychiatric disorders was dominated by insulin shock and electroshock. But for many patients, he used what he described as "a diluted kind of psychoanalytic approach, with psychoanalytic reasoning and analysis of etiology, and so on. In the course of those two years, I had a patient who actually got well!

I was so shaken by this, I really got interested. I thought at the time that psychoanalysts did not care about the brain or where it was. But I was sure mental disease had something to do with the brain. What in the world happens to the brain when all I did was listen as she talked and that made her better?"[3]

On his discharge from the Army in 1949, Sokoloff returned to Philadelphia to work with Kety at the Graduate School of Medicine. His discussions with Kety were not limited to research. Kety was critical of psychoanalytic psychiatry and Sokoloff, on the basis of his Army experience, felt compelled to defend it. "Both Kety and I must have been persuasive," Sokoloff wrote later, "because I eventually gravitated deeper into basic science and Kety drifted toward psychiatry with his studies on the genetics of schizophrenia."[4]

Sokoloff's first project in Kety's lab was a study of the effects of hyperthyroidism on cerebral blood flow and oxygen consumption. Since an increase in the body's metabolic rate characterizes the overactive thyroid state, Sokoloff and his group expected to find increased oxygen utilization in the brain. To their surprise, however, there was no increase in cerebral oxygen consumption.

That negative result was a challenge to Sokoloff because hyperthyroidism is defined clinically by hypermetabolism. The results of their study were not published until 1953. By that time, Sokoloff had moved to NIMH with Kety, but the thyroid conundrum stayed with him. If the brain did not participate in the hypermetabolism, perhaps the increased oxygen consumption of other organs had to do with increased protein synthesis.

At NIH, however, Sokoloff continued to work primarily on cerebral metabolism. He thought the thyroid problem required biochemical skills beyond his reach. However, one of the advantages of the NIH setup was the luxurious supply of experts with diverse skills. In an adjacent laboratory Seymour Kaufman was working on problems related to phenylketonuria, a metabolic disorder that causes mental retardation. One day, Sokoloff gave a seminar on the thyroid problem and explained why he thought it might have to do with protein synthesis. After the lecture Kaufman said that he, too, had come to a similar conclusion and that they should work on the problem together. Both were preoccupied with other projects and it was not until 1955 that they attacked the problem.

As Sokoloff later wrote: "He then offered to collaborate with me, provide the biochemical expertise, and supervise and train me in biochemistry. I accepted and this began my career in biochemistry."

Together they developed an assay system for protein synthesis, found that this synthesis was indeed stimulated by thyroid hormone in thyroid-sensitive tissues but not brain, suggesting that the rise in oxygen consumption was related to the stimulation of protein synthesis, which was much more active in heart, liver, and kidney – but not the brain.

Sokoloff faced another challenge from observations made during the cerebral blood flow and metabolism studies. It was known that cerebral metabolism decreased in conditions that lowered consciousness, but they had found no changes in particular states of brain activity – performance of mental tasks (arithmetic problems), tranquilization, or slow wave sleep. A likely explanation was the gross nature of the measurement, because changes in specific parts of the brain could occur without being detected by a method that evaluates the entire brain.

A method for measuring local cerebral metabolism was needed. The 1953 studies of local cerebral blood flow in the cat (as described in the biography of Seymour Kety) provided a turning point.

Those experiments showed that local cerebral blood flow could be measured, that it was a function of local neural activity (increasing blood flow with stimulation of specific brain pathways), and that autoradiography was a useful quantitative method. Sokoloff saw the promise of extending those studies.

Sokoloff pursued the problem of local cerebral metabolism by experimenting with carbon-labeled glucose, but the rapid catalysis to lactate and carbon dioxide removed the label too fast for measurements to be made. In a 1957 conversation with Donald Tower, he learned about deoxyglucose, a compound that is phosphorylated just as glucose is, but its product is not further metabolized down the glycolytic pathway. Instead, it accumulates in the brain.

Sokoloff thought the product might be trapped and used to measure local metabolism. He began to use deoxyglucose in trial experiments, but the time was not yet ripe for further development.

One of Sokoloff's students was Martin Reivich, a neurologist who joined the laboratory in 1964 to work on different tracers for the radioautographic measurements of local cerebral blood flow. Reivich, together with Kety and Sokoloff, adapted the radioautographic local blood flow method for use with the ^{14}C-labeled tracer ^{14}C-antipyrine before he left in 1966 to return to his home base at Penn. This made ^{14}C radioautography possible He soon asked Sokoloff if they could work together to develop the method involving ^{14}C-deoxyglucose.

Their early efforts showed that more information was needed before they could create the key operational equation. In 1968, Sokoloff went on sabbatical leave to Paris to work on the thyroid problem in the laboratory of Jean Roche. There, he immersed himself in learning more about enzyme kinetics. With his new knowledge, he revised the mathematical equations used in the deoxyglucose measurements and solved the problem. The time was finally ripe for measurements of local cerebral metabolism and the use of deoxyglucose as a tracer of nerve tracts.

When Sokoloff returned to NIH in late 1969, he once again set out to develop the deoxyglucose method with Charles Kennedy and others in his laboratory. The first animal experiment was done in 1971; animal experiments were reported in 1974, and published in 1975. The results showed clearly the functional activation or depression in specific pathways. For instance, with visual stimulation, they delineated the ocular dominance columns of active cells in the visual portion of the occipital cortex, even demonstrating the representation of the blind spots of the eye in the cortex of the brain. That is truly local cerebral metabolism.

Sokoloff recognized the value of collaborative research: "One person cannot be expert in all the disciplines that go into neuroscience," he said. "And the way to attack a multidisciplinary problem is to have a multidisciplinary team, with an expert in each discipline working together with a common goal."[4]

Sokoloff was an exemplary leader of cooperating investigators. The deoxyglucose method provided "massive amounts of data derived from laborious and tedious manual densitometric analyses of the autoradiograms. Quantification was therefore limited to a relatively few selected structures and valuable information in the autoradiograms was being lost." To solve this problem, Sokoloff worked with Charles Goochee and Wayne Rasband, a computer scientist, to develop a computerized method for reconstructing the quantitative autographic results in a color photo. In 1978, Charlene Jarvis presented a report at the Society for Neuroscience, describing the first use of color-coded metabolic maps, another innovation. The beautiful figures were featured on the cover of *Chemical & Engineering News.*

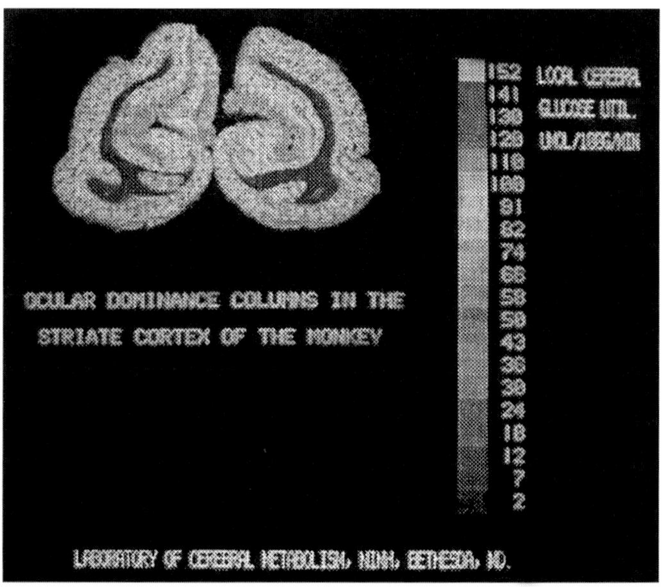

DEOXYGLUCOSE AUTORADIOGRAPH OF THE STRIATE CORTEX FROM A RHESUS MONKEY

Following up on Sokoloff's breakthrough, in the late 70s, Reivich and Sokoloff initiated deoxyglucose studies in humans, using detection methods being developed by David Kuhl at Penn. Alfred Wolf, at the Brookhaven National Laboratory, cooperated with them by synthesizing[18] fluorine-labeled deoxyglucose, which eliminated the need for radioautography and provided the necessary radioactive tag for external detection. Fluorodeoxyglucose is still a favored isotopic substrate for imaging studies in humans.

These early attempts grew into positron emission tomography, functional magnetic resonance imaging, and a new neuroanatomy based on functional pathways illuminated by deoxyglucose. Through the years, Sokoloff has maintained an active laboratory, continuing the monumental level of his fundamental contributions to cellular chemistry in the brain.

1 Sokoloff L. In Squire LR, ed. *The History of Neuroscience in Autobiography*, vol. 1. Washington, DC, Society for Neuroscience, 1996:456-497.

2 Sokoloff L. In vitro veritas: probing brain function through the use of quantitative in vivo biochemical techniques. *Annu Rev Physiol* 2000;62:1-14.

3 Sokoloff L. Interview with author, June 27, 2000.

4 Sokoloff L. In Squire LR, ed. *The History of Neuroscience in Autobiography*, Washington, DC, Society for Neuroscience, 1996:478.

CHAPTER FIFTEEN

NANCY S. WEXLER, PH.D.

Albert Lasker Public Service Award, 1993

Awarded to Nancy S. Wexler, Ph.D., for her groundbreaking work in the scientific and public arenas towards finding a cure for Huntington's disease and for increasing awareness of all genetic diseases.

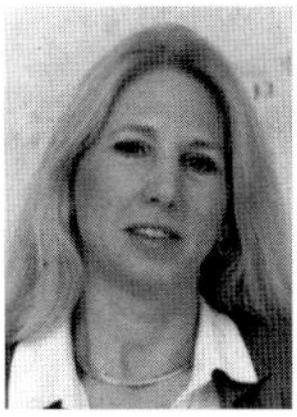

NANCY S. WEXLER, PH.D.

Nancy Sabin Wexler was given the Albert Lasker Public Service Award in 1993. Her four major achievements were unique and all related to Huntington disease (HD). She was executive director for the influential Congressional Commission on the Control of Huntington's Disease and Its Consequences. She organized expeditions to a remote region in Venezuela to study a large HD-affected population, and then led a multi-institutional group of investigators in the search for the gene. Wexler has now become an authority and public voice in ethical and practical discussions of presymptomatic diagnosis of diseases that are not yet remediable.

The diagnosis of HD is based on three clinical characteristics: personality change with behavioral disorders; dementia; and involuntary movements called chorea (from the Greek word meaning "dance"). Clinical diagnosis is accurate and can be buttressed by finding evidence of atrophy of the caudate nucleus in brain CT or MRI. The progressive deterioration takes a decade or more before it is fatal.

The disease was first described by George Huntington in 1872 and, from that time, has been known to be an autosomal dominant disease (or *homozygous*, meaning that only one gene from one parent is required). In this pattern of inheritance, every affected person has one affected parent, and any child born to a parent carrying the gene has a 50:50 chance of inheriting the gene and developing HD. HD has assumed a place in the history of medical research because, in 1983, work by James Gusella at Harvard on HD established the validity of *positional cloning*, the DNA method of mapping the gene for a disease without knowing the gene product.

Dr. Wexler did not know that the disease affected her family until she was 21 years old and her mother was diagnosed with HD. At the same time, she also learned about her own 50:50 risk of having the disease in the future. Nancy's only sibling, Alice Wexler, has provided a moving history of the impact of the diagnosis on the family.[1] By the time she learned her mother's diagnosis, Nancy was a graduate student in psychology at the University of Michigan. After she was awarded her doctorate in 1974, she took a teaching position at the New School for Social Research (now New School University) in New York City and was in private practice. She joined with Marjorie Guthrie in the Committee to Combat Huntington's

Disease. Her father, Milton Wexler, a psychoanalyst in Los Angeles, had already started the California chapter of the Committee, which later became the Hereditary Disease Foundation.

In 1968, Milton Wexler initiated a series of workshops for scientists for discussions of new research ideas. In a pattern that was later to prove eminently fruitful, he invited the few clinicians and pathologists who were experts in the disease. In an unconventional mode, he also invited scientists who previously had had no direct connection with HD. Among them were Julius Axelrod (before he won the Nobel Prize), immunologist William Dreyer, and molecular biologist Seymour Benzer. Later, they were joined by neuroscientist Edward Kravitz and worm geneticist Robert Horvitz. This group recommended an emphasis on young scientists to encourage their training and attendance at future meetings. They recruited Ronald Konopka, a Benzer postdoctoral fellow, to organize future meetings.

One of the workshops was held in 1972, in connection with a larger international conference to honor the centennial of the birth of Dr. Huntington. After that, the movement accelerated and NIH responded to the increasing interest. In 1976, Donald B. Tower, director of what was then NINCDS, and Thomas N. Chase, director of intramural research at NINCDS, appointed Nancy Wexler as executive director of the Congressional Commission for the Control of Huntington's Disease and Its Consequences, which was based within the institute.

Marjorie Guthrie chaired the commission. She was the widow of the fabled folk singer Woody Guthrie, who had died of HD, and mother of the renowned singer Arlo Guthrie. Wexler's father was co-chair, and Charles Mackay of NIH was deputy director. Among the members were Stanley Aronson, Dean of Medicine at Brown University; actress Jennifer Jones Simon; Alice Pratt of the Wills Foundation; and Guy McKhann, then Chair of Neurology at Johns Hopkins University.

The Commission held hearings[2] and submitted its report[3] in 1977. Among the recommendations were several that were Wexler's personal wishes: to explore the Lake Maracaibo cluster of HD in Venezuela, map the gene (no disease of unknown gene product had yet been mapped), train young investigators, create a voluntary patient registry and a brain bank, and develop programs for genetic counseling. All of these suggestions were subsequently adopted.

One recommendation, however, went unheeded – a call for national health insurance, including chronic care. The commission noted that, in the United States, a diagnosis of HD or even being at genetic risk for the disease, precludes access to private health insurance. In contrast, the national health program in neighboring Canada covers all citizens regardless of diagnosis.

The commission also recommended the creation of HD Centers Without Walls for patient care and research. This was adopted – with historic results.

The acknowledgement in the report included this appreciation: "To Executive Director, Dr. Nancy Wexler, our very special and warmest thanks. Her deep personal commitment and her intelligence, graced with wit, are a force which can make all things possible."

Nineteen seventy-eight was a turbulent year for the Wexler family. Nancy's mother died, her work with the commission had been completed, and she was appointed health science administrator in the extramural program of NINCDS under the supervision of Jack Brinley. Her assignments included the management of grants for dementia research.

At the centennial meeting in Columbus, Ohio, in 1972, a Venezuelan psychiatrist, Ramón Ávila-Girón, had shown a film about the high prevalence of HD on the shores of Lake Maracaibo in a remote region of Venezuela. The cluster of cases had been discussed in detail at commission hearings. Wexler decided it was time to arrange a trip to Maracaibo in search of homozygous people, those who have inherited two genes, one from each parent. Wexler's reasoning was that if one dose of the mutated gene sufficed to cause HD, then a double dose could be expected to cause a more severe manifestation of the disease. In a genetic isolate like Maracaibo, there had to be more than the usual frequency of marriage among relatives and it would be likely that two people carrying the mutation might marry.

Later investigations traced the disease back 200 years, to a woman who may have inherited it from European traders. If so, all of the affected people in the same generation are either siblings or cousins, all descended from one person, the so-called founder effect.

Wexler made her first trip to Lake Maracaibo in 1979, accompanied by Thomas Chase. He was still in charge of intramural research at NINCDS and had a special interest in movement disorders, including HD. They went to learn whether the disease was truly HD and whether the people there could cooperate for studies. Their exploratory survey gave promise and Wexler returned the following year with Jack Brinley, who made the necessary formal contractual arrangements between NINCDS and the University of Zulia. Wexler has returned to Venezuela for 2 months each year since then.

At first, the trips were financed by discretionary funds from the extramural program. By 1982, however, they were reviewed by an external committee of experts and given high scores. The grant is now entering its third 5-year cycle at NINDS.

Wexler's first goal was achieved readily. She and her associates found homozygous people and learned that the disease was no more severe in them than in others who had inherited the gene from only one parent. One mutated gene was enough to cause the disease, a true autosomal dominant condition.[4] This was the first time such a condition had been documented genetically: one dose of the mutated gene could cause the disease; having two was no worse. In other words there was no "dose effect." Any theory about the disease would have to accommodate this fact.

Then it was recognized that this extended family, now including more than 16,000 people, could serve as the model of a large family needed for gene mapping. Almost 3,000 children carried the gene. In 1978, Milton Wexler had induced Allan Tobin of Cal Tech to take over the scheduling of workshops and he, in turn, contacted David Housman of MIT. Nancy played an increasing role. Housman was a champion of the then-new theory that the gene for a disease could be mapped if there were a sufficient number of DNA markers.

According to Nancy Wexler,[5] Housman provided another kind of leadership – unselfishness. For instance, when they were assigning pieces of a chromosome for mapping, some portions were more promising than others. Housman would let others pick first, keeping the most unpromising piece for himself because "it is one project and we are all doing it together." All three Wexlers – Nancy, Alice, and Milton – worked with Allan Tobin to keep the group together, buoyed by their interactions and, soon, real progress.

The year 1980 provided another landmark. Two HD Centers Without Walls were established – one at Harvard, the other at Hopkins. The center at Harvard began when Joseph Martin, then chair of neurology, called Housman to ask if molecular biology might play a role in HD research. Housman replied with his customary zeal for mapping. More than that, he provided one of his postdoctoral students to work on the project. That was how James Gusella came to work on HD.

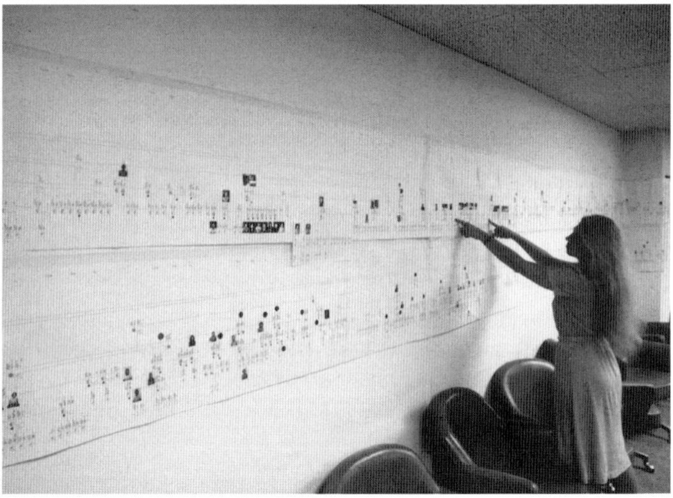

NANCY WEXLER WITH THE EXTENSIVE "FAMILY TREE" OF HUNTINGTON DISEASE IN THE COMMUNITY OF LAKE MARACAIBO, VENEZUELA

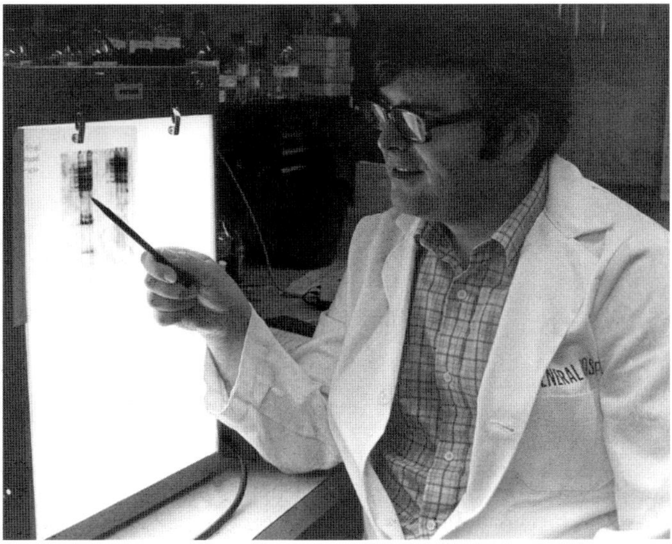

Jim Gusella, M.D., points to an X-ray showing a sequence of DNA from a patient with Huntington disease

Using DNA from Maracaibo families and from a family in Indiana studied by Michael Conneally, Gusella mapped the gene to the end of the short arm of chromosome 4. This was a historic first – vindicating those who believed in positional cloning. The success of the program was important itself, because it took much less time than skeptics predicted. The paper announcing the results came within 3 years of starting the project.[6] It took another decade to clone the gene[7] and to identify the mutation as an expansion of a *trinucleotide repeat*, a category of mutations that was beginning to be found in several different neurodegenerative diseases.

Their paper had 58 authors, including several truly illustrious investigators. The research groups were led by Gusella, Hans Lehrach, David Housman, Francis Collins, and Peter Harper. Each group made essential contributions over the decade-long search but the gene itself emerged in the laboratory directed by Gusella. Later developments from several groups included a transgenic mouse model of HD, a *Drosophila* fruitfly model, recognition of cytoplasmic inclusions that contain protein aggregates, and the beginning of therapy for these cellular or animal models.

In the meantime, the Maracaibo pedigrees keep increasing in size. Although there is still no effective treatment, controlled trials of possibly efficacious drugs are being planned for the people in Venezuela.

Throughout all of this, Wexler has become an expert in another daunting area, the ethics of presymptomatic diagnosis for incurable diseases.[8-10] With an accurate DNA test available, some people at risk opt to be tested. What they hope for is reassurance they will not get the disease themselves or transmit the gene to their children. But about half of those tested prove to carry the gene, which is tantamount to saying they will have the disease some day. It is easy to understand why many do not want to be tested until there is an effective treatment.

As a result of her personal and organizational experience, Wexler became a spokesperson for the field – on television, in print media, and in government. When the National Human Genome Research Institute was founded at NIH, one of the first actions of the first director, James Watson, was to establish the ELSI program – the Ethical, Legal and Social Implications of the genome project. Wexler chaired the working group of the Joint NIH/Department of Energy Working Group from 1989 to 1995. She has performed similar service for the Institute of Medicine and the Society for Neuroscience. With the continuing Maracaibo project, too, Wexler is much in demand.

1 Wexler A. *Mapping Fate. A Memoir of Family, Risk, and Genetic Research.* New York: Times Books, Random House, 1995.

2 U.S. Congress. Senate. Committee on Appropriations. *Hearing before a Subcommittee of the Committee on Appropriations*, 95th Cong., 1st sess., Special Oversight Hearing. U.S. Government Printing Office, Washington, DC, 1977.

3 *Report: Commission for the Control of Huntington's Disease and Its Consequences.* vol. 1, Overview. U.S. Department of Health, Education, and Welfare, Public Health Service, National Institutes of Health, October 1977.

4 Wexler NS, Young AB, Tanzi R, Travers H, Starosta-Rubenstein S, Penney JB, Snodgrass SR, Shoulson I, Gomez F, Ramos-Arroyo MA, Penchaszadeh GK, Moreno H, Gibbons K, Faryniarz A, Hobbs W, Anderson MA, Bonilla E, Conneally PM, Gusella JF. Homozygotes for Huntington's disease. *Nature* 1987;326:194-197.

5 Wexler N. Recorded interview, May 5, 2000.

6 Gusella JF, Wexler NS, Conneally PM, Naylor SL, Anderson MA, Tanzi RE, Watkins PC, Ottina K, Wallace MR, Sakaguchi AY, Young AB, Shoulson I, Bonilla E, Martin JB. A polymorphic DNA marker genetically linked to Huntington's disease. *Nature* 1983;306:234-238.

7 The Huntington's Disease Collaborative Research Group. A novel gene containing a trinucleotide repeat that is expanded and unstable on Huntington's disease chromosomes. *Cell* 1993;72:971-983.

8 Wexler NS. Genetic jeopardy and the new clairvoyance. In Bearn A, Childs B, Motulsky A, eds. *Progress in Medical Genetics*, New York: Praeger Books, 1985.

9 Wexler NS. The Tiresias complex: Huntington's disease as a paradigm for late-onset disorders. *FASEB Journal* 1992;6:2820-2825.

10 Wexler NS. Genetics session: the human genome. Prognostications and predispositions. *Ann NY Acad Sci*, June 30, 1999;882:22-31.

CHAPTER SIXTEEN

ROSCOE O. BRADY, M.D.

Lasker Award for Clinical Research, 1982

> *For his original and creative contributions to our understanding of a group of hereditary disorders called lipid storage diseases, and for the development of genetic counseling procedures and the initiation of possible treatment methods for these diseases.*

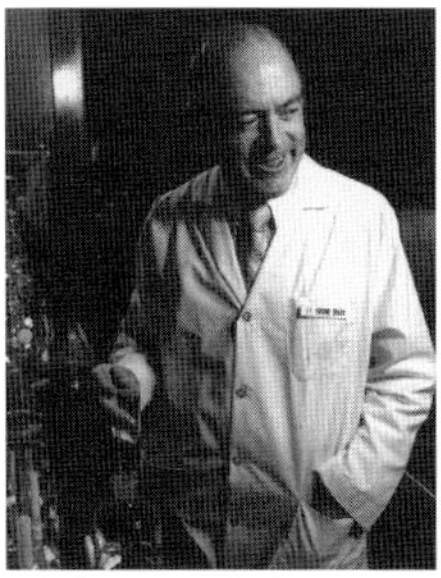

ROSCOE O. BRADY, M.D.

Before molecular genetics, there was biochemical genetics. Roscoe Brady is one of the few M.D.-investigators who have made major contributions in both eras.

Brady was in the first cohort recruited to NIH by Seymour Kety in 1954. Like Louis Sokoloff, Brady first knew Kety at the University of Pennsylvania. The complete integration of the NIMH and NINDB programs was evident when Kety appointed Sokoloff to NIMH and Brady to NINDB; their laboratories were close together.

A pioneer in disease-oriented research, Brady won the 1982 Albert Lasker Clinical Medical Research Award. The above citation continued:

> Because of a metabolic defect, the body tissues of persons afflicted with these disorders begin to accumulate and store an excessive amount of fatty materials called lipids. The accumulating lipids may cause enlargement of the spleen and liver, damage to the bones and kidneys, failure of major organs, severe mental retardation, and often early death.
>
> In a series of elegant experiments, Dr. Brady discovered the precise metabolic defect – a particular missing enzyme – that causes the lipids to build up and destroy body tissues. In demonstrating this to be the case for such disorders as found in Gaucher disease, Niemann-Pick disease, Fabry disease, and Tay-Sachs disease, Dr. Brady solved an enigma that had confounded medical practitioners for nearly a century.
>
> Dr. Brady's discoveries now provide the basis for the early diagnosis of the diseases, for the identification of those who might pass on the disorders to their children, and for the detection of the diseases prenatally.
>
> The present and continuing thrust of Dr. Brady's investigations deal with the treatment of the disorders. In his efforts to find a promising treatment, Dr. Brady is attempting to learn how to replace the missing enzyme, thus reducing the buildup of destructive lipids and preventing the damage they cause.

Roscoe Brady was born in 1923 and raised in Ambler, a suburb of Philadelphia. His father was a pharmacist and his mother worked in the pharmacy. Brady[1] has said his father was an "imaginative" pharmacist who concocted therapeutic mixtures that were popular with his clientele. As a child Brady was impressed with the ambience of the store and the rows of chemicals. His interest in science was evident while he was still in elementary school; for a novel creation, he won a prize magic collection from the A.C. Gilbert Company, renowned maker of the Erector Set.

Brady did his undergraduate work at Pennsylvania State College and received his M.D. degree from Harvard in 1947. In medical school his research interests were whetted by an opportunity to work with W.W. Westerfeldt, evaluating a new "miracle" touted as "vitamin N," which could cure alcoholism. Rats were induced to drink alcohol instead of water by depriving them of vitamin B. Vitamin N, a yeast extract, temporarily eliminated their preference for alcohol. But controlled experiments with other vitamins had the same effect. After 3 weeks all the animals began to drink alcohol again – no matter what the prior treatment. Vitamin N soon disappeared from the scene. For this muckraking achievement, Brady won the Borden Award for research by a medical student and he published his first peer-reviewed paper.[2]

In his senior year at medical school, he worked with Rulon Rawson, a thyroid investigator who combined clinical and laboratory work. That combination of skills in clinical investigation fired Brady's imagination.

After graduating from Harvard in 1947, he interned in medicine at the Hospital of the University of Pennsylvania and started to work in the Department of Biochemistry with Samuel Gurin, a biochemist who later became dean of the medical school. Brady had a fruitful experience with Gurin. From 1948 to 1952, Brady was supported by fellowships from the National Research Council and the U.S. Public Health Service, while he was introduced to the use of radioactive isotopes in studying the biosynthesis of testosterone, fatty acids, and cholesterol. One of his early successes was recognition of the role of gonadotrophin on testosterone synthesis, one of the first indications that hormones could be important in the creation of steroids, which are constituents of many key compounds in the body.

Brady and Gurin also started to work on the biosynthesis of long-chain fatty acids; using pigeon liver, they developed the first enzyme system for this pathway. As the number of successful projects increased, so did Brady's commitment to a research career.

Those were heady years for chemists and biochemists because isotopes had just become available after World War II. Using radioactive labels, investigators elucidated the biosynthesis of large molecules, including nucleic acids, cholesterol, and hemoglobin. These were crowning achievements of the new era. With this new understanding, metabolic pathways were unraveled and, with understanding of the synthesis of nucleic acids, DNA was identified as the stuff of genes. Compared to pre-World War II biochemistry, this was a true revolution.

For 2 years, Brady did military service when he was in charge of the clinical chemistry laboratory at the U.S. Naval Hospital in Bethesda. Busy with routine work, he had little time for research. Then, in 1954, Brady became Chief of the Section on Lipid Chemistry in the Laboratory of Neurochemistry at NINDB. By then, his lifework had been defined.

Kety[3] wanted a biochemistry program which would focus on elucidating the lipid coverings of nerves. A lipid-protein complex called *myelin* is the major component of the nerve sheaths and was already known to be the target of demyelinating diseases, which included multiple sclerosis and some peripheral nerve diseases. The lipids are important in all cell membranes and in normal brain functions. Kety knew they would be important in diseases, too. Brady had already demonstrated his interest in lipids and his talent was evident.

Brady responded to the challenge with a series of papers on the essential chemistry of lipids. He did not publish his first paper on a disease until 1960.[4] After the years of chemical and biochemical preparation, Brady directed his attention increasingly to a group of rare metabolic diseases in which normal constituents of the nerves accumulate in abnormally increased amounts that are incompatible with normal function. The chemistry of these compounds was being worked out to define what are called lipid storage diseases.

Gaucher disease was the first lipid storage disease that captured Brady's attention. In one type of Gaucher disease, the brain and nerves are spared, but the accumulated material swells the liver and spleen. Distortion of the bones causes pain and disability. Blood

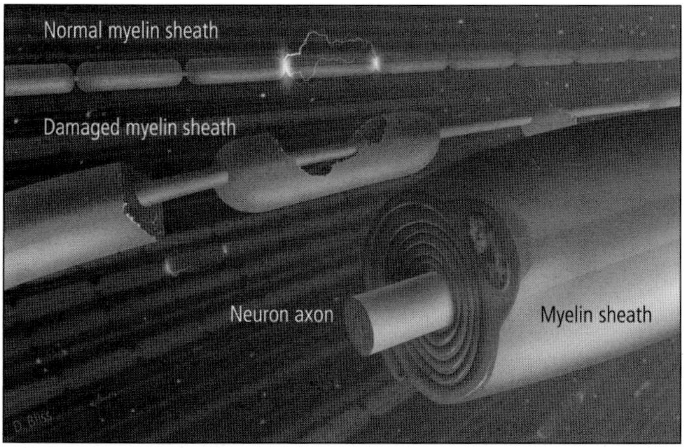

MYELIN SHEATH AND NERVE FIBER

clotting is impaired, making the person susceptible to repeated bruising. In types 2 and 3, the brain and nerves are affected in addition to liver and spleen. Type 2 is the most severe; affected children die before age 2. Type 3 begins later and is more slowly progressive, but is still debilitating and life shortening.

The chemical nature of the accumulating substance had been worked out in the 1920s and 1930s. The compounds have several components and their names are arcane. In Gaucher disease, the villain is called *cerebroside*, a complex molecule that includes fatty acids, sugars, and an amino-alcohol called *sphingosine*. The sugars, *glucocerebrosides*, are the familiar glucose and a related but slightly different sugar called *galactose*. The largest class comprises what are called *sphingolipids* and the diseases are *sphingolipidoses*.

All of this was known. However, there was no explanation for the failure of the cerebroside to follow normal metabolic pathways and, instead, stuff the cells in noxious amounts. One possibility was that affected individuals could not make a form of cerebroside in which the sugar is galactose (galactocerebroside) and, instead, make too much of the glucose-containing glucocerebroside. In other words, if normal pathway A is blocked, the body may revert to abnormal pathway B. To evaluate the possibility that galactose metabolism might be abnormal, it was necessary to learn how galactose and fatty acids are normally activated to combine to form the finished product as cell membranes are created.

Brady and his colleagues gave galactose to normal people and to some with Gaucher disease, following the rise and fall of blood levels. They found no difference in the patients' metabolism of this sugar. Another opportunity allowed them to check out galactose metabolism. Splenomegaly not only distorts the abdomen and causes discomfort, but it causes the spleen to function abnormally. A standard treatment is therefore surgical excision of the organ, which is a safe procedure. For Brady, that practice provided spleen tissue, making it possible to measure the synthesis of cerebroside, which proved to be normal, no matter whether they started with radio-labeled glucose or galactose. The abnormality was not in the starting materials – there was no abnormality in the usage of either glucose or galactose.

Brady shifted sights. The problem might be a failure in the breakdown of glucocerebroside. To evaluate that possibility, they had to synthesize labeled cerebroside and follow the rate of enzymatic loss of the label. However, cerebroside had never been synthesized previously, with or without an isotope label. Using a crude method, they succeeded in labeling the compound without direct chemical synthesis, but the product proved unsatisfactory for purposes of assay.

At about that time, Brady saw a paper describing the chemical synthesis of sphingomyelin by a chemist, David Shapiro, who had been working at the Weizmann Institute in Israel. Brady therefore asked Shapiro if he could synthesize the substance with a radioisotope label. Shapiro replied that he had no experience with radioactive tracers. Brady soon made arrangements for Shapiro to come to NIH and they synthesized radiolabeled glucocerebroside.

With this new reagent, they found that glucocerebroside was degraded by an enzyme (*glucocerebrosidase*) in extracts of any organ from a normal person. They then tested preparations of spleen, expecting to find no activity in the patients' material. Instead, they found that the residual activity was about 15 percent of normal. The deficit in total enzymatic activity was sufficient to account for the accumulation; there was not enough enzyme to dispose of all the cerebroside that was being synthesized.

Looking ahead, the 15 percent residual enzyme protein proved to be fortunate. Because there was some protein, the body did not make antibodies. If there had been no enzyme at all, there would have been a problem in developing treatment. People make antibodies against proteins they have not previously encountered. Because of the presence of residual enzyme, it seemed less likely that patients would develop antibodies if they were injected with supplemental glucocerebrosides. If a treatment included administration of the enzyme protein, and if there were no residual enzyme, the body would have created antibodies that neutralize the therapeutic preparation. Because of this view, many experts told Brady that it would be impossible to administer the enzyme for treatment.

Immunology was not the stumbling block, but it took 8 years to purify the enzyme in amounts sufficient to give to two patients. Brady and his group did a liver biopsy with a small needle, gave the enzyme by vein, and then repeated the biopsy a few days later. In that second biopsy, they found a 26 percent reduction in the content of the stored glucocerebroside.

Even so, they were greeted with skepticism. Normally, there is some variation in enzyme activity at different sites in an organ. This normal variation, the skeptics said, could account for the differences in the content of cerebroside in the two biopsies. But Brady tested and excluded that possibility by taking multiple samples from different sites of normal liver they obtained at autopsy.

He adduced other evidence. In the liver, cerebroside content increases about 200 times normal. In the blood the increase is three or four times. In both patients under study, these blood levels returned to normal within a few days after the infusion of enzyme. Even more encouraging was the observation that levels remained normal for 3 months, making it possible to think about effective treatment. In fact, blood levels remained lower than the original value for more than a year.

This treatment has become standard and has improved. Patients are not cured of their symptoms, but they have less pain and much less disability. Liver and spleen enlargement decreases and the abnormalities of blood clotting are ameliorated. Genetically engineered enzyme is now replacing the tedious and expensive process of extracting it from placentas.[5]

It was 1965 when Brady and his team identified the enzymatic defect in Gaucher disease as a lack of the cerebroside-degrading enzyme, glucocerebrosidase.[6] Then, using the same methods of synthesizing labeled substrates and developing enzyme assays, he found the genetic faults in other lipid storage diseases. The reports followed annually to include Niemann-Pick disease,[7] Tay-Sachs disease,[8] and Fabry disease.[9,10] Following the enzyme treatment of Gaucher disease,[11] Brady initiated similar intravenous replacement therapy for Fabry disease,[12,13] which causes skin lesions, strokes, heart attacks, and renal failure in young people.

As with Gaucher disease, the early evidence that injecting the enzyme intravenously could help Fabry disease patients was followed by a long hiatus – from 1967 to 1991 – while they tried to produce enough enzyme to give treatment continuously to assure true enzyme replacement. Genetically engineered skin fibroblasts in culture became the factory to manufacture the enzyme.

Throughout all this time, Brady's group continued to make important observations about the basic biochemistry of the normal and abnormal functions and cell structures involved in these diseases. They developed simplified biochemical tests for diagnosis and for identifying carriers of the genes (who usually have no symptoms), and they worked on prenatal diagnosis.

In the era of molecular genetics, the genes for these diseases have been mapped but gene therapy has not yet been feasible. Brady thinks that Fabry disease may be a better candidate for gene therapy than Gaucher disease. The Gaucher enzyme remains within cells and does not circulate in the blood; therefore the synthesizing cells would have to be corrected. In Fabry disease, however, the enzyme is released by the cells and circulates in the blood and fewer transduced cells have to be modified, perhaps 25 percent of all those making the enzyme. In transgenic mice the gene is rendered non-functional and the "knockout" mice lack the necessary enzyme, making them a useful test object in the quest for new treatments.[14,15] Brady and his group have also shown that it is possible to insert the missing gene into bone marrow stem cells from Fabry patients and to correct the metabolic abnormality of cultured skin fibroblasts from patients.[16] These findings open the possibility for successful gene therapy.

There is still much to be done in this field.[17] Not only is improved gene therapy needed but also the success of replacement therapy is limited because the enzyme circulating in the blood does not readily enter the brain. New delivery methods are being sought.[18]

Roscoe Brady considers his experience as one that could only have been achieved at NIH. It took 5 years to discover the enzyme defect, 8 more years to get enough enzyme for the first Gaucher trials, and then another 16 years to make enough enzyme for effective treatment of many patients. NIH was designed, he thinks, for that kind of high-risk, long-term research as opposed to the short-range, quick publication projects needed by university investigators to qualify for tenure and obtain grants. He is an outstanding model of the physician-investigator.

1 Brady RO. Interview with author, October 5, 2000.

2 Brady RO, Westerfeld WW. The effect of B-complex vitamins on the voluntary consumption of alcohol by rats. *Q J Studies on Alcohol* 1947;7:499-505.

3 Brady RO. Interview with author, March 27, 2000.

4 Trams EG, Brady RO. Cerebroside synthesis in Gaucher's disease. *J Clin Invest* 1960;39:1546-1550.

5 Brady RO, Murray GJ, Barton NW. Glucosylceramide lipidosis: Gaucher disease. In Rosenberg RN, Prusiner SB, DiMauro S, Barchi RL, eds. *The Molecular and Genetic Basis of Neurological Disease,* 2nd ed., Boston: Butterworth-Heinemann, 1997:405-420.

6 Brady RO, Kanfer J, Shapiro D. Metabolism of glucocerebrosides. II. Evidence of an enzymatic deficiency in Gaucher's disease. *Biochem Biophys Res Comm* 1965;18:221-225.

7 Brady RO, Kanfer J, Mock MB, Fredrickson DS. The metabolism of sphingomyelin. II. Evidence of an enzymatic deficiency in Niemann-Pick disease. *Proc Natl Acad Sci USA* 1966;55:366-369.

8 Kolodny EH, Brady RO, Volk BW. Demonstration of an alteration of ganglioside metabolism in Tay-Sachs disease. *Biochem Biophys Res Commun* 1969;37:526-531.

9 Brady RO, Gal AE, Bradley RM, Martensson E, Warshaw AL, Laster L. Enzymatic defect in Fabry's disease. *N Engl J Med* 1967;276:1163-1167.

10 Barton NW, Brady RO, Dambrosia JM, DiBisceglie AM, Doppelt SH, Hill SC, Mankin HJ, Murray GJ, Parker RI, Argoff CE, Grewal RP, Yu K-T. Replacement therapy for inherited enzyme deficiency – macrophage-targeted glucocerebrosidase for Gaucher's disease. *N Engl J Med* 1991;24:1464-1470.

11 Brady RO, Penchev PG, Gal AE, Hibbert SR, Dekaban AS. Replacement therapy for inherited enzyme deficiency: use of purified glucocerebrosidase in Gaucher's disease. *N Engl J Med* 1974;291:989-993.

12 Brady RO, Tallman JF, Johnson WG, Gal AE, Leahy WE, Quirk JM, Dekaban AS. Replacement therapy for inherited enzyme deficiency: use of purified cramidetrihexidase in Fabry's disease. *N Engl J Med* 1973;289:1-4.

13 Schiffmann R, Murray GJ, Treco D, Daniel P, Sellos-Moura M, Myers M, Quirk JM, Zirzow GC, Borowski M, Loveday K, Anderson T, Gillespie F, Oliver KL, Jeffries NO, Doo E, Liang TJ, Kreps C, Gunter K, Frei K, Crutchfield K, Selden RF, Brady RO. Infusion of alpha-galactosidase A reduces tissue globotriaosylceramide storage in patients with Fabry disease. *Proc Natl Acad Sci USA* 2000;97:365-370.

14 Oshima T, Murray GJ, Swain WD, Longnecker G, Quirk JM, Cardarelli CO, Sugimoto Y, Pastan I, Gottesman MM, Brady RO, Kulkarnia AG. α-Galactosidase A deficient mice: a model of Fabry disease. *Proc Natl Acad Sci USA* 1996;93: 15266-15271.

15 Takenaka T, Murray GJ, Qin G, Quirk JM, Ohshima T, Qasba P, Clark K, Kulkarni AB, Brady RO, Medin JA. Long-term enzyme correction and lipid reduction in multiple organs of primary and secondary transplanted Fabry mice receiving transduced bone marrow cells. *Proc Natl Acad Sci USA* 2000;97:7515-7520.

16 Brady RO, Schiffmann R. Clinical features and recent advances in therapy for Fabry disease. *JAMA* 2000;284:2771-2775.

17 Brady RO. Therapy for sphingolipidoses. *Arch Neurol* 1998;55:1055-1056.

18 Zirzow GC, Sanchez OA, Murray GJ, Brady RO, Oldfield EH. Delivery, distribution, and neuronal uptake of exogenous mannose-terminal glucocerebroside in the intact rat brain. *Neurochemical Res* 1999;24:301-305.

CHAPTER SEVENTEEN

D. CARLETON GAJDUSEK, M.D.

The Nobel Prize in Physiology or Medicine, 1976

Awarded jointly to Baruch S. Blumberg and D. Carleton Gajdusek for their discoveries concerning new mechanisms for the origin and dissemination of infectious diseases.

Neuroscientists have been well represented among the Nobel Prizes for Physiology or Medicine. The list starts with Santiago Ramón y Cajal and Camillo Golgi in 1906. Naming others creates a landmark history of brain research: Julius Wagner-Jauregg, Lord Edgar Adrian, Sir Charles Sherrington, Sir Henry Dale, Otto Loewi, Albert von Szent-Györgi, Joseph Erlanger, Herbert Gasser, Walter Hess, Georg von Békésy, Sir John C. Eccles, Alan Hodgkin, Andrew Huxley, Egas Moniz, Ragnar Granit, Haldan Kiefer Hartline, George Wald, Julius Axelrod, Sir Bernard Katz, Ulf von Euler. D. Carleton Gajdusek, Allan Cormack, Godfrey Hounsfield, Roger Sperry, David Hubel, Torsten Wiesel, Rita Levi-Montalcini, Stanley Cohen, Erwin Neher, Bert Sakmann, Stanley Prusiner, Arvid Carlsson, Paul Greengard, and Eric Kandel.

Of the 34, only Wagner-Jauregg, Moniz, and Prusiner were neurologists when they made their discoveries. Only Gajdusek was in the intramural program of NINDS. Axelrod's appointment was in NIMH.

Gajdusek and Prusiner are joined forever in one of the great stories of modern medicine. Seeking the nature of an obscure disease of sheep and an obscure disease of people in remote New Guinea, the investigators were led to recognize new forms of a human disease caused by an agent that could be considered a new form of life. The story has many implications, including an appreciation of the

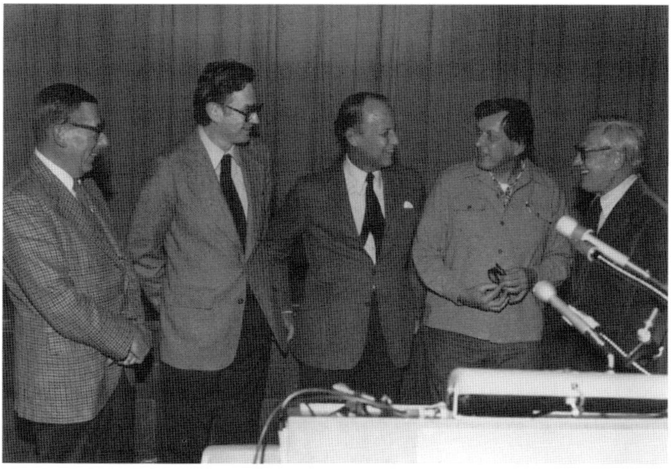

(FROM LEFT) DONALD TOWER (DIRECTOR OF NINDS), MARSHALL NIRENBERG (NHLBI, 1968 NOBEL LAUREATE), DONALD FREDRICKSON (DIRECTOR OF NIH), CARLETON GAJDUSEK (NINDS, 1976 NOBEL LAUREATE), JULIUS AXELROD (NIMH, 1970 NOBEL LAUREATE)

value of clinical research – the direct study of human disease – for basic science. And it also illustrates the importance of veterinary medicine for understanding human disease. The story involves revolutionary medical concepts of slow viruses and neologistic *prions*; it includes cannibalism, mad cows, and a colorful cast of diverse research investigators. The story perhaps never would have begun had it not been for the curiosity of a veterinarian who wrote a letter to the editor of a medical journal.

The modern history of the story begins with *scrapie*, a disease of sheep that had been known to farmers for hundreds of years. Affected animals rubbed against trees or posts; they did this vigorously enough to scrape off their fur, as though they had to relieve constant itching. After several years, the animals would show evidence of a neurological disorder that was ultimately fatal. In 1936, French scientists reported that grinding up the spinal cord of a sick sheep and injecting it into a normal animal could transmit the disease. This remarkable observation, however, was greeted by skepticism because the symptoms did not appear for a year or two after the injection. No known viral disease took that long; viral diseases were acute infections, like measles, with incubation periods of a few days after exposure.

In 1939, however, William Gordon, at the Moredun Research Institute in Scotland, repeated the experiment and confirmed the years-long period of latency.[1] In 1939 Gordon was made director of the United Kingdom's Institute for Research for Animal Health at Compton, which became the center for scrapie research. There, Ian Pattison found the disease could be transmitted from sheep to goats by intracerebral injection or by feeding. Within the next few years they determined that the organism was not destroyed by formalin, which kills most viruses. Unlike viruses, the agent caused no inflammation in the brain and elicited no antibodies in the blood. It was also smaller than any other known virus and no signs of nucleic acid were found, also unlike known viruses.

Only a small audience knew all of this. Britons had eaten mutton for centuries and no connection to scrapie was evident. Only sheep farmers were harmed, and their problem was economic, not medical; they lost money when their sheep died.

Enter Carleton Gajdusek. Born in 1923 in Yonkers, New York, he was interested in science from childhood.[2,3] Like other famous medical scientists of his generation, he was a juvenile devotee of Paul de Kruif's *Microbe Hunters*; he inscribed the names of the heroes of the book on the stairs in his home. He was precocious in school and, at age 19, he graduated from the University of Rochester with a degree in biophysics.

After receiving his medical degree at Harvard Medical School in 1946, Gajdusek was trained in pediatrics in an itinerant fashion that presaged his itinerant research; the 4-year program incorporated three leading hospitals: Babies Hospital in New York, and Children's Hospitals in Cincinnati and Boston. He was a research fellow with Linus Pauling and Max Delbrück at the California Institute of Technology and with John Enders at Harvard; all three were Nobel laureates. Enders recommended Gajdusek to Joseph Smadel, who at that time directed the laboratory of virus and rickettsial diseases at the Walter Reed Army Institute of Research.

In 1954, under Smadel's direction, Gajdusek traveled to investigate acute viral infections in India, Iran, Turkey, the Middle East, and Afghanistan. He studied hemorrhagic fever in Korea when he served in the Army Medical Corps. In these travels he nourished an appetite for anthropology and became fluent in German, French, Spanish, Russian, and Slovak; he reported "limited" skills in Persian, Bahasa Indonesian, and Dutch languages. He corresponded voluminously with Smadel[4] and prepared ten papers on these studies in the one year of 1956. His inquisitiveness, industry, and talents for anthropology, virology, learning new languages, and writing all served him well later.

In 1955 he found his fourth Nobel-Prize winning mentor, Macfarlane Burnet, in Melbourne, Australia. After 2 years in Australia, he was scheduled to return to the United States. He planned to stop in New Guinea on the way home, on another anthropologic foray. He intended to continue studies of "child growth and development and disease patterns in isolated" populations.[5] His guide was Vincent Zigas, an Estonian who had migrated to Australia during World War II and then became an Australian public health officer in charge of the area in New Guinea that included the Fore people. It was Zigas who first introduced Gajdusek to *kuru*, a neurological disease of the Fore. In the local language, the word meant "trembling." Zigas had first encountered the disease there in 1955, sending specimens to a virology laboratory in Melbourne.[6]

Together, Zigas and Gajdusek engaged the local people to help build a hospital and a small house with a thatched roof for Gajdusek. For more than a year, they examined more than 200 patients with kuru, including 50 children; almost all the rest were women. Adult men were almost totally spared from the disease. Finding patients involved extended treks through forests and over mountains. Zigas could speak the pidgin English of the area and Gajdusek learned to speak the local language. Gajdusek kept a detailed journal. They made a film about the disease. They delineated the clinical syndrome, a combination of cerebellar signs, parkinsonism, and mutism, but not dementia. Their first paper was published in 1958.[7]

Without special training in pathology, Gajdusek and Zigas carried out autopsies themselves and sent the brains for examination to either Melbourne or Washington, DC, where an NINDB neuropathologist, Igor Klatzo, noted the similarity of the degeneration of the brain in kuru to that in Creutzfeldt-Jakob disease,[8] a condition so rare at the time that it had hardly been mentioned in American publications. Another neuropathologist, Meta Neumann, also noted the similarity. In 1958, Gajdusek returned to the United States. By then, Smadel had become Associate Director of NIH and he arranged an appointment for Gajdusek in NINDB. One of Gajdusek's first tasks was to prepare an exhibition of photographs and text for a traveling display about the clinical patterns and pathology of kuru.

That exhibit proved to have unique consequences because of another American investigator who happened to be working at the Compton scrapie laboratory in England. His name was William Hadlow, a veterinarian by training, and self-taught in neuropathology. He had worked as a veterinary neuropathologist in the Rocky Mountain laboratory in Montana for 7 years. A bit restive, he had then accepted an offer from the U.S. Department of Agriculture to join a British group working on scrapie, a disease he knew very little about.[9] He arrived at Compton in the spring of 1958. Within a few months he had done complete brain examinations on many of the animals that died. He saw widespread vacuolation of neurons, sponginess of gray matter, and astrogliosis (scarring). In June, a friend told Hadlow that he would be interested in Gajdusek's exhibition, now in London. Hadlow took the train to London and viewed the unique poster presentation.

He "found the overall resemblance of kuru and scrapie to be uncanny." He wondered if, like scrapie, kuru might be transmissible. Within a week, on July 18, 1959, Hadlow sent a letter to the editor to the British medical journal *Lancet*,[10] but he feared publication might be delayed by a printers' strike and therefore also sent a copy of the letter to Gajdusek.[11] In the last sentence, Hadlow wrote that "it might be profitable, in view of veterinary experience with scrapie, to examine the possibility of the experimental induction of kuru in a laboratory primate, for one might surmise that the pathogenic mechanisms involved in scrapie – however unusual they may be – are unlikely to be unique in the province of animal pathology." In his response Gajdusek mentioned "poor luck with inoculation experiments" but he had not yet tried primates.

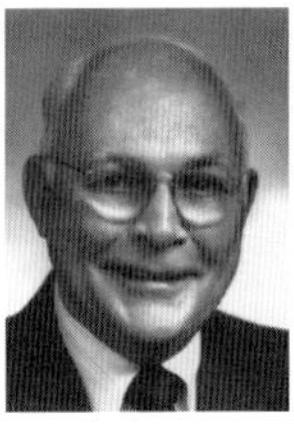

CLARENCE "JOE" GIBBS, JR., PH.D.

Clarence J. Gibbs, Jr., a virologist and son of a veterinarian, had been working under Smadel at the Walter Reed Army Medical Service Graduate School where he developed a vaccine for Rift Valley fever. In 1959, he left to take a position in the Laboratory of Tropical Virology of the National Institute of Allergy and Infectious Diseases, but the future of that laboratory seemed uncertain and, in 1961, he was about to accept a fellowship to work on arthropod-borne viruses in Brazil. He paused long enough to seek Smadel's advice,[12] which was unequivocal: "Goddam it Gibbs; you're not going to

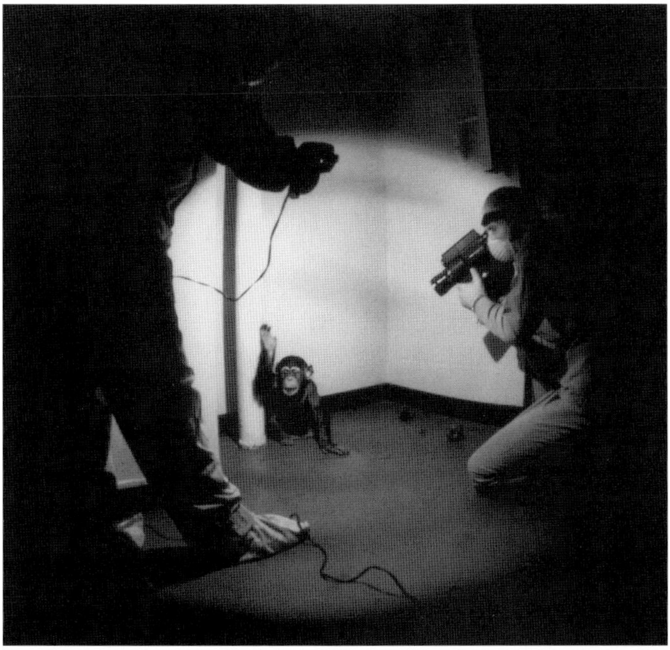

DR. HERBERT AMYX FILMS BEHAVIORAL CHANGES IN A CHIMPANZEE INOCULATED WITH KURU

Brazil!" Instead he would be going to the Patuxent Wildlife Research Center in Laurel, Maryland, to work on scrapie and to transmit kuru to chimpanzees under the direction of Gajdusek. Smadel predicted they would have "golden results," either positive or negative.

They did not inject the first chimpanzee with kuru brain material, however, until 1963. Instead, scrapie brains were injected into mice. By the end of the year, Gibbs had injected "10,000 mice, 7 chimpanzees, and 75 smaller non-human primates." While this was going on, Gajdusek was back in New Guinea carrying out field studies on kuru. Also in 1963, the pair organized the first meeting on slow virus infections. The proceedings were not published for 2 years,[13] just enough time to include an addendum to a paper by Gibbs[14] reporting that two of the first chimpanzees injected with kuru had come down with the disease. The proceedings also recorded a new animal disease, transmissible encephalopathy of mink, which had many similarities to scrapie. The full report of kuru transmission came later,[15,16] documenting the first slow virus disease of humans.

Smadel, so important in the background, never saw the "golden results" he had predicted. He died in 1963 at the age of 56. Sponsoring Gajdusek and Gibbs was only one of his numerous contributions to viral diseases throughout the world. For that work, he won a Lasker Award himself in 1962. His other achievements gave Smadel a place in history.[17]

Others played important roles in the elucidation of kuru. Elisabeth Beck, a British neuropathologist, documented the similarities of brain pathology in kuru patients, chimpanzees with transmissible kuru, and animals with scrapie. She also noted the variations in the spongiform condition and the similarities to Creutzfeldt-Jakob disease (CJD), another human disease that the group also transmitted to primates.[18] Later, they transmitted a third condition with similar pathology, the Gerstmann-Scheinker-Sträussler disease.[19] Paul Brown, another major contributor to the NINDS program, followed the clinical patterns of CJD in France and the United States, providing more accurate diagnostic criteria.

Michael Alpers was an Australian neurologist who had worked in New Guinea with Gajdusek, recording the clinical findings and conducting autopsies. He was the one who made the connection between kuru and the Fore practice of cannibalism of dead tribe members – enacted primarily by women of the tribe, according to custom. Later, Alpers reviewed the case records and noted the precipitous drop in the incidence of new cases of kuru in children after 1961.[20] He saw that this change coincided with the end of cannibalism among the Fore, a practice that had been documented in detail by anthropologists Robert and Shirley Glasse (who later became Shirley Lindenbaum).[21] This explained the preponderance of kuru among women and their children; they were last to feed, and consumed the brains of people who had died of kuru. The men ate other parts of the body in honor of the deceased.

In less than a decade, Gajdusek, Gibbs, and their colleagues had found three transmissible human diseases with incubation periods of years, even more than a decade, and with no signs of inflammation in cerebrospinal fluid or central nervous system but unique spongiform pathology. The causative agent differed from viruses in resistance to formalin and radiation and lacked evidence of nucleic acids. They recognized that some cases were both familial and transmissible.

Carleton Gajdusek taking medical histories in the New Hebrides in 1972

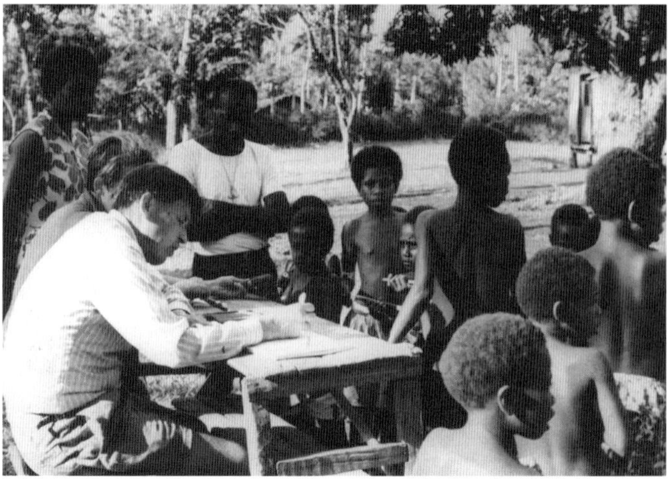

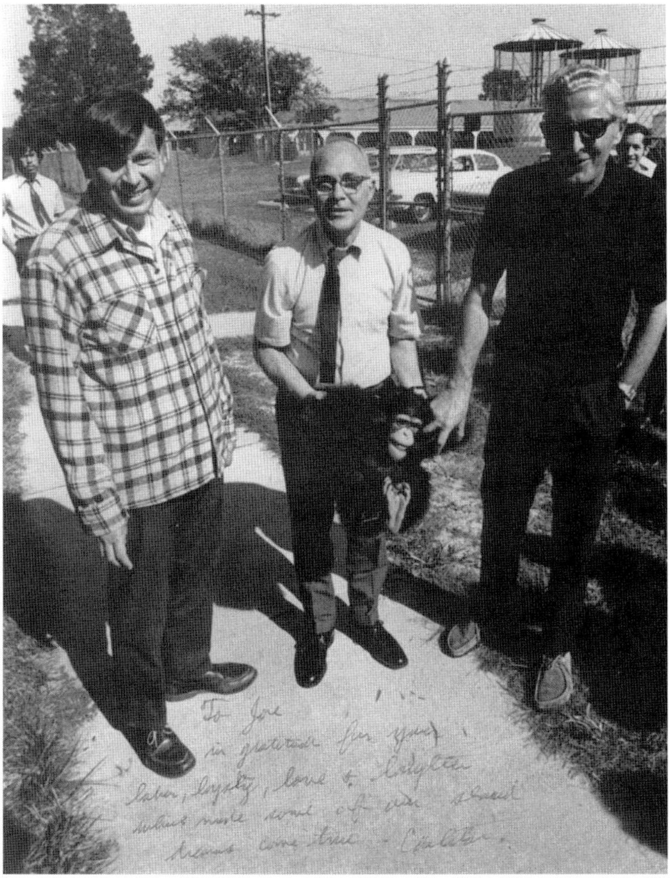

A photo of Carleton Gajdusek, Joe Gibbs, and Vin Zigas at Patuxent that hung on the wall in Gibbs' office. The inscription, from Gajdusek, reads: "To Joe, in gratitude for your labor, loyalty, love & laughter which made some of our shared dreams come true — Carleton"

Gajdusek and his colleagues also provided an international diagnostic service when transmission was the ultimate criterion for diagnosis. That gave them experience with more than 200 cases by the time of Gajdusek's Nobel Lecture in 1976,[2] followed by another hundred in the next two decades.[22] The diagnostic service led to the development of a test for a protein in the cerebrospinal fluid (the "14-3-3" protein);[23] identification of that protein has proved to be a relatively specific and most sensitive diagnostic laboratory test,[24] an important advance in the diagnosis of rapidly advancing dementia, but it still leaves some uncertainty. With more accurate diagnosis there has been more clinical interest in the disease and it does not seem so rare any longer.

One major practical effect of these studies was the identification of other slow virus diseases, especially subacute sclerosis panencephalitis (SSPE), a fatal form of persistent infection with measles virus that was identified by another NINDS investigator, John Sever. Just as the end of cannibalism eliminated kuru, so measles vaccination eliminated SSPE. Another important slow virus infection is progressive multifocal leukoencephalopathy, which is seen in immunocompromised people with malignant tumors or HIV infection.

A side issue emerged when it was found that CJD had been transmitted in the course of a corneal transplant. This was followed by other reports of iatrogenic transmission (disease originating unintentionally by the actions of physicians) through neurosurgical operations on the brain or through injections of human growth hormone prepared from homogenates of human pituitary glands.[25,26]

In later years, the NINDS investigators contributed to the recognition and characterization of a new prion disease, familial fatal insomnia (FFI). This new condition affected concepts of inherited diseases, that is, information about fatal insomnia partially explained what is called allelic heterogeneity, how mutations in the same gene can cause different clinical conditions. This phenomenon is usually attributed to the indirect effects of other genes or to environmental factors, none ever identified previously. Here, it was found that normal variants in the structure of the prion DNA determine whether the disease will have the features of CJD or FFI. The same variation or *polymorphism* determines whether a person is susceptible to sporadic or iatrogenic CJD. The team also became immersed in the debates about mad cow disease.

The Bethesda group contributed to the diagnosis of the only celebrity to have died of CJD, George Balanchine, who was probably the greatest ballet-master in history. He died in 1983 and official biographies record the autopsy diagnosis of CJD.[27,28] However, the results of that examination have not yet been published. The pathological diagnosis was made by Philip Duffy, then Director of the Division of Neuropathology at the Columbia-Presbyterian Medical Center in New York. (Duffy was the one who first described iatrogenic disease in the recipient of a corneal transplant from a donor who later developed CJD.[29])

In 2000, James Goldman, Duffy's successor in the position, confirmed the histological diagnosis. He reviewed the microscopic sections and wrote:[30]

> There is no question that he suffered from a transmissible spongiform encephalopathy. The neocortex is affected focally, ranging from severely to mildly, thalamic nuclei also severely affected, and most of the other deep nuclei show moderate degrees of spongiform changes. The cerebellum contains typical "kuru" plaques in the internal granule layer.

Gibbs[31] later reported that material from Balanchine had transmitted disease to a chimpanzee.

The research of Gajdusek and Gibbs and their colleagues surely opened a new world, one in which more wonders and more diseases were soon to follow.

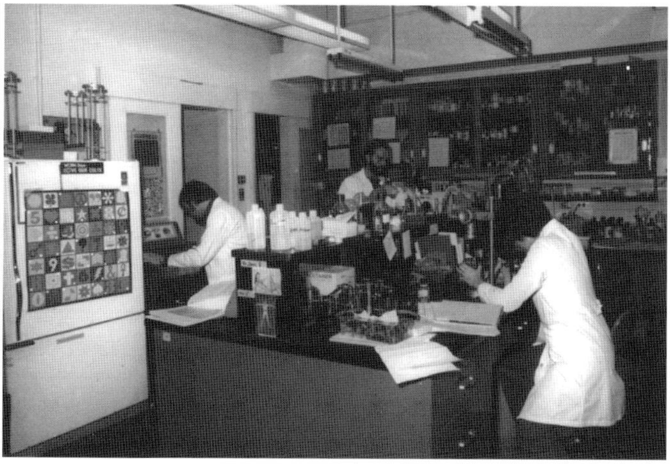

THE INFECTIOUS DISEASE LABORATORY AT NINDS, 1974

Gajdusek's contributions were widely applauded when he won the Nobel Prize. Gibbs was such an integral part of the project that many people thought he should have shared the Nobel Prize. Asked if he felt slighted because he did not share the award,[32] Gibbs said he had made peace with that but he wished that Hadlow had been more appreciated. That kind of modesty was characteristic of Joe Gibbs, who died in February 2001, at age 76.[33]

1 Pattison IH. A sideways look at the scrapie saga: 1732-1991. In Prusiner SB, Collinge J, Powell J, Anderton B, eds. *Prion Diseases of Humans and Animals.* New York: Ellis Horwood, 1992:1-21.

2 Gajdusek DC. Unconventional viruses and the origin and disappearance of kuru (Nobel Prize Lecture). *Science* 1977;197:943-960.

3 Rhodes R. *Deadly Feasts. The "Prion" Controversy and the Public's Health.* New York: Simon & Schuster, 1997.

4 Gajdusek DC, ed. Correspondence on the Discovery and Original Investigations on Kuru. Smadel-Gajdusek Correspondence, 1955-1958. Study of Child Growth and Development and Disease Patterns in Primitive Cultures. NINCDS, National Institutes of Health, Bethesda, MD, 1975. Copy in Library of the National Institutes of Health, Bethesda, MD, RC 394 K8 G145 1975.

5 Gajdusek DC. Observations on the early history of kuru investigation. In Prusiner SB, Hadlow WJ, eds. *Slow Transmissible Infections of the Nervous System.* New York: Academic Press, 1979:7-36.

6 Zigas V. Origin of investigations on slow virus infections in man. In Prusiner SB, Hadlow WJ, eds. *Slow Transmissible Infections of the Nervous System.* New York: Academic Press, 1979:3-6.

7 Gajdusek DC, Zigas V. Kuru. Clinical, pathological and epidemiological study of an acute progressive degenerative disease of the central nervous system among natives of the eastern highlands of New Guinea. *Am J Med* 1959;26:442-469.

8 Klatzo I, Gajdusek DC, Zigas V. Pathology of kuru. *Lab Invest* 1959;8:799-846.

9 Hadlow WJ. The scrapie-kuru connection: recollections of how it came about. In Prusiner, et al., eds. *Prion Diseases of Humans and Animals*, pp. 40-46.

10 Hadlow WJ. Scrapie and kuru. *Lancet* 1959;2:289-290.

11 Gajdusek DC. Kuru and scrapie. In Prusiner, et al., eds. *Prion Diseases of Humans and Animals*, pp. 47-52.

12 Gibbs CJ, Jr. Spongiform encephalopathies – slow, latent, and temperate virus infections – in retrospect. In Prusiner, et al., eds. *Prion Diseases of Humans and Animals*, pp. 53-62.
13 Gajdusek DC, Gibbs CJ, Jr., Alpers M, eds. *Slow, Latent, and Temperate Virus Infections*. NINDB Monograph No. 2 Public Health Publication No. 1378, Washington, DC: Government Printing Office, 1965.
14 Gibbs CJ, Jr., Gajdusek DC. Attempts to demonstrate a transmissible agent in kuru, amyotrophic lateral sclerosis, and other subacute and chronic progressive nervous system degenerations of man. In Gajdusek DC, Gibbs CJ, Jr., Alpers M, eds. *Slow, Latent, and Temperate Virus Infections*, pp. 39-48.
15 Gajdusek DC, Gibbs CJ, Jr., Alpers M. Experimental transmission of a kuru-like syndrome to chimpanzees. *Nature* (London) 1966;209:794-796.
16 Gajdusek DC, Gibbs CJ, Jr, Alpers M. Transmission and passage of experimental kuru to chimpanzees. *Science* 1967;155:212-214.
17 Woodward TE. Joseph E. Smadel, 1907-1963. *Trans Assoc Am Phys* 1964;87:29-32.
18 Gibbs CJ, Jr, Gajdusek DC, Asher DM, Alpers MP, Beck E, Daniel PM, Matthews WB. Creutzfeldt-Jakob disease (spongiform encephalopathy): transmission to the chimpanzee. *Science* 1968;161:388-389.
19 Masters CL, Gajdusek DC, Gibbs CJ, Jr. Creutzfeldt-Jakob disease virus isolations from the Gerstmann-Sträussler syndrome with an analysis of the various forms of amyloid plaque deposition in the virus-induced spongiform encephalopathies. *Brain* 1981;104:559-588.
20 Alpers M. Reflections and highlights: A life with kuru. In Prusiner, et al., eds. *Prion Diseases of Humans and Animals*, pp. 66-76.
21 Glasse R, Lindenbaum S, Fieldwork in the South Fore: the process of ethnographic inquiry. In Prusiner, et al., eds. *Prion Diseases of Humans and Animals*, pp. 77-91.
22 Brown P, Gibbs CJ, Jr., Rodgers-Johnson P, et al. Human spongiform encephalopathy: the National Institutes of Health series of 300 cases of experimentally transmitted disease. *Ann Neurol* 1994;35:513-529.
23 Hsich G, Kenney K, Gibbs CJ, Jr., et al. The 14-3-3 brain protein in cerebrospinal fluid as a marker for transmissible spongiform encephalopathies. *N Engl J Med* 1996;335:924-930.
24 Lemstra AW, van Meegen MT, Vreyling JP, et al. 14-3-3 Testing in diagnosing Creutzfeldt-Jakob disease: a prospective study in 112 patients. *Neurology* 2000; 55:514-516.
25 Brown P, Gajdusek DC, Gibbs CJ, Jr., Asher DM. Potential epidemic of Creutzfeldt-Jakob disease from human growth hormone. *N Engl J Med* 1985; 313:728-731.
26 Gibbs CJ, Jr., Joy A, Heffnerr R, et al. Clinical and pathological features and laboratory confirmation of Creutzfeldt-Jakob disease in a recipient of pituitary-derived human growth hormone. *N Engl J Med* 1985;313:734-738.
27 Taper B. *Balanchine. A Biography*. New York: The New York Times Book Co., 1984:387.
28 Wickham, RD. In Mason F. *I Remember Balanchine: Recollections of the Ballet Master by Those Who Knew Him*. New York: Doubleday, 1991:604.
29 Duffy P, Wolf J, Collins G, et al. Possible person to person transmission of Creutzfeldt-Jakob disease. *N Engl J Med* 1974:290:692.
30 Goldman H. E-mail Communication to author, September 29, 2000.
31 Gibbs CJ, Jr. Telephone Conversation with author, October 2, 2000.
32 Gibbs CJ, Jr. Recorded Interview with author, March 22, 2000.
33 Obituary for Clarence "Joe" Gibbs, Jr., NIH Scientist. *The Washington Post*, March 14, 2001.

CHAPTER EIGHTEEN

STANLEY B. PRUSINER, M.D.

The Nobel Prize in Physiology or Medicine, 1997

Awarded to Stanley Prusiner for his discovery of prions – a new biological principle of infection.

Albert Lasker Award for Basic Medical Research, 1994

For landmark, revolutionary work that established the existence of an entirely new class of infectious agents, and which opened new understanding of the pathogenesis of several baffling neurodegenerative diseases.

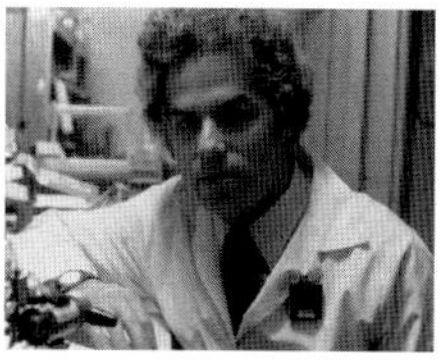

STANLEY PRUSINER, M.D., IN HIS LAB AT THE UNIVERSITY OF CALIFORNIA, SAN FRANCISCO IN 1985

Stanley Prusiner won the Lasker Award in 1994. Three years later, he gained both the Louisa Gross Horwitz Prize and the Nobel Prize. He was recognized for elucidating the nature of the agents that cause scrapie, kuru, and other diseases. In the process he defined the *prion* as a new form of life. There is no better example of how the pursuit of rare human diseases can contribute to basic science.

Born in 1942, Prusiner grew up in the Midwest, spending time in Des Moines and Cincinnati. In a brief autobiography,[1] he gave no indication of a childhood interest in science. Instead, he credited his undergraduate experience at the University of Pennsylvania for the start of his scientific career. Nevertheless, he majored in chemistry, undoubtedly indicative of an earlier interest.

In 1963, between his junior and senior undergraduate years, he worked on a research project to understand how the low body temperature of hypothermia alters the body's metabolism. To continue this work, he decided to remain at Penn for medical school and there he met Britton Chance, the pioneer physical chemist of oxidative phosphorylation – the chemical events that provide energy for life processes.

One of the key questions Prusiner wanted to answer was how animals maintain body temperature when they hibernate. He asked Chance if he could work on the surface fluorescence of brown fat, a special structure of the Syrian hamster and important for hibernation. Continuing these experiments, he spent much of his fourth year of medical school in Sweden, still working on brown fat.

He returned to Philadelphia to graduate with his M.D. in 1968 and then interned at the University of California in San Francisco. Moving to NIH, he spent 3 years in the biochemistry laboratory of Earl Stadtman at the National Heart and Lung Institute. This concentrated training period established his skills in protein chemistry and enzymology and confirmed his interest in a research career. He then had to decide whether to take a neuroscience fellowship or a residency in neurology. Opting for neurology, he returned to San Francisco in July 1972. Within 2 months, Prusiner was assigned a patient who was to transform his life – and the world, too.

The patient was a young woman who had been diagnosed with Creutzfeldt-Jakob disease (CJD). By then, the diagnosis was not so esoteric, largely because of the work of the Gajdusek team. CJD was one of several human diseases attributed to a *slow virus*, a term introduced by Björn Sigurdsson,[2] an investigator of scrapie in Iceland, to account for a latent period of years, rather than the interval of days that characterized the more familiar viruses of childhood infections such as measles and chickenpox. Other human slow virus diseases included kuru and Gerstmann-Sträussler-Scheinker (GSS) disease. A fourth, familial fatal insomnia, was added later.[3,4] CJD was usually sporadic but about 10 percent of the cases were familial. GSS was more often familial. Rapidly progressive dementia and involuntary movements dominated CJD, whereas GSS was manifested mostly by ataxia (a severely unsteady gait) before dementia appeared. Both were fatal within a year of onset.

The Gajdusek team had established the pathological criteria for diagnosis, especially a Swiss cheese-like appearance of parts of the brain, which when translated into medicalese, came out as *spongiform encephalopathy*. Among the major characteristics were large accumulations of a protein-carbohydrate complex called *amyloid*. Transmission to chimpanzees of kuru first, then CJD, established the group as infectious diseases. But the nature of the presumed slow virus was still unknown. Research attention was directed to the scrapie agent because the disease in sheep was typical of this class of diseases and also because the agent was so amenable to study.

Prusiner learned the beliefs of the day. The causal *slow virus* differed from typical viruses in that it elicited neither antibodies in the blood nor white blood cells in the spinal fluid. He learned that the virus was atypical in its physical properties, too. These esoteric and incomprehensible features fascinated him; he read everything he could. The more he read, the more he became fixated on the idea of solving the riddle, of elucidating the nature of the causative agent. After his self-styled "abbreviated residency" in 1974, he was appointed an Assistant Professor of Neurology at the University of California, San Francisco, in the department chaired by Robert A. Fishman (who is renowned, among his other talents, for recognizing and nourishing talent in others).

In his new laboratory Prusiner was soon funded by NIH to work on glutamate metabolism in the choroid plexus, a brain organ that participates in the formation of cerebrospinal fluid. He was grateful for the grant but thought he had received it largely because of his earlier experience in the field. He was disappointed when an application to NIH for scrapie research was turned down; he really wanted to work on slow viruses.

To comply with criticisms of the study section that he had had no training in virology, he sought collaboration with William Hadlow and Carl Elkund at the Rocky Mountain Laboratory in Montana for a joint project on the scrapie agent. They worked together well enough, but their teamwork generated only more problems. In studying the sedimentation properties of the agent, for instance, Prusiner expected to find evidence of a virus of low molecular weight, but instead he found that the weight was even lower than anticipated and, like others before him, he found no evidence of nucleic acids, which should have been anticipated in a virus. The material seemed to contain only protein, a finding both paradoxical and inexplicable.

Matters became worse. He was told that financial support from the Howard Hughes Medical Research Institute would cease and that he would not be given tenure. Fortunately the tenure decision was reversed; private funds and continued NIH support carried him through a difficult period, but it was not to be his last travail.

In 1982, after 8 years of work, Prusiner wrote a review[5] that included a neologism in the abstract; it was the first public appearance of the word *prion*. The title of the paper used the more complicated term "novel proteinaceous infectious particles cause scrapie." The new word was a compound – from "protein" and "infectious;" in correct sequence, it would have been "proin," but that could be slurred to one syllable. Prusiner therefore made the transposition to "prion" and he set the pronunciation to rhyme with *pree*-on, not Zion.

In the paper he propounded three heretical views. Most important was the concept that the infectious agent contained no nucleic acid, differentiating it from all known viruses. Second, was the notion that a disease could be both hereditary and infectious (transmissible). Third, he concluded that the causal protein might be self-replicating. This was the most difficult for his peers to accept; the dogma of the day stated that DNA directed the synthesis of RNA and that RNA, in turn, was translated into the amino acid sequence that determined a protein. Without DNA or RNA, it was believed, there could be no creation of new protein.

Each of these proposals had been made earlier by others[6-10] and those earlier investigators surely deserve credit, but their suggestions had been insufficiently substantiated and were made at a time when many different and competing proposals were in the air. Prusiner[11] listed 24 unproven possibilities from that early era. The power of Prusiner's 1982 paper was the detailed description of the experimental results that led to an inexorable conclusion. The work defined Prusiner's achievements – prodigious labor, unflinching acceptance of unexpected or conflicting evidence, clever experiments based on up-to-date techniques from different fields of science, and fruitful collaborations.

To identify the causal agent, Prusiner first needed a new and improved method to purify it. Originally, tissue extracts from affected animals had to be injected into sheep or goats. After an interval of more than a year, sometimes 3 years, the animal's brain could be tested for infectious particles. In 1961, scrapie was transmitted to mice but it still took 18 months to find out whether the animals had been infected. With hamsters, the time was reduced to 200 days, and then, with Prusiner's new incubation time method, to 60 days.

Being able to follow the infection, investigators could purify preparations from infected animals to analyze the structure of the scrapie agent. Again, physical measurements showed the presence of protein, but not nucleic acid. Exposure of extracts to chemicals and enzymes that destroyed proteins also inactivated the agent, but chemicals that destroyed nucleic acids did not.

Exposure to ultraviolet light inactivates DNA or RNA viruses, a technique that has been used practically to kill a virus and render it harmless; the residue acts as a vaccine by eliciting long-lasting antibodies to the virus, which prevents infection. But neither ultraviolet light nor ionizing radiation had much effect on the scrapie agent. Moreover, viruses elicit antibodies, which are not found in scrapie or other prion diseases. The list of these differences from viruses seemed endless and the results were always consistent. Nucleic acids have still not been found reproducibly in preparations of scrapie agent.

Prusiner and his associates worked as hard as their predecessors and critics to find the hypothetical nucleic acid, but they failed, again. The results were not watertight; absence of proof is not proof of absence. There could have been a tiny amount of DNA within a protective protein coat or some other structure. If not, it would mean that the information for reproduction of the agent would have to be contained within the host cell (a *host-encoded protein*) or in the agent itself (a virus). Starting on the publication day in 1982, the concepts of prions and prion diseases in Prusiner's paper were hotly debated.

In Prusiner's[1] words, "the paper set off a firestorm. Virologists were generally incredulous and some investigators working on scrapie and CJD were irate. The term prion, derived from protein and infectious, provided a challenge to find the nucleic acid of the putative 'scrapie virus.' Should such a nucleic acid be found, then the word prion would disappear! Despite the strong convictions of many, no nucleic acid was found. The personal attacks of the naysayers at times became very vicious."

To top off the problems, Prusiner suffered a back injury and had a laminectomy in the winter of 1983, while the "torrent of criticism" was increasing. The literature of the next decade includes many attempts to disprove the prion hypothesis, even criticizing the name *prion* because it was merely a new word for old observations. The word was not even new, it had already been used to name an obscure Antarctic bird. The debate has had some lasting effects. Some investigators continue to call the diseases *transmissible spongiform encephalopathies.* That term came first and therefore has the weight of tradition behind it, as well as technical accuracy. But it is a tongue twister. Others prefer the simpler *prion diseases*, which is not only easier to say but has a molecular basis.

Despite the criticism, Prusiner came up with more and more powerful evidence.[12,13] With Leroy Hood, he determined the amino acid sequence of the prion protein (PrP).[14] With Charles Weissmann, the gene was cloned.[15] These two papers made a great leap forward in proving the prion theory. There was also a major practical advance. Once the protein had been purified, specific antibodies could be raised for further experiments and to provide a crucial diagnostic demonstration of PrP in people with CJD, an observation made first in two patients by the Prusiner group[16] and then almost simultaneously in larger numbers of patients by both the Prusiner and Gajdusek teams.[17,18]

The diagnostic antibody test is called the Western blot; proteins are extracted from fresh or frozen tissue, from a brain biopsy, or a postmortem examination. The proteins are separated in a gel by applying an electric gradient (gel electrophoresis) and then labeled antibodies are applied to the gel to identify the specific protein of interest. Similarly, a labeled antibody can be applied to a microscopic section of a brain biopsy or other tissue specimen (immunocytochemistry) to identify the protease-resistant PrP.

With the antibody now available, it was also possible to confirm the PrP identity of rod-shaped particles from preparations enriched in scrapie infectivity; these particles had the staining characteristics of amyloid, which was known to accumulate in the brains of people with CJD; the antibody reaction proved that the amyloid was a characteristic of PrP, not some other virus or host protein.

Another major advance came from the PrP gene. Once it had been cloned, transgenic mice were constructed. Among the other achievements of these mice, it was shown that the *species barrier* could be crossed. Normal mice were resistant to inoculation with hamster scrapie protein. However, transgenic mice carrying the hamster PrP gene were susceptible to the disease when they were challenged with scrapie PrP from hamsters, showing that the species barrier can be crossed if the recipient animal carries the PrP gene from the donor.

Knockout mice were prepared by inactivating the PrP gene; the animals therefore totally lacked PrP. They seemed to be perfectly normal animals even though this presumably important protein was absent, but they resisted infection from any source of abnormal PrP. If the brain of the recipient animal did not have its own normal PrP, it could not be infected with abnormal PrP from any species.

Once the gene had been cloned, it was possible to test people for the inherited forms of prion disease. In 1989, the Prusiner team and others found the first PrP mutation in a patient with GSS disease.[19] They then reproduced an animal model of the neurological disease by inserting the mutant gene into transgenic mice, with not only symptoms of brain dysfunction but also typical spongiform changes in the brain. More than 20 different mutations have been found in familial forms of CJD, FFI, or GSS. There is no doubt now that abnormal prion protein can cause a disease.

These cases explain how the diseases can be inherited and they provide strong evidence that the agent is a protein encoded in the PrP gene, which is located on human chromosome 20. Showing a mutation can also provide key information in the differential diagnosis of mid-life dementia. To prove the diagnosis, it was once necessary to inject tissue from the patient into the brain of an animal, which was a cumbersome and time-consuming test. Now the diagnosis of an inherited prion disease can be made by DNA analysis on a sample of blood or tissue. Also, in either inherited or sporadic cases, tagged specific antibodies to PrP can be applied to an extract of tissue. The trick here is to differentiate the normal PrP – which is sensitive to digestion by a specific enzyme which chews up proteins so they can be removed from the tissue being tested – from the altered form of the enzyme, which resists this treatment (protease-resistant). The abnormal form is called PrP-scrapie and abbreviated as PrP^{Sc}, which accumulates in cells, forms amyloid plaques, and exerts a toxic effect. This presumably leads to the spongiform pathology and cell death. However, it is not known how the abnormal PrP exerts its noxious effect.[20]

Prusiner's work had so far explained two of the three heretical views, that the agent was a protein and that it was both infectious and hereditary. But there was still the issue of replication. If the prion protein was present in normal brains, where it was not only innocuous but also presumably useful, how did it get converted to the abnormal toxic form? Another mystery was added when Prusiner and his colleagues found the same amino acid composition in both the normal and abnormal forms.

The difference seems to lie in the three-dimensional structure of the proteins. The normal PrP exists in a spiral configuration called the alpha helix; the abnormal protease-resistant form is physically different, composed largely of what are called *beta sheets*. The difference is one of "conformation" and can be detected only by sophisticated techniques of physical chemistry, including x-ray diffraction. This discovery was yet another heretical view because it had long been believed that the three-dimensional structure or conformation of a protein was an automatic result of the amino acid sequence. Yet normal and abnormal PrP have the same amino acid sequence.

These discoveries by Prusiner and his associates quieted the "vicious" attacks, which came mostly from journalists who seemed to provoke competing researchers to express their antagonisms. There has not been much debate, however, since Prusiner piled on the evidence for which he won award after award through the decade of the 90s. The criticisms almost disappeared after the 1997 Nobel Prize, though civilly stated questions remain.[21]

The challenge now for Prusiner and other investigators studying prions is to determine how the change from normal to abnormal comes about. In iatrogenic disease, seeding the brain with abnormal PrP by a dural graft or a surgical instrument converts the normal protein to the abnormal. How does the abnormal version induce the change from normal to pathologic?

These questions are particularly relevant today because of the specter of bovine spongiform encephalopathy (BSE) or "mad cow disease" and what may be its human form, called *variant CJD* or vCJD. This epidemic raises many scientific questions as well as social concerns. It is the ultimate question about the species barrier – how a disease of sheep became a disease of cows and then a human disease.

The disease in cows was attributed to faulty industrial practices.[22] It has long been a practice to feed cows the remains or offal from sheep; even if the animals had been affected, the process of rendering eliminated the PrP. However, in 1981 a new rendering method omitted a solvent that extracted fat in the process. Elimination of that solvent proved to be disastrous. The first cases of mad cow disease were reported in 1986. Feeding cattle bone meal or offal was banned in 1988 and at least 160,000 possibly infected cows were slaughtered in the United Kingdom, with a subsequent decline in frequency there. Nevertheless, the epidemic has still spread throughout the meat farms of Europe. So far, the United States has been spared.

The economic consequences were immense but the health consequences became even more urgent when the first cases of human vCJD were identified in 1995. The syndrome differed from typical CJD because the patients were younger (between ages 20 and 40 rather than older than 50), because symptoms diverged (psychiatric disorders more often preceded the dementia), and the pathology differed, with more prominent clumps of abnormal PrP in a pattern that resembled the changes in kuru rather than sporadic CJD. Eighty cases had been recognized in the United Kingdom by September 2000.[23]

Variant CJD is considered a form of BSE because the strains of PrP seem to be identical in incubation periods, and the brain pathology is similar when infected human brain tissue is injected into laboratory animals. Prusiner and his team have provided "compelling evidence" that human vCJD and bovine agents are the

Theoretical progression of the transmission of bovine spongiform encephalopathy (BSE or "mad cow" disease) from cattle to humans via BSE prions

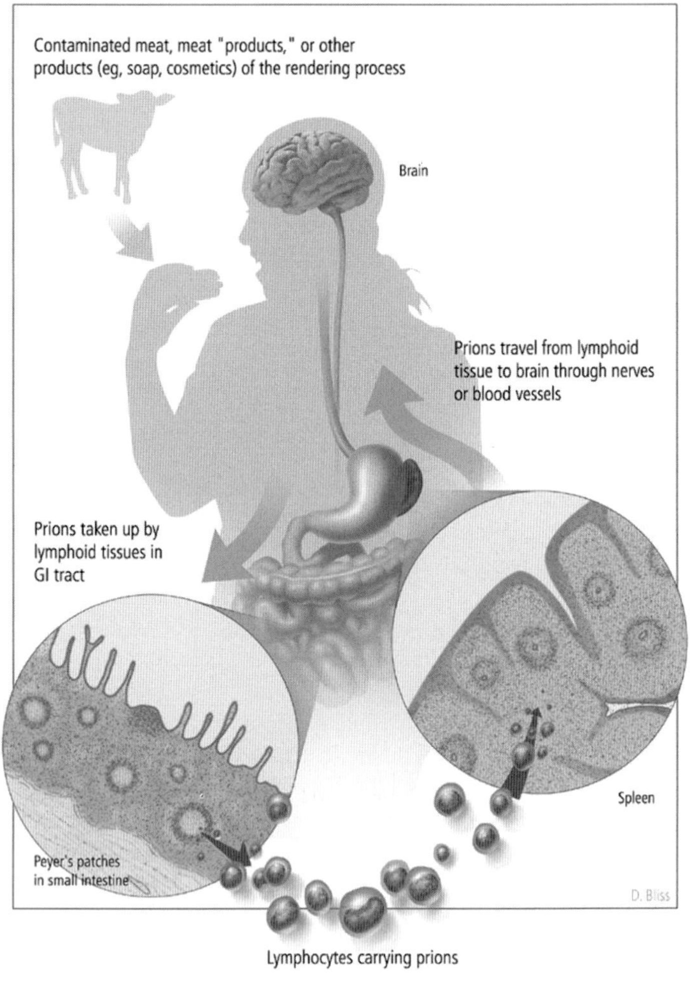

same.[24] In transgenic mice bearing the cow-PrP, they have found identical features of disease, including the incubation period, pathology, and physical properties of agent after injection of human vCJD brain or bovine PrP-scrapie. Transmission by ingestion of food harks back to kuru, but how that actually happens is not known. It raises concerns about possible transmission by blood transfusion, still more of a fear than a fact, because there has been no example of blood-borne transmission.[25] Perhaps most important, vCJD makes more urgent the development of treatment.

Clearly, there is much yet to be done. For instance, the normal functions of the prion protein are not known. Similar proteins have been found in yeast, making it clear that they have been conserved in the long process of evolution from simple organisms to humans since they are presumably important in normal cells. The transgenic experiments do not explain transmissibility – how the disease can appear in laboratory animals after injection of tissue from an affected person or another animal. There is no clear explanation for observations of strains of PrP that differ in the incubation times of the disease in animals, or in the clinical features of the disease. The species barrier and self-replication are challenges. Another question is how sporadic CJD starts in the first place. And it is not clear how the nature of the amino acid at one locus in the gene (codon 129) affects the physical structure of the protein and so determines whether the clinical manifestations are those of fatal insomnia or CJD.[26]

Prusiner's major concerns now are the development of a diagnostic test for BSE, the development of effective treatment, and the elucidation of the role of an abnormal protein in causing an age-related degenerative disease of the brain. Knowing how this works in prion diseases might offer a clue to similar mechanisms in Alzheimer and other dementing diseases, Parkinson disease, and amyotrophic lateral sclerosis (Lou Gehrig's disease). Abnormal proteins are important in those diseases, too. Working to solve these problems ought to keep Prusiner productively occupied for many years.

1 Autobiography of Stanley B. Prusiner. [www.nobel.se/laureates/medicine-1997-1-autobio.html].

2 Sigurdsson B. Rida, a chronic encephalitis of sheep with general remarks on infections which develop slowly and some of their special characteristics. *Brit Vet J* 1954;110:341-354.

3 Prusiner SB. The prion diseases. *Brain Pathol* 1998;8:499-513.

4 Johnson RT, Gibbs CJ, Jr. Creutzfeldt-Jakob disease and related transmissible spongiform encephalopathies. *N Engl J Med* 1998;339:1994-2004.

5 Prusiner SB. Novel proteinaceous infectious particles cause scrapie. *Science* 1982;216:136-144.

6 Alper T, Haig DA, Clarke MC. The exceptionally small size of the scrapie agent. *Biochem Biophys Res Comm* 1966;22:278-284.

7 Alper T, Cramp WA, Haig DA, Clarke MC. Does the agent of scrapie replicate without nucleic acid? *Nature* 1967;214:764-766.

8 Griffith JS. Self-replication and scrapie. *Nature* 1967;215:1043-1044.

9 Gajdusek DC. Unconventional viruses and the origin and disappearance of kuru. *Science* 1977;197:943-960.

10 Gibbs CJ, Jr, Gajdusek DC, Latearjet R. Unusual resistance to ionizing radiation of the viruses of kuru, Creutzfeldt-Jakob disease and scrapie. *Proc Natl Acad Sci USA* 1978;75:6268-6270.

11 Prusiner SB. Development of the prion concept. In Prusiner SB, ed. *Prion Biology and Diseases*. Cold Spring Harbor, NY: Cold Spring Harbor Laboratory Press, 1999, p. 70.

12 Prusiner SB. Nobel Lecture: Prions. *Proc Natl Acad Sci USA* 1998;95;13363-13383.

13 Prusiner SB, Collinge J, Powell J, Anderton B, eds. *Prion Diseases of Humans and Animals*. London: Ellis Horwood, 1992.

14 Prusiner SB, Groth DF, Bolton DC, Kenet SB, Hood LE. Purification and structural studies of a major scrapie prion protein. *Cell* 1984;38:127-134.

15 Basler K, Oesch B, Scott M, Westaway D, Walchi M, Gdroth DF, McKinley MP, Prusiner SB, Weissmann C. Scrapie and cellular PrP isoforms are encoded by the same chromosomal gene. *Cell* 1986;46:417-426.

16 Bockman JM, Kingsbury DT, McKinley MP, Bendheim PE, Prusiner SB. Creutzfeldt-Jakob disease prion proteins in human brains. *N Engl J Med* 1985; 312:73-78.

17 Brown P, Coker-Vann M, Pomeroy K, et al. Diagnosis of Creutzfeldt-Jakob disease by Western blot identification of marker protein in human brain tissue. *N Engl J Med* 1986;314:547-551.

18 Bockman JM, Prusiner SB, Tateishi J, Kingsbury DT. Immunoblotting of Creutzfeldt-Jakob disease prion proteins: host species-specific epitopes. *Ann Neurol* 1987;21:589-595.

19 Hsaio KK, Baker HF, Crow TJ, et al. Linkage of a prion protein missense variant to Gerstmann-Sträussler syndrome. *Nature* 1989; 338:342-345.

20 Prusiner SB. Interview with author, November 30, 2000.

21 Chesebro B. Prion protein and the transmissible spongiform encephalopathy diseases. *Neuron* 1999;24:503-506.

22 Prusiner SB. Prion diseases and the BSE crisis. *Science* 1997;278:245-251.

23 Balter M. Tracking the human fallout from "mad cow disease." *Science* 2000; 289:1452-1454.

24 Scott MR, Will R, Ironside J, Nguyen HOB, Tremblay P, DeArmond SJ, Prusiner SB. Compelling transgenetic evidence for transmission of bovine spongiform encephalopathy prions to humans. *Proc Natl Acad Sci USA* 1999;96:15137-15142.

25 Brown P, Cerrvenakova L, McShane LM, Barber P, Rubenstein R, Drohan WN. Further studies of blood infectivity in an experimental model of transmissible spongiform encephalopathy, with an explanation of why blood components do not transmit Creutzfeldt-Jakob disease. *Transfusion* 1999;39:1169-1178.

26 Parchi P, Zou W, Wang W, et al. Genetic influence on the structural variations of the abnormal prion protein. *Proc Natl Acad Sci USA* 2000;97:10168-10172.

CHAPTER NINETEEN

CELEBRATING THE SYNAPSE

Although their awards were made 30 years apart, there is a direct link between the discoveries of Julius Axelrod, the 1970 Nobelist, and the year 2000 trio of Arvid Carlsson, Paul Greengard, and Eric Kandel. Prior awards also recognized their interconnected research. For example, Axelrod, Carlsson, and Greengard shared the 1989 Bristol-Myers Squibb Award. Also, in 1997, Kandel and Greengard shared The Charles A. Dana Award. The honors acknowledged their fundamental contributions to concepts of synaptic transmission: how one nerve cell transmits information to another neuron, or to a muscle or gland.

Axelrod was a permanent NIH staff scientist, first in the Heart Institute, then in the combined NIMH-NINDB program led by Seymour Kety. The other three were transient investigators at NIH – in three different institutes – Carlsson and Greengard in the Heart Institute, and Kandel in Kety's NIMH-NINDB program. Early in his career, Greengard was supported by a postdoctoral fellowship from NINDB. Later, Greengard and Kandel received extramural support from both NIMH and NINDS. Their experience illustrates the overlap of neuroscience research regardless of the institute involved.

Carlsson's research in the Heart Institute came from investigations of high blood pressure and, unintentionally, proved to be more important for brain science than for cardiology. He came to the Heart Institute to learn the methods of modern pharmacology. His experience there led him to work on psychosis; in doing so, he made a fundamental contribution to a neurological disorder.

Some called the 2000 Nobel Prize in Medicine "a celebration of the synapse."[1] Carlsson's work led to treatment of Parkinson

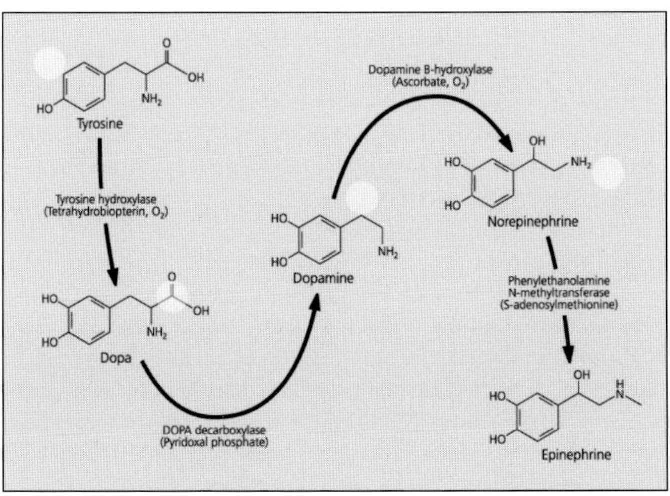

CHEMICAL STRUCTURE OF THE MAJOR NEUROTRANSMITTERS DOPAMINE, NOREPINEPHRINE, AND EPINEPHRINE

disease and to a major theory of the pathogenesis of schizophrenia, as well as the development of a new class of drugs, the serotonin re-uptake inhibitors, which are prescribed to treat depression. Greengard elucidated the mechanism of action of these drugs, and Kandel explored the role of synaptic changes in learning and memory, giving promise of pharmacological therapy for memory loss and dementia.

To understand their contributions, it is helpful to consider the concept of chemical neurotransmitters,[2] which are chemicals released by one cell to activate another. In the 1930s, Otto Loewi found that stimulation of the vagus nerve released acetylcholine from nerve terminals in the heart and acted to control the heart rate. This is a form of "cholinergic" transmission. Although a person can control motion of the limbs (a "voluntary" system), the heart rate cannot be willfully modified. Instead it is "involuntary" or "autonomic." Other involuntary muscles are found in the bowel, bladder, and blood vessels.

Soon thereafter, Sir Henry Dale, in England, found autonomic nerve systems where the transmitter was "adrenergic," not cholinergic, The transmitter in these nerves is adrenalin (also known as epinephrine) or noradrenalin (norepinephrine). Norepinephrine is a precursor of epinephrine; they are chemical look-alikes, differing only in the addition of a methyl group (CH_3).

One characteristic of neurotransmitters is that they are released from the nerve cell and act on an effector cell in the immediate vicinity, separated by only a microscopic gap. In contrast, hormones such as epinephrine are released by one organ into the blood and carried to a remote receiving system in a second organ of the body. As a hormone, epinephrine is synthesized in the adrenal gland, secreted into the blood, and widely circulated to prepare an individual under stress for "fight or flight."

Compared to epinephrine, norepinephrine is more often a neurotransmitter than a hormone and, as described in the chapter about Julius Axelrod, is found mostly in nerve terminals. In the 1930s, Dale and his associates found that transmission from nerve to skeletal muscle is also cholinergic. By 1950, it was generally accepted that transmission from nerve to muscle – voluntary or autonomic – is chemical, not electrical.

Chemical transmission at these sites involves two cells – either two neurons (nerve cells) or one neuron and a muscle cell. The junction between them is the synapse, a word derived from a Greek term meaning "to clasp." The first nerve cell is "presynaptic" and the second, "postsynaptic." The flow of information is one-way. In later years, it was learned that the process comprises four steps: synthesis of the transmitter; storage and release of the transmitter; interaction of the transmitter with a specific receptor on the postsynaptic membrane; and removal of transmitter from the synaptic cleft. Each of these steps was to prove important in the design of drugs and in the understanding of human diseases.

However, evidence of chemical transmission was limited to "peripheral" transmission in the autonomic nervous system or at the neuromuscular junction for voluntary muscle. There was still debate about communication between nerve cells in the brain – whether it was electrical or chemical. As late as 1963, a prominent investigator could claim that no transmitter other than acetylcholine was known to serve in the brain or spinal cord.[3] That was not precisely true because, in 1946, von Euler, a Swiss investigator, had discovered norepinephrine in the brain and shared the 1970 Nobel with Axelrod (even though the function of that transmitter in the brain was not yet known). Also, the findings of Arvid Carlsson had already started in the mid-1950s and were essential in proving the chemical theory. As often happens, however, it took almost a decade for general acceptance of his data and his theory.

Axelrod and Carlsson both provided information to support the theory of chemical transmission in the central nervous system (CNS). Axelrod proved that the transmitter activity of norepinephrine begins when it is released from nerve terminals, and is terminated by re-uptake into the same nerve terminals. At about the same time, Carlsson found that another substance, dopamine, acted similarly – but in different parts of the CNS. Greengard's contribution was to delineate the chemical events in the postsynaptic neuron that respond to the presynaptic message. And Kandel showed how changes in the synapse (synaptic plasticity) provide the molecular basis of memory.

It is convenient to describe the work of this modern quartet of NINDS-linked investigators in historical sequence. Axelrod's work on transmission started in 1955, when he moved from the Heart Institute to Seymour Kety's research program in NIMH and NINDB. Just at that time, Carlsson arrived in the laboratory of Bernard Brodie, from which Axelrod had just departed. That brief visit transformed Carlsson's research, which he elaborated in the next decade and thereafter. Greengard's work on neurotransmission can be dated to 1969, more than a decade after Axelrod and Carlsson had started. Kandel's work overlapped all the other three.

1 Balter M. Celebrating the synapse. *Science* 2000;290:424.

2 Schwartz JH. Neurotransmitters. In Kandel ER, Schwartz JH, Jessell TM. *Principles of Neural Science*, 4th ed. New York: McGraw-Hill, 2000:280-297.

3 Carlsson A. Perspectives on the discovery of central monoaminergic neurotransmission. *Ann Rev Neurosci* 1987:10:19-40.

CHAPTER TWENTY

JULIUS AXELROD, PH.D.

The Nobel Prize in Physiology or Medicine, 1970

Awarded jointly to Julius Axelrod, Sir Bernard Katz and Ulf von Euler for their discoveries concerning the humoral transmitters in the nerve terminals and the mechanism for their storage, release and inactivation.

Dr. Julius Axelrod's *discoveries concern the mechanisms which regulate the formation of this important transmitter in the nerve cells and the mechanisms which are involved in the inactivation of noradrenaline, partly under the influence of an enzyme discovered by himself.*

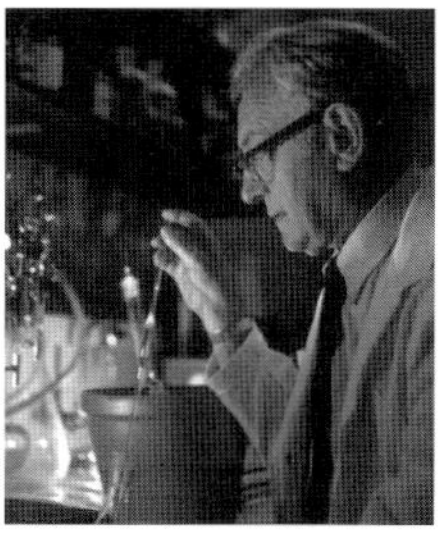

JULIUS AXELROD IN THE LABORATORY AT NIMH, 1976

Julius Axelrod won the 1970 Nobel Prize with two other neuroscientists, Bernard Katz of London and Ulf von Euler of Stockholm. All three had elucidated the mechanisms of synaptic transmission, how one nerve cell communicates with another neuron or with a muscle. Their work was essential in proving that transmission in most synapses is chemical, not electrical. In the process they facilitated the development of biological psychiatry. Axelrod's work paved the way for the prize-winning research of 2000, which provided the details of chemical transmission, led to treatment for Parkinson disease, and led to the development of serotonin re-uptake inhibitors for the treatment of depression.

Axelrod's career was marked by unforeseen twists and turns. He was born in New York in 1912. His parents were poor immigrants who spoke Yiddish, not English. He attended a public high school and was admitted to New York University (NYU), a private college. He could not afford to stay there and transferred to City College, an excellent academic school with no tuition for New York residents. Like so many of his generation, he was lured to medical research by Paul de Kruif's *Microbe Hunters* and he wanted to go to medical school.

But when he graduated in 1933, there was a strict 10 percent quota for Jews in most American medical schools and the private schools mostly declined to admit students from City College. Worse, the United States was in the depths of the Depression and the unemployment rate was 20 percent. Axelrod felt fortunate to obtain a position as a laboratory assistant at NYU with a salary of $25 a month.

Two years later that position terminated for lack of funds and he transferred to a laboratory related to the New York City Department of Health. He stayed there until 1946, testing the truth of labeling claims that vitamins had been added to foods. He gained experience in laboratory methods that had been described in biochemical journals. The laboratory subscribed to the *Journal of*

Biological Chemistry, which he read avidly. He gained an M.S. degree in chemistry by taking courses at night. He married and had two children. He was deferred from Army service during World War II because a laboratory accident had left him blind in his left eye.

In 1946, his laboratory was commissioned by drug manufacturers to investigate the problem of methemoglobinemia, a condition that prevents hemoglobin from carrying oxygen. Depending on the severity of the condition, an affected person becomes cyanotic (the skin turns from healthy pink to an ominous blue) because there is insufficient oxygen in the blood. The disorder was seen in some people who used common over-the-counter non-aspirin painkillers that included acetanilide or phenacetin. Axelrod's boss, George Wallace, suggested that he consult with Bernard Brodie, who had been doing research on antimalarial drugs at Goldwater Memorial Hospital (now Coler-Goldwater). Wallace and Brodie knew each other because they had been in the Pharmacology Department together at NYU.

James Shannon, who was later to become a Director of NIH, led the laboratory at Goldwater. Among Shannon's many talents was a gift for picking talented young scientists, including Bernard Brodie, who loomed like a gigantic scientific shadow over Axelrod and Carlsson. As we will see, Brodie affected Greengard's career even though they never worked together. At Goldwater, Shannon's team included a future director of the Heart Institute and a Dean at Yale (Robert Berliner), a leader of the Association of American Medical Colleges (John Sherman), a tinkerer who developed an instrument essential for Axelrod and Carlsson (Robert Bowman), and an outstanding biochemist (Sidney Udenfriend).

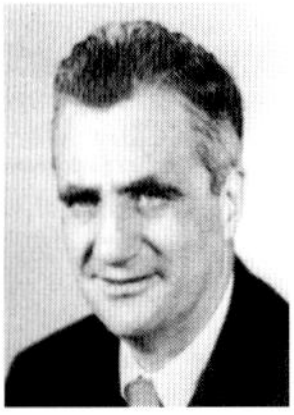

Bernard Brodie, M.D. (NHLBI)

Their urgent mission started at Goldwater during World War II. It was imperative to develop new malaria treatments besides quinine, since the Japanese had captured most of the world's supply. Shannon assigned the project to Brodie.

Looking back later, Axelrod[1] said that what Brodie did "was really revolutionary for that time. He measured plasma levels of drugs. And to do that he devised methods to measure the antimalarial drugs." Atabrine was the only available substitute for quinine, but there was virtually no quantitative information about the drug. It was taken by mouth, but what happened in the body was totally unknown. American troops were non-compliant; atabrine turned their skin yellow and had other unpleasant effects. Malaria was deadly. Something had to be done.

Brodie's team developed a method to measure the amount of the drug in body fluids and tissues. They could track blood levels after a single dose and determine the patterns of peak levels after taking different amounts. With that information they could recommend a new dosing schedule that was much more effective in treating symptomatic malaria or in preventing attacks. It was also more acceptable to soldiers. The effort was a huge success practically and theoretically; it also enhanced the reputations of both Shannon and Brodie.

Brodie was a powerful figure who garnered a Lasker Award in 1967. He is still recognized as the pioneer of *pharmacokinetics*, the study of the distribution of drugs in the body, transformations of the drug into other compounds, and medical actions of the drug and its derivatives.[2] Many expected him to share the Nobel Prize with Axelrod, and Axelrod nominated Brodie for the prize three times.[3]

Bernard Brodie was called "Steve" after the noted saloon-keeper who had jumped from the Brooklyn Bridge on a bet. Brodie had worked his way through medical school playing poker. Then he became a champion boxer in the Canadian army. He took his chances in science, too – and he mostly won.

At the suggestion of George Wallace, Axelrod went to see Brodie for technical advice. Their first conversation lasted several hours. Axelrod was entranced by Brodie's knowledge and imagination. Brodie pointed out that many drugs are transformed in the body and may be converted into other active or toxic derivatives. That view profoundly affected Axelrod.

Brodie asked him to draw the structure of acetanilide on the blackboard, which Axelrod did quickly. Brodie immediately saw that one of the products of the drug could be aniline, a derivative of benzene that was used to make industrial dyes. Aniline was already known to be toxic to hemoglobin. Brodie invited Axelrod to join his laboratory and work on the problem. Axelrod, skilled in chemical methods from his experience with vitamins, soon developed a way to measure small amounts of aniline, which he found in the plasma and urine of volunteers who took the drugs. They also found a direct relationship between blood levels of aniline and the amount of methemoglobin, implying cause-and-effect.

In doing that work, Axelrod and associates made another important observation. Seeking other products of acetanilide metabolism, they identified acetaminophen as the major effective pain-relieving derivative of the original drug. In their published report, Brodie and Axelrod noted that this product might itself be an effective analgesic.

Acetaminophen is now called Tylenol, the popular non-prescription pain reliever. In that less commercial era, however, scientists were not concerned with entrepreneurial opportunities. Axelrod never filed a patent and later said that he "never made a penny" on the discovery.[4] But that was his first scientific paper and by then he was committed to research. He knew he had the skills for laboratory investigation.

In his autobiographical essays,[5-7] Axelrod was consistently deferential to Brodie and acknowledged his indebtedness to his mentor. He called Brodie magnetic, stimulating, and charismatic.[1] In a 1996 interview,[1] however, he also said:

> I published many papers with Brodie but I got only one senior authorship although I initiated and did most of our work. And I realized I had very little chance getting any place in an academic institution with a Master's degree. I needed a Ph.D. I was married with two children. Either I didn't want to or was afraid it would be too difficult to get a Ph.D. I didn't want to think about it.
>
> I saw an item in *The New York Times* – Dr. Shannon has been appointed the Director of the National Heart Institute in Bethesda. I wrote to him for a position and he offered me one. He also persuaded Brodie to come to Bethesda and when I went there I was assigned to Brodie's laboratory. I worked for a year or two and then I was offered a position in a drug company. When I told Brodie I would like to leave, Dr. Brodie asked me what would make me stay. I told him I wanted to do my own research. Brodie agreed and asked me to stay.

It seems as though Axelrod had tried to escape from Brodie – or, at least, tried to become independent of Brodie – by applying to NIH through Shannon, only to find out that Shannon was moving the whole Goldwater team to NIH and Axelrod would once again be under Brodie. Nevertheless, he became an independent investigator and began to work on caffeine. Even without the doctorate he was elected to membership in the prestigious American Society of Pharmacology in 1953.

At that time he became interested in the *sympathomimetic amines*, chemicals that have effects similar to those of stimulation of the autonomic (sympathetic) nervous system – which controls the heart, blood vessels, blood pressure, intestines, and bladder. Among the compounds were amphetamine, mescaline, and ephedrine, which also have behavioral effects. Axelrod found that all were subject to diverse metabolic conversions – and that the pathways differed in different species, implying a genetic component in controlling the different routes. It was not so clear at the time but drugs, behavior, and genes were going to come together some day.

When Axelrod studied the fate of amphetamine in rabbits, it "disappeared without a trace," suggesting that it might be degraded by an enzyme. His biochemistry advisor was Gordon Tomkins, who worked at an adjacent laboratory bench and told him that all "you need for that kind of study is a method to measure amphetamine, an animal liver, and a razor blade for making thin tissue slices." Axelrod found that adenosine triphosphate (ATP) and other co-factors were needed. If a single one was omitted the reaction would not work.

At about that time, other investigators were developing methods to isolate some of the particulate components of cells – surface membranes, mitochondria, nuclei, and other organelles. Axelrod found that none of the fractions worked if separated from the others, but when small cellular particles called microsomes were combined with the cell fluids, amphetamine rapidly disappeared when the co-factors were added.

Some characteristics of the reaction implied that this was a unique phenomenon. By heating the fractions separately to inactivate the enzyme, he soon determined that the enzyme was in the microsomes, not the cell fluids. By the end of June 1953 he concluded that he had found a new enzyme, localized in the microsomes, requiring a co-factor called TPNH and oxygen. (TPNH is triphosphopyridine nucleotide reduced form.) It could add or remove amino and methyl groups from drugs.

Other members of the laboratory found similar reactions in the metabolism of other drugs, including several different biochemical reactions: the oxidation of barbiturates, removing a methyl group from ephedrine, and removing an amino group from amphetamine. There were still other reactions and the diversity made Axelrod realize that he had come to a major discovery. This enzyme system proved to be important in the disposition of many different and commonly used drugs. The microsomes are effective defense systems that protect the body by the enzymatic disposal of drugs and other foreign chemicals after they enter the body. Axelrod considered "the discovery of the microsomal enzymes among the best work I did."[2]

He extended his work to include narcotics and developed a theory for the development of tolerance, namely that continuous interaction between the drugs and the microsomal enzymes could inactivate the enzymes. Alternatively, the decreased response to narcotic drugs might result from unavailability of the drug receptors.

Despite his productive studies of caffeine, amphetamine, ephedrine, and the microsomal enzymes, Axelrod realized that, without a doctoral degree, he could not be promoted to higher rank in the Heart Institute, nor shake free of Brodie's control. He made arrangements to use his research for a doctoral dissertation and took the required courses at George Washington University. He was awarded the Ph.D. in 1955, at age 42.

In the next move in Axelrod's career, he worked in the laboratory of Edward Evarts, who was working under Seymour Kety. Evarts, a psychiatrist and physiologist, later became famous for the first intracellular recordings of nerve cells in the motor cortex of waking animals. At the time of Axelrod's move, he was working with the street hallucinogen, LSD. A 1996 interview[1] makes it clear that the transition was more than a straightforward recruitment. In Axelrod's words:[1]

> I submitted two abstracts on the enzymatic metabolism of amphetamine and ephedrine for the usual meeting of the American Society of Pharmacology and Therapeutics. Brodie

saw these later and was upset. He knew it was an important discovery and he set the whole laboratory to work on this problem. I hate to tell you this, I owe a great deal to Brodie, but this was something that upset me very much. Brodie wished to write a paper on this group of enzymes, the microsomal enzymes, as they are called now, with himself as the senior author. [Axelrod later said that Brodie told team members that their names would appear alphabetically. Then, realizing that A comes before B, he added: "But my name comes first."]

I now thought I had to get my Ph.D. and leave Brodie's lab. To get a Ph.D., I took a year off and went to George Washington Medical School. By the time I got my Ph.D., Shannon had become head of the entire NIH.

I sent applications to both the National Cancer Institute and the National Institute of Mental Health and I received a call from Seymour Kety, who was at that time Director of the intramural program of the NIMH. He interviewed me for the position. I knew he was interested in me. He sent my application to several laboratories in the Institute. There was one laboratory I wanted to work in and that was Giulio Cantoni's, a well-known biochemist who discovered S-adenosylmethionine, but I didn't get to work with him. I was hired by Ed Evarts, a neurophysiologist and psychiatrist.

Evarts was a lovely man. He was the Head of a Laboratory of Clinical Science and he did a lot of fundamental work on the central control of motion. At that time, Evarts was interested in biological psychiatry. He saw my papers on amphetamine and asked me to come and work in his laboratory. This was just as I was taking my Ph.D. He was working on LSD at that time. In my spare time, while going to class, I was working on the metabolism of LSD. We published a paper in *Nature* in 1955. We developed a fluorescent method for measuring it and found that incredibly small amounts of LSD in the brain could cause behavioral effects.

The philosophy of Seymour Kety in the NIMH was to hire the best people you can and leave them alone because they are in the best position to know what problems are important, doable, and possibly relevant to the institution. This was a great philosophy for me. I knew nothing about neuroscience or the brain. I had worked in the Heart Institute and I felt almost intimidated by these bright physiologists and psychiatrists working on these electrical phenomena. They were all very good talkers – especially Kety.

Kety warned Axelrod that working with Cantoni might reproduce his experience with Brodie, another reason for his choice of Evarts.

The freewheeling independent atmosphere fostered by Kety and Evarts was a world away from the tightly controlled and aggressively competitive attitude of Brodie. Axelrod quoted Kety as reassuring him that he did not have to do "psychiatric" research by saying: "Good science is better than conspicuous relevance."

Naturally, there is another side to the story – Brodie's. However, it is difficult to find an autobiography or an oral history by Brodie. To this day, Axelrod acknowledges his debt to Brodie, but the split was irrevocable. The most detailed telling of the story is recorded in a book, "*Apprentice to Genius.*"[8] The author, Robert Kanigel, gave a balanced interpretation of the tensions. When, at age 88, Axelrod was asked if he liked the Kanigel book, Axelrod answered: "Of course. I still have five copies."

In an autobiography,[2] Axelrod described his entry into brain chemistry. He said he "thought that a study of LSD would be an appropriate problem for my new laboratory at the NIMH. LSD was then used as an experimental drug by psychiatrists to study abnormal behavior." Close to home, Evarts had been giving the hallucinogen to volunteers.

One of the many bright lights on Brodie's team was Robert Bowman, who had just developed a new instrument that could be useful for measuring infinitesimally small amounts of chemicals in tissue and blood. Axelrod borrowed Bowman's spectrophotofluorometer and developed a sensitive assay for LSD. He credited the new device for advancements made in measuring epinephrine, dopamine, and serotonin, among other compounds. He recognized that these methods "were crucial in the subsequent rapid expansion in neurotransmitter research."

Axelrod and his associates[9,10] found that LSD was distributed widely in the body, including the brain and cerebrospinal fluid; the distribution suggested that it passed the blood-brain barrier. Tiny amounts in the brain of a cat created the well-known behavioral effects. The drug was metabolized, not excreted, and the only organ in the body involved in that degradation was the liver. As with his earlier experience with amphetamine, the microsomal enzyme system was responsible for an oxidation reaction that transformed LSD.

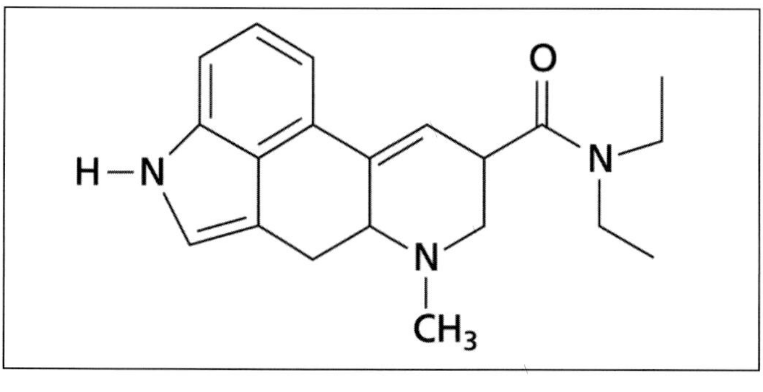

CHEMICAL COMPOSITION OF LSD

PROTOTYPE OF THE SPECTROPHOTO-FLUOROMETER

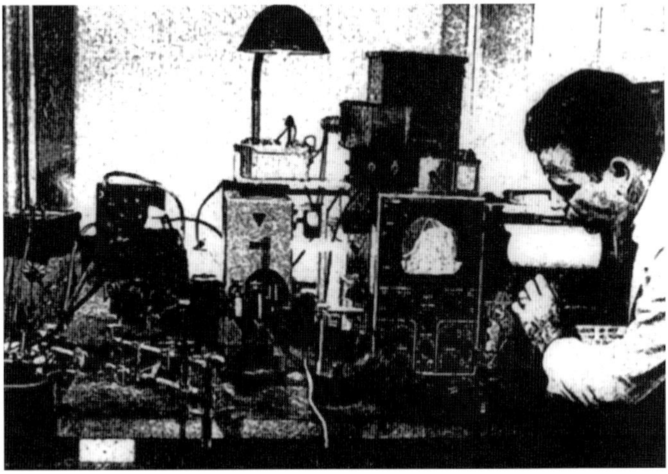

His published papers established that the disappearance of LSD was slowed by serotonin, reserpine, and chlorpromazine (Thorazine), all key agents in the emergence of psychopharmacology.

These were Axelrod's first papers after he joined NIMH and they were the first reports to show the power of the spectrophotofluorometer. The sensitivity of that instrument to miniscule amounts of a transmitter or a drug made it possible to find out where these chemicals were in the nervous system, or elsewhere in the body, and how the drug acted; Bowman's technical advance opened a new era of neuroscience.

At the same time that Axelrod was studying LSD at NIMH, Brodie was experimenting with the compound in the Heart Institute. Brodie had just completed work showing that reserpine blocked the action of LSD on serotonin. Within weeks, Arvid Carlsson arrived in the Brodie laboratory and started the work that led to his Nobel Prize in 2000. It is uncertain if Axelrod told Brodie about LSD, Brodie told Axelrod, or both had the idea independently and simultaneously. Their experiments, however, transformed Carlsson's research, as described in the next chapter.

Roscoe Brady[11] believes that he himself was the one who brought LSD to Axelrod's attention. Thinking that degradation of LSD might result from the action of an enzyme he was evaluating, Brady initiated the studies and sought to collaborate with Axelrod, who already had experience with so many drugs. When they worked together, the enzyme turned out to be not Brady's but, once again, Axelrod's microsomal system.

Axelrod made yet another important contribution in his early days at NIMH. Just before he left the Heart Institute, a chance meeting with biochemist Jack Strominger led to discovery of the enzymes involved in the conjugation of drugs and metabolites to compounds called glucuronides. In the process they discovered the enzymatic defect in a congenital form of jaundice. Also, with Rudi Schmid, they identified the mechanism of metabolism of bilirubin, which is formed in the liver and is responsible for the jaundice in people with gallstones. A side project for Axelrod had wide-ranging effects.

After LSD, Axelrod tuned his attention to his masterwork. It started when Kety gave a departmental seminar about a report by two psychiatrists who noted that if adrenalin was exposed to air on a piece of filter paper, a pink spot appeared. The new product was called adrenochrome and, when it was taken by mouth in tiny amounts, the resulting symptoms were like those of schizophrenia. The psychiatrists suggested that schizophrenia might be caused by adrenochrome, which they thought was the product of an abnormal metabolism of epinephrine.

Axelrod reviewed the literature and found that almost nothing was known about the metabolism of epinephrine. If the normal pathways were not known, it would not be possible to attribute schizophrenia to malfunction of the system. Epinephrine was thought to be inactivated by an enzyme, monoamine oxidase (MAO), which was the target of the then-new psychotropic drugs, the MAO-inhibitors. However, even when MAO was inhibited, the physiological actions of epinephrine still terminated and other enzymes had to be involved in the process of inactivation.

After several months of failed experiments in a search to find adrenochrome as a product of epinephrine, one day Axelrod's eye was caught by an abstract reporting the finding of an unusual compound in the urine of people with a rare adrenal tumor that overproduces another catecholamine. (A catecholamine consists of a benzene ring with two adjacent hydroxyl groups and an amine on an ethyl side-chain.) The structure of that overproduced compound included a methyl group on the oxygen of what had originally been a hydroxyl group. Axelrod wondered if epinephrine might undergo that kind of reaction.

That very afternoon, Axelrod incubated epinephrine with rat liver homogenate, ATP and methionine (an amino acid known to be a donor of methyl groups). In the process, the epinephrine rapidly disappeared.

To prove the nature of the reaction, Axelrod obtained S-adenosylmethionine from a postdoctoral fellow in the laboratory of Giulio Cantoni, who had already shown that this compound was the activated intermediate for methylation reactions (adding a CH_3 group to a chemical or a protein). Cantoni was protective of his compound, but happened to be out of town that day. The postdoc gave some to Axelrod, who then found that, as predicted, S-adenosylmethionine sufficed to substitute for the ATP and methionine.

Axelrod asked another laboratory neighbor, Bernhard Witkop, if it were possible to obtain some of the presumed product of the methylation reaction. Within a few days, a chemist in Witkop's group had synthesized it and Axelrod could take the next step. With the synthetic product in hand, they could positively identify the product of the enzymatic reaction.

Soon they found that the same enzyme worked equally well on other catecholamines – norepinephrine, dopamine, and levodopa – which were to return again in Carlsson's studies. They called the enzyme catechol-O-methyltransferase (COMT), which translates to mean "the enzyme that puts a methyl group on the oxygen that had been part of a hydroxyl group." Nevertheless, when this enzyme was inhibited, the action of epinephrine was still terminated, and it also ended when MAO was inhibited. If neither of these enzymes was involved, enzymatic transformation was ruled out. Some other system had to be involved.

Just at that time, Kety wanted to test the possibility that epinephrine metabolism was involved in schizophrenia and he ordered the synthesis of radiolabeled epinephrine from a commercial company. He gave some of the precious material to Axelrod and a visiting scientist, Hans Weil-Malherbe. When they injected it into cats they were puzzled to find that the radioactive epinephrine persisted unchanged in different organs long after its physiological effects had subsided. A similar pattern was seen for norepinephrine in organs rich in sympathetic nerves – heart, spleen, and salivary glands. They thought this might be explained by a previously unknown mechanism, uptake and retention of the catecholamines by sympathetic nerves.

Another visitor to the laboratory did the simple and crucial experiment. Georg Herting from the University of Vienna removed the sympathetic nerves on one side of a cat, causing unilateral degeneration of the nerves to the eye muscles and salivary glands on that side. When they injected the radioactive norepinephrine, the radiolabel accumulated on the normal side and not on the side with the degenerated nerves. This implied that the nerves were gathering up the isotopically labeled material.

Herting and Axelrod proved that hypothesis by stimulating the nerves electrically and finding that the radioactive substance was released from the nerve terminals. They concluded that norepinephrine was rapidly inactivated by re-uptake into the nerves. Later it was learned that this re-uptake mechanism, not enzymatic transformation, is the dominant method for the inactivation of neurotransmitters.[12]

Where in the nerve terminals was the norepinephrine? Lincoln Potter joined Axelrod, and gave labeled norepinephrine to rats. They then fractionated heart muscle and found that the three essential elements traveled together in the same cellular organelles: the labeled norepinephrine, the natural unlabeled catecholamines, and the enzyme that converts dopamine to norepinephrine. This experiment and electron microscopy showed that the transmitter had accumulated in vesicles; other experiments showed that the vesicles were emptied by nerve stimulation.

These results formed the basis of current views about neurotransmitters – that they are synthesized in the cell body and transported down the long, slender nerve processes to the terminals where they are stored in vesicles. Each vesicle contains a pool of transmitters, which are brought to the surface membrane when the nerve is activated by a nerve potential. At the surface, the vesicle is emptied of its contents, which are released into the cleft between the two cells and then act on receptors in the postsynaptic neuron. To terminate the action, the transmitter may be degraded by an enzyme (which is characteristic of the neuromuscular transmitter, acetylcholine) or by re-uptake into the nerve terminals (as Axelrod had shown for norepinephrine and Carlsson did later for dopamine).

Axelrod noted the irony of events. His work with catecholamines was started by Kety, but was fruitful and led to the Nobel Prize. Kety himself, however, ended with a negative result; he found no abnormality of epinephrine metabolism in schizophrenia. The adrenochrome theory was put to rest.

Axelrod then pursued the pineal gland, which is rich in sympathetic nerves[13] but was then the only organ in the body without known functions. At about that time, Aaron Lerner, at Yale, had identified melatonin as the hormone of the pineal. The chemical structure of melatonin suggested to Axelrod that it was synthesized from serotonin.

With Richard Wurtman,[14] Solomon Snyder,[15] and others, he worked out the synthesis of melatonin; the hormone is synthesized by the enzymatic condensation of the amino acid tryptophan and serotonin. They identified serotonin and melatonin-synthesizing enzymes in the gland and found that the amounts varied with the time of day, which is a circadian rhythm. They found that these rhythms were regulated by the release of norepinephrine from the ample supply of sympathetic nerves. For instance, when they again removed the superior cervical ganglion in the neck, removing that nerve supply to the pineal, the circadian rhythm of serotonin was abolished. It also disappeared if the rats were kept constantly in the light, but it persisted if the animals were kept in the dark, indicating there was an intrinsic clock.

These rhythms paralleled changes in the release of norepinephrine from the sympathetic nerves – low levels during the day and high levels at night. The sensitivity of the receptors varied in the opposite direction. When the release of norepinephrine was reduced, the sensitivity of the receptors increased and vice versa. In other words, in daytime, release of the transmitter is at a low level and the receptors become more sensitive. At night, the receptors are supersensitive, but the release of the transmitter increases in its circadian fluctuation, amplifying the action. There was also a corresponding increase in the synthesis of the enzyme that makes melatonin.

The circadian rhythm of melatonin is not an isolated peculiarity. Many body functions vary with the time of day (especially endocrine hormone levels) or the time of the month (as in menstrual cycles) and similar mechanisms are involved.

Axelrod was pleased with the pineal studies because each experiment seemed to bring new information. In contrast to other projects, where failed experiments were the norm, everything Axelrod did with the pineal seemed to bear fruit. For that reason, he regarded the pineal as his "personal antidepressant."[3] The pineal effort was valuable in and of itself but it also exemplifies Axelrod's role as teacher. He was a magnet for young investigators who themselves became outstanding neuroscientists, more than 60 in all.

The discovery of the microsomal enzyme system for metabolizing drugs might have sufficed for a Nobel Prize. The demonstration of nerve re-uptake of neurotransmitters, however, was an even greater landmark in the history of science and had major ramifications. Some parts of Axelrod's works related to the research of all three Nobelists in 2000. Other parts led to the development of antidepressive drugs that block re-uptake of serotonin. At age 88, Axelrod still has a vital interest in the achievements of the neuroscience he did so much to create.[3]

1 Healy D. *The psychopharmacologists.* London: Chapman & Hall, 1996:29-50.
2 Costa E. *Neurochemical pharmacology – a tribute to B. B. Brodie.* New York: Raven Press, 1989.
3 Axelrod J. Interview with author, January 3, 2001.
4 Stevens C. The man who saved himself. *Washingtonian.* June 1993.
5 Axelrod J. In Squire LR, ed. *The History of Neuroscience in Autobiography,* vol. 1. Washington, DC: Society for Neuroscience, 1996:50-79.
6 Axelrod J. Doing research in the intramural program of the National Institutes of Health. *Persp Biol Med* 1986;29:S131-S137.
7 Axelrod J. An unexpected life in research. *Ann Rev Pharmacol Toxicol* 1988; 28:1-23.
8 Kanigel R. *Apprentice to Genius: The Making of a Scientific Discovery.* Baltimore: Johns Hopkins University Press, 1986.
9 Axelrod J, Brady RO, Witkop B, Evarts EV. Metabolism of lysergic acid diethylamide. *Nature* 1956;178:143-144.
10 Axelrod J, Brady RO, Witkop B, Evarts EV. The distribution and metabolism of lysergic acid diethylamide. *Trans New York Acad Sci* 1957;66:435-444.
11 Brady RO. Recorded Telephone Conversation with author, December 5, 2000.
12 Axelrod J. Neurotransmitters. *Sci Am* 1974;230:56-71.
13 Axelrod J. Catecholamine neurotransmitters, psychoactive drugs, and biological clocks: the 1981 Harvey Cushing Oration. *J Neurosurg* 1981;55:660-677.
14 Wurtman RJ, Axelrod J. The pineal gland. *Sci Am* 1965:221:50-60.
15 Snyder SH, Zweig M, Axelrod J, Fischer JE. Control of the circadian rhythm in serotonin content of the rat pineal gland. *Proc Natl Acad Sci USA* 1965;53:301-305.

CHAPTER TWENTY ONE

ARVID CARLSSON, M.D.

The Nobel Prize in Physiology or Medicine, 2000

Awarded jointly to Arvid Carlsson, Paul Greengard, and Eric Kandel for their discoveries concerning signal transduction in the nervous system.

***Arvid Carlsson** is rewarded for his discovery that dopamine is a transmitter in the brain and that it has great importance for our ability to control movements. His research has led to the realization that Parkinson's disease is caused by a lack of dopamine in certain parts of the brain and that an efficient remedy (L-dopa) for this disease could be developed. Arvid Carlsson has made a number of subsequent discoveries, which have further clarified the role of dopamine in the brain. He has thus demonstrated the mode of action of drugs used for the treatment of schizophrenia.*

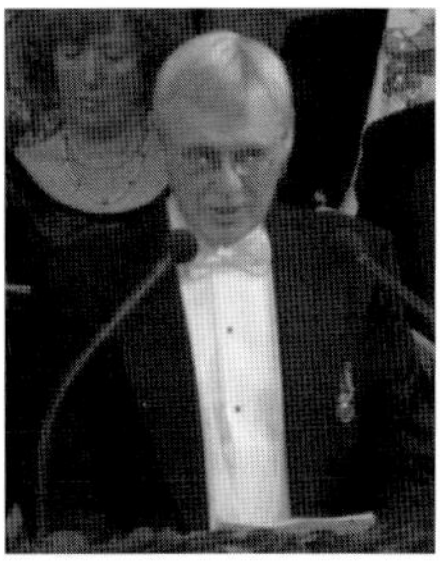

ARVID CARLSSON, M.D., GIVING NOBEL SPEECH

It was during a 6-month sabbatical leave at NIH in 1955, that Nobel winner Arvid Carlsson first began to work with the neurotransmitters that were soon to command his attention for decades. Out of this brief visit came the first truly effective treatment for Parkinson disease and a major class of antidepressant drugs. Some have wondered why it took so long for Carlsson to be recognized by the Nobel Committee.

The basis of Arvid Carlsson's work was a gift of herbal folk medicine, reserpine, a substance extracted from the leaves of the Rauwolfia plant. It had been used for centuries in India to treat snakebite and bowel disease. In 1931, Sen and Bose[1] recorded its use to treat hypertension and psychosis, but their paper in an Indian journal went unnoticed until 1949 when another paper appeared in a British journal. By 1954, American psychiatrist Nathan Kline was using it to treat psychotic patients, although by then it had been noticed that some of the patients developed symptoms of parkinsonism.

This adverse effect turned the world of movement disorders upside down. Back in the late 1940s, Fred Mettler at Columbia University and his students, Malcolm Carpenter and John Whittier, had been busy trying to assign each different type of movement disorder to a specific neuronal structure – chorea to the caudate, ballism to the subthalamic nucleus, and others to be elucidated. Their work led to modern surgical and stimulation therapy for abnormal movements.

But Houston Merritt (and undoubtedly others) opined that the parkinsonian effects of reserpine could only mean that Parkinson disease had to be a biochemical disease, not an anatomical disorder.

It was Carlsson's work that initiated the investigations proving the truth of the biochemical theory. His work – as we shall see – was totally independent but overlapped with Axelrod's in time, place, and theory.

Arvid Carlsson was born in 1923 in Uppsala, Sweden. His father was a professor of history. His mother was a model homemaker of the time, raising her children and assisting her husband in his research. She was a formidable woman. When Carlsson's father died, his mother was 71 years old. She continued her research on the legal status of women in Sweden in the middle ages, published books and articles, and gained a Ph.D. some years later.

Carlsson considered science more "useful" than the liberal arts, but was not involved in science at an early age. He received the equivalent of the M.D. and Ph.D. degrees from the University of Lund in 1951. From that time on, he was involved in laboratory research, first in Lund, and then, in 1959, he became Chair of Pharmacology at the University of Göteborg.

At first Carlsson worked on calcium metabolism and vitamin D, using the then recently introduced radioisotopic tracers. He had started the work with his own doctoral dissertation in 1951 and supervised the dissertations of two students. He was beginning to be recognized, but in 1955 he was a candidate for promotion to associate professor and "the expert committee let me know that in their opinion calcium metabolism did not occupy a central position in pharmacology."[2]

Carlsson asked Sune Bergström, a Nobel laureate, for help in contacting an outstanding American laboratory in biochemical pharmacology. The request ultimately reached Bernard Brodie and led to a 6-month sabbatical leave in Brodie's laboratory in the National Heart Institute. At the time, in 1955, Robert Bowman had just introduced the spectrophotofluorometer for the measurement of biological chemicals that are present in blood and tissues in minute amounts. This instrument, previously unknown to Carlsson, proved to be important to him, ultimately replacing cumbersome biological assays for the neurotransmitters that were soon to command his attention.

The spectrophotofluorometer linked Carlsson to Julius Axelrod, who had just moved from Brodie's laboratory in the Heart Institute to NIMH. In fact, the findings of Axelrod and Carlsson combined to explain the function of neurotransmitters, and their studies of LSD (lysergic acid diethyamide) led to identification of serotonin as a neurotransmitter. In his autobiography, Axelrod[3] wrote:

> I thought that a study of the metabolism and distribution of LSD would be an appropriate problem for my new laboratory in NIMH. LSD was then used as an experimental drug by

psychiatrists to study abnormal behavior. Bob Bowman at the NIH was in the process of building a spectrophotofluorometer. He was kind enough to let me use his experimental model, which allowed me to develop a very sensitive fluorometric assay for LSD. This made it possible to measure the nanogram amounts found in brain and other tissues.

LSD and the fluorometer involved the laboratories of both Axelrod and Brodie, just at the time when Carlsson was visiting. Serotonin was a substance being studied in both labs.

How serotonin was first discovered in the brain is a story that involves a cast of colorful figures[4] whose work sets the background for Carlsson's. Vittorio Erspamer, a professor at the University of Pavia in Italy, discovered serotonin in rabbit intestine in the 1930s and named it enteramine. Irvine Page was the scintillating leader of a team at the Cleveland Clinic that was in search of vasoconstrictive substances that might cause high blood pressure; he hired Maurice Rapport, an organic chemist, and Arda Green, a biochemist. Together, they found the substance in blood and named it "serotonin" to record its origin in serum and its constrictive or "tonic" properties. In 1951, Betty Twarog found that serotonin was the relaxing neurotransmitter in the forceful muscle that clamps shut the shell of a clam. Then came Dilworth W. Wooley, blind from diabetic retinopathy, but having the remarkable capacity to see in his mind's eye that the chemical structure of serotonin was contained within the structure of LSD. His experiments with rat uterus showed that LSD could block the effects of serotonin.

Until he joined NIMH in 1955, Axelrod had been a subordinate in Brodie's laboratory. According to Axelrod, both his laboratory at NIMH and Brodie's in the Heart Institute began to work on LSD independently.[5] But, even though Axelrod borrowed the Bowman spectrophotofluorometer from Brodie's laboratory, they did not discuss LSD. By that time, however, Brodie knew that Irvine Page in Cleveland had identified serotonin as a normal constituent of the brain, as had John Gaddum in England. Wooley and Shaw[6] had noted that serotonin antagonists, including LSD and amphetamines, induced mental aberrations. Wooley found that serotonin could prevent the psychotic behavior of mice given LSD.[7] Gaddum, too, noted the antagonism between LSD and serotonin.

In 1955, 2 months before Carlsson's arrival in his laboratory, Brodie's team reported that reserpine blocked the action of LSD in the brain.[8] Brodie concluded that serotonin "acts to keep us sane."[9] Since reserpine was thought to have an antipsychotic action, Brodie's group gave the drug to animals and then analyzed the brain content of serotonin. They found a major depletion of serotonin in the brains and other organs of animals given reserpine.[10] In Carlsson's words: "For the first time, one could talk about a bridge between neurochemistry and psychiatry."

It is uncertain how the experiment with reserpine in Brodie's lab was conceived. Brodie was a clever and vigorous lab chief. As domineering as he may have been, he nevertheless attracted many postdoctoral fellows who were themselves destined to become leaders and had independent thoughts.[11] The science writer Robert Kanigel[12] credits one of them, Parkhurst Shore, with the idea of studying reserpine.

Like others, Shore was struck by the chemical similarities between reserpine and serotonin. He therefore injected the drug into a dog, collected the urine, and asked lab colleague Herb Weissbach to analyze it. Weissbach, who was already working with Sidney Udenfriend in Brodie's laboratory on the metabolism of serotonin, found large amounts of a serotonin metabolite. Reserpine was somehow releasing serotonin from its storage sites and the overflow was ending up in the urine. Axelrod later gave equal credit to Weissbach[2] for this major discovery.

It is difficult now to realize how recent is the concept of chemical neurotransmission in the central nervous system. When Carlsson arrived at NIH in 1955, some neuroscientists still thought that messages in the brain were conveyed from one cell to another by electric signals.[13] In 1954, however, Marthe Vogt had discovered large amounts of norepinephrine and epinephrine in the brain, compounds called "catecholamines," which consist of benzene rings with two hydroxyl (—OH) groups on adjacent carbon atoms and an amino group (—NH_2) elsewhere.

Carlsson therefore proposed a study of the effects of reserpine on brain catecholamines, but Brodie was "not very interested." Despite this rejection, Carlsson considered Brodie "the father of modern biochemical pharmacology." However, Brodie erred in his conviction that serotonin, not catecholamines, was the key to the effects of drugs on the brain. For once, Brodie, known as a gambler, had bet on the wrong horse. Even so, the report generated excitement and opened a new field. Postdocs came to Brodie in droves.

The only paper Carlsson wrote during his 6-month fellowship at NIH concerned the release of serotonin in blood platelets exposed to reserpine. But his attention had been drawn to reserpine and he had learned how to use the spectrophotofluorometer. Although that sabbatical leave transformed Carlsson's scientific life, investigation of the other neurotransmitters had to await his return to Lund. There, he teamed with Swedish colleagues Nils Hillarp and Bengt Falck. Even before he left Bethesda, he had already written to Hillarp, proposing a collaborative study of the problem.

When Carlsson returned to Sweden, he and his collaborators gave reserpine to rabbits. The catecholamines were depleted as dramatically as serotonin was. They also found that sympathetic nerves – those that control blood vessels, bowel contractions, and heart actions – no longer responded to electrical stimulation, implying that peripheral catecholamine functions were not working, which could explain why blood pressure levels fell. But there was also evidence that the brain itself was affected; the reserpine-treated animals were immobile.

To counteract the possible depletion of catecholamines, Carlsson's team injected the rabbits with DOPA (dihydroxyphenylalanine), a precursor in the biological synthesis of norepinephrine. DOPA was not known to have any function other than to serve as a step in the formation of norepinephrine. Within 10 minutes, the immobility and sedation disappeared; the animals were again frisky.[14]

Because the animals had recovered from the effects of reserpine when given DOPA, the precursor of norepinephrine, the researchers expected to find normal levels of norepinephrine in the brain. They used the spectrophotofluorometer to measure small amounts of catecholamines in tissues, using methods they had devised for the new instrument. When they analyzed the brains, after the animals had recovered, they expected to find that the levels of norepinephrine had been brought back to normal by the injection of DOPA. To their surprise, they found no norepinephrine in the brain; it had not been restored. However, in the pathway of norepinephrine synthesis they knew another compound had to be considered because DOPA could also be converted to dopamine, which in turn could be converted to norepinephrine. Carlsson and his group modified the fluorometric method to include dopamine; it was the first specific method for this substance.

In doing so, the researchers made a key observation. When the rabbits recovered motion, brain levels of dopamine returned to normal. Therefore, recovery of movement paralleled the return of normal levels of dopamine. For the first time, dopamine was identified as a normal constituent of the brain. Accordingly, they concluded that dopamine must itself be a neurotransmitter, not merely a precursor in the biosynthesis of norepinephrine.

Carlsson and his group also found that restoring serotonin levels by administering a precursor did not reverse the clinical syndrome caused by reserpine, a death blow to theories about the centrality of serotonin in explaining the effects of reserpine.

In 1958,[15] Carlsson formally presented his theory that dopamine was involved in the control of motor functions. The evidence included the presence of large amounts of dopamine in the basal ganglia, the parkinsonian picture caused by reserpine, and the ability of

Dopamine pathways in the brain

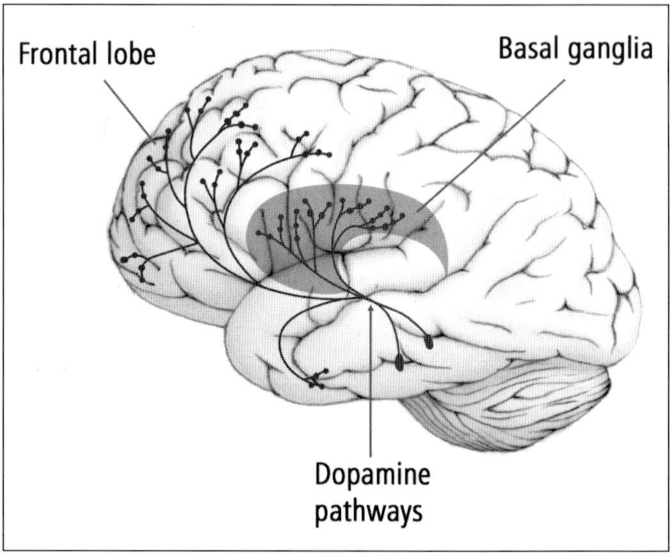

DOPA to reverse the motor effects of reserpine.[16] Carlsson and his colleagues mapped out the distribution of the cells that produce DOPA, which they found in basal parts of the brain – the nigrostriatal pathway that is severely affected in Parkinson disease.

Following up on Carlsson's findings, in 1960, the Austrian investigator Oleh Hornykiewicz[17] found that levels of dopamine were depleted in the particular part of the human brain that is affected in Parkinson disease; the substantia nigra showed marked loss of nerve cells. These findings, in turn, led to the introduction of levodopa treatment for Parkinson disease.

At first, several investigators in different countries noted limited benefit from small doses of levodopa, but it was George Cotzias, at the Brookhaven National Laboratory on Long Island, who used amounts larger than any one else – with correspondingly more dramatic benefit. Unfortunately, experience has shown that the benefits of levodopa therapy cannot be sustained indefinitely because the drug ultimately causes new involuntary movements. The search for better treatment continues, but nevertheless, levodopa is still the mainstay of treatment for Parkinson disease.

Carlsson's team continued to examine other psychotropic drugs that caused parkinsonian symptoms as adverse side effects. In 1963, they found that, in contrast to reserpine, these antipsychotic drugs did not deplete the catecholamines but, instead, blocked dopamine receptors. Regardless, a parkinsonian syndrome resulted in either case – whether as the result of too little dopamine, or from blocking the transmitter's receptors. Both actions impede the normal action of dopamine, which causes the parkinsonian manifestations.

As happens too often, a major scientific discovery is first greeted with incredulity. At a 1960 meeting on catecholamines, Carlsson encountered skepticism about the role of these catecholamines in the brain, primarily because electrical activity was still held responsible for transmission of messages. The formidable Nobel laureate, Sir Henry Dale, led the opponents. Several other distinguished luminaries expressed disbelief and Carlsson was bruised. He wrote:

> In his concluding remarks Gaddum stated that at this meeting nobody had ventured to speculate on the relation between catecholamines and the function of the brain. But this was what I had insisted upon throughout the meeting, so the clear message to me was that I was nobody!

Hillarp was at that meeting and, on the trip back to Sweden, Carlsson and he planned to free Hillarp from teaching responsibilities so he could do research fulltime. A grant from the Swedish Medical Research Council provided the means.

Carlsson had just been appointed to the Chair at Göteborg; Hillarp arrived in the autumn. Together, they developed fluoroscopic methods to show the microscopic location of the amines in the brain as well as the sympathetic nerves. They found that the amines were stored in granules within the nerve terminals, an observation that "contributed very much to a general acceptance of chemical transmission in the brain as it had already been recognized in the peripheral nervous system." Their histological methods opened the way for detailed study of the mechanisms involved in transmitter actions, a major contribution to neuroscience and drug development. (It also paralleled the observations of Axelrod that epinephrine was stored in similar vesicles.)

Five years later, in 1965, the world of transmitter research was vastly different from the rejection Carlsson had met with originally. Now, at another international symposium, the chairman's introductory remarks included the statement that "these amines play an important role as chemical mediators in the peripheral and central nervous system." No one demurred.

Carlsson turned his attention to the actions of drugs called neuroleptics, from Greek words meaning to "seize the nerves." These drugs did not deplete the amine transmitters but antagonized their stimulating actions. In 1963, Carlsson and his team reported that the drugs blocked the postsynaptic receptors for the amines, including chlorpromazine (Thorazine). After exposure to the drugs, there was compensatory overaction of the presynaptic neurons and the tissue levels of the catecholamines actually increased, even though there was no observable effect on the animal.

In the course of these studies Carlsson and his team described the three basic neural mechanisms that drove their observations on dopaminergic transmission: reserpine blocks the uptake of amines via the intracellular storage granules (or vesicles); chlorpromazine acts on the postsynaptic receptors to block the action of dopamine; and imipramine acts on a pump to block re-uptake of the amines into the vesicles. The molecular basis of each drug action is different, but all three mechanisms impede the actions of a transmitter on its receptors.

In something of a turnaround, Carlsson also re-evaluated the importance of serotonin. He introduced the very first serotonin re-uptake inhibitor (SSRI) drug, zimelidine, which was not a marketable success because of an autoimmune side effect, but which led to the later development and widespread use of other SSRI drugs such as fluoxetine (Prozac)[18] and sertraline (Zoloft).

In 1975, other investigators found a correlation between the average clinical dose of neuroleptic drugs and the affinity of each drug for dopamine receptors, validating Carlsson's theory about the effects of these drugs on dopamine and its receptors. Since the same drugs helped the symptoms of schizophrenia, these observations spurred the hypothesis that dopamine has a key role in the development of schizophrenia, a theory still in play but unproven.[19]

In the meantime, Carlsson was active on a related but different front. Julius Axelrod won a Nobel Prize in 1970 for his work at NIMH on the synthesis and pharmacology of norepinephrine. He had shown that tricyclic antidepressant drugs blocked the uptake of catecholamines by nerve endings. In 1968, Carlsson reported that the same drugs also blocked the uptake of serotonin. Some of the drugs were more active with norepinephrine and others were more active with serotonin. The tricyclic drugs have been largely supplanted by the SSRI drugs for the treatment of depression.

Since then, Carlsson has continued to work on the biochemistry of both Parkinson disease and schizophrenia in the quest for better drug therapies.[2,20] Few scientists have made such important contributions to two major public health problems, and few have had the chance to show so convincingly that clinical progress depends on "basic" research.

1 Sen G, Bose KC. Rauwolfia serpentina, a new Indian drug for insanity and high blood pressure. *Indian Med World* 1931;2:194-201.

2 Carlsson A. A half-century of brain neurotransmitter research: impact on neurology and psychiatry. Nobel Lecture, 2000.

3 Axelrod J. In Squire R, ed. *The History of Neuroscience in Autobiography.* Washington, DC: Society for Neuroscience, 1996:50-79.

4 Whitaker-Azmita PM. The discovery of serotonin and its role in neuroscience. *Neuropsychopharmacology* 1999;21:2S-8S.

5 Axelrod J. Interview with author, January 3, 2001.

6 Wooley DW, Shaw E. A biochemical and pharmacological suggestion about certain mental disorders. *Science* 1954;119:587-588.

7 Wooley DW. Production of abnormal (psychotic) behavior in mice with lysergic acid diethylamide, and its partial prevention with cholinergic drugs and serotonin. *Proc Natl Acad Sci USA* 1955;41:338-344.

8 Shore PA, Silver SL, Brodie BB. Interaction of reserpine, serotonin, and lysergic acid diethylamide in brain. *Science* 1955;122;284-285.

9 Carlsson A. Early psychopharmacology and the rise of modern brain research. *J Psychopharmacol* 1990;4:120-126.

10 Pletscher A, Shore PA, Brodie BB. Serotonin release as a possible mechanism of reserpine action. *Science* 1955;122:374-375.

11 Costa E, ed. *Neurochemical Pharmacology. A Tribute to B.B. Brodie.* New York: Raven Press, 1989.

12 Kanigel R. *Apprentice to Genius: The Making of a Scientific Dynasty.* Baltimore: Johns Hopkins University Press, 1986:99.

13 Carlsson A. Birth of neuropsychopharmacology – impact on brain research. *Brain Res Bull* 1999;50:363.

14 Carlsson A, Lindqvist M, Magnusson T. 3,4-Dihyroxyphenyl alanine and 5-hydroxytryptophan as reserpine antagonists. *Nature* 1957;180:1200.

15 Carlsson A. The occurrence, distribution, and physiological role of catecholamines in the nervous system. Symposium on catecholamines. Bethesda, MD, October 16-18, 1958. *Pharmacol Rev* 1959;11:490.

16 Carlsson A. Basic concepts underlying recent developments in the field of Parkinson's disease. In McDowell FH, Markham C, eds. *Recent Advances in Parkinson's Disease.* Contemporary Neurology Series, vol. 8, Oxford: Oxford University Press, 1971:1-31.

17 Hornykiewicz O. Parkinson's disease: from brain homogenate to treatment. *Fed Proc* 1973;32:183-190.

18 Carlsson A, Wong DT. A note on the discovery of selective serotonin reuptake inhibitors. *Life Sci* 1997;61:1203.

19 Carlsson A. The current status of the dopamine hypothesis of schizophrenia. *Neuropsychopharmacology* 1988;1:179-186.

20 Carlsson A, Waters N, Waters S, Carlsson ML. Network interactions in schizophrenia – therapeutic implications. *Brain Sci Rev* 2000;31:342-349.

CHAPTER TWENTY TWO

PAUL GREENGARD, PH.D.

The Nobel Prize in Physiology or Medicine, 2000

Awarded jointly to Arvid Carlsson, Paul Greengard, and Eric Kandel for their discoveries concerning signal transduction in the nervous system.

Paul Greengard is rewarded for his discovery of how dopamine and a number of other transmitters exert their action in the nervous system. The transmitter first acts on a receptor on the cell surface. This will trigger a cascade of reactions that will affect certain "key proteins" that in turn regulate a variety of functions in the nerve cell. The proteins become modified as phosphate groups are added (phosphorylation) or removed (dephosphorylation), which causes a change in the shape and function of the protein. Through this mechanism the transmitters can carry their message from one nerve cell to another.

Paul Greengard was born in 1925 and grew up in New York City. His mother died in childbirth when he was born and he therefore knew little about her family. His father's family had emigrated from Koenigsberg (now Gdansk) during the mid-19th century movement of Central European Jews.

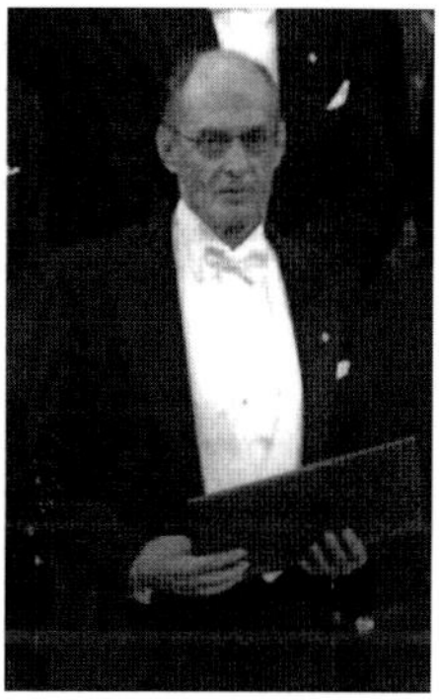

PAUL GREENGARD, PH.D., RECEIVING NOBEL AWARD

The first three generations of Greengard's family lived in St. Louis, but his grandfather moved to upstate New York. His father had careers in show business and cosmetics sales, then worked as a civilian purchasing agent for the army, and finally for large companies. Greengard's father remarried when Paul was a year old. His new stepmother was Episcopalian; from that time on, the family celebrated only Christian holidays.

Greengard attended public schools in Brooklyn and Queens, gradually recognizing his aptitude for mathematics and quantitative thinking. During World War II, he spent 3 years in the Navy as an electronics technician. In one assignment, he was part of a team at the Massachusetts Institute of Technology, developing an early-warning system to intercept kamikaze suicide planes. After the war, in 1948, he graduated from Hamilton College in upstate New York with a degree in physics and mathematics.

He would have considered a career in physics, but he was dissuaded from heading in that direction because the only fellowships available were directed to armaments. This was, he said,[1] "right after dropping the atom bombs. And I thought I didn't want to be involved in that kind of research, which could lead to more weapons of mass destruction."

Then Greengard heard about the emerging field of biophysics. He had thought there were only two kinds of physicists in medicine:

those who did electrophysiology and those who worked with radioisotopes. Since the University of Pennsylvania was the center for training in biophysics, he went there to study with Detlev Bronk. After a year, however, Bronk left to become President of Johns Hopkins University and he took Haldan Hartline with him; Hartline later won a Nobel Prize for his work on vision. Greengard moved to Hopkins and worked briefly with Hartline, but the experience did not much affect his career.

Greengard was headed for a degree in neurophysiology when, in the second year, Alan Hodgkin gave a lecture about the ionic shifts involved in the generation of nerve potentials. Even though Hodgkin described what was later to be a Nobel prize-winning discovery, Greengard concluded.[1] "It would be a long time before any further advances could be made by limiting one's investigations to the biophysical measurements of nerve cell properties." He decided to study biochemistry.

Greengard had a clear vision of what he wanted to do, although the way to get there was murky. What he wanted to do was difficult, because in the 1950s there was no such thing as a "neuroscientist." Instead, neurophysiologists dominated brain research and they were restricted to electrophysiology. But Greengard wanted to know how electrical signals were generated in the cell, and what was the cell biology. That called for knowledge of biochemistry, but then there was no such thing as a "neurochemist" either. The biochemists who did use the brain did so as they would any other organ of the body – because a particular enzyme or transmitter was concentrated there. They did not necessarily want to find out how the brain worked.

In graduate school, Greengard found himself in a bind because no single faculty member could encompass his interests in both physiology and biochemistry. Bronk was no longer directly involved in his studies. Greengard was lucky enough to find two willing sponsors – Frank Brink, a well-known physiologist, and Sidney Colowick, a famous biochemist. They encouraged his approach to a brand new field – what would later become "neuroscience" or "neurobiology." Where Greengard was headed, there would not be a clear division between physiology and chemistry. Instead, scientists would use whatever techniques were needed for the problem at hand.

Currently, those techniques involve not only traditional physiology and biochemistry but also molecular genetics, transgenic mice, and analysis of receptors – as Greengard's career illustrates. But, 50 years ago, few crossed the boundaries in the way Greengard did.

In 1953 Greengard received his Ph.D. and went to England, where he worked with several pioneer neurochemists. The first was Henry McIlwain, at the Maudsley Hospital in London. McIlwain was stimulating brain slices and measuring oxygen consumption, but the technique was not penetrating into nerve cells and would not help Greengard discover what he needed to know. He moved to Cambridge to work with E.C. Slater, an early investigator of mitochondria who was measuring energy metabolism in the brain. But 6 months later, in an eerie repetition of his earlier experience at Penn, Slater left for a new appointment in Amsterdam. Greengard followed. Once there, Greengard realized he needed both physiological and biochemical equipment. The only departments that had both were in pharmacology.

After another 6-month stint, Greengard left Amsterdam and returned to London, this time to work at the National Institute for Medical Research at Mill Hill, London, in the laboratory of Wilhelm Feldberg, who had earlier been a close colleague of Henry Dale, discoverer of one of the first neurotransmitters. Greengard worked there for 3 years until Sir Hans Krebs, another Nobel laureate, offered him a position at Oxford. It was a flattering and attractive opportunity.

Greengard was offered an endowed position to head a new section on neurochemistry, but he had reservations about accepting it. The mid-1950s were a time of severe restriction in England. For instance, Greengard needed a fluorometer to measure concentrations of neurotransmitters – but there was no money to buy one. He had to construct it himself, a formidable task that took a full year. As a result of these limitations, many British scientists were leaving for the United States, a true "brain drain." There were personal considerations for Greengard as well; he was married and had two children in school. And he was dissuaded also by a conversation he had with Krebs, who admitted that even though he was a professor at Oxford, a Nobel laureate, and a knight, he still felt himself an outsider, unaccepted by British society – not because he was Jewish but because he was a foreigner. Greengard decided to return to the United States, where Congress, spurred by Sputnik and the Cold War, was increasing funds for scientific research.

Greengard had spent 5 years in Britain and was gaining recognition. His publications included studies of the metabolism of nerves. The work had been supported partly by a fellowship from NINDB.

Bernard Brodie had loomed large in the lives of Axelrod and Carlsson, Greengard's Nobel Prize co-winners. He entered the picture once again and indirectly affected Greengard.[1] One of the productive scientists in Brodie's group was Sidney Udenfriend, who had come to NIH from St. Louis to rejoin the original team of pharmacologists from Goldwater Memorial Hospital. Like others in the laboratory, Udenfriend was not entirely happy. He was on the verge of accepting a position as head of research at the Geigy Pharmaceutical Company. To avoid losing Udenfriend, the Director of NIH offered him his own laboratory, which would liberate him from Brodie. Udenfriend accepted the offer and set up his own projects independently. He then told Greengard about the Geigy position, which Greengard accepted, welcoming the opportunity to develop new therapeutic drugs.

However, the company laboratories were not yet fully installed, so when he returned to the States in 1958, Greengard worked in Udenfriend's new labs at NIH for a year. Udenfriend had the idea that the entry of amino acids into the brain might be an "active" process – which meant it would require the participation of adenosine triphosphate (ATP), a chemical that serves as a source of energy. Some substances cross cell membranes by diffusion; others require the participation of ATP for "active transport." Working together that year, Greengard and Udenfriend did find the first evidence of an active amino acid transport system into the brain; Udenfriend found others later.

After his year with Udenfriend, Greengard moved to the Geigy Research Laboratories in Westchester, New York, as Director of the Department of Biochemistry. There, for the next 8 years, his task was to develop antidepressant drugs. During that time, he was also a professor at the Albert Einstein College of Medicine.

Greengard discovered that corporate science had limits. He found it frustrating to have to induce his staff to develop new drugs. Chemists were kings at pharmaceutical companies in those days, but they still tended to avoid taking chances with new ideas. Their preference was to make an imitative "me-too" variation of another company's successful drug. Looking back,[1] Greengard said he learned a lot in those days but it was mostly about drug metabolism and chemistry, not much that influenced his subsequent career.

"I thought . . . there would be great resources within the company," said Greengard. "But, in all that time, chemists dominated research. Every director of research was a chemist. The biologist was basically there as a servant to assay their new compounds."

In 1967, Greengard left Geigy and joined Murdoch Ritchie, a physiologist at the Albert Einstein College of Medicine in New York. They tried to determine how local anesthetics block pain sensation, which they found involved blocking sodium channels within the nerve membranes; the secret was a transformation of the anesthetic, which entered the nerve in one form, changed to another form inside the cell and altered the channels from within. Greengard was back on track – unraveling the cell biology of neural functions. He was almost ready for his prize work.

Greengard had maintained a close relationship to Sidney Colowick, one of his thesis advisors at Hopkins. For years, both he and Colowick had been impressed by – and often discussed – the research of Earl Sutherland, a biochemist who had been trying to find out how a hormone called glucagon works. Secreted by the pancreas, it acts on the liver. Sutherland's key discovery was the function of a compound called cyclic adenine monophosphate or cAMP, which is produced from the ubiquitous ATP by an enzyme, adenyl cyclase. Sutherland found that glucagon, a pancreatic hormone, acts on liver cells to increase the formation of cAMP from ATP. Then cAMP, in turn, stimulates enzymes to convert cell stores of the inactive glycogen into usable glucose. In effect, cAMP is a second messenger; glucagon is the first messenger. This and other second messenger systems are now known to be widespread in many organs, and function as a kind of amplification system. One molecule of the first messenger can induce the formation of many molecules of the second messenger, which then set off a blast of biochemical reactions.

In 1967, Colowick was at Vanderbilt and Greengard had an opportunity to work there for 6 months, this time with Sutherland himself. At the end of that visit, just before Greengard left for Yale, Edward Krebs (no relation to Sir Hans Krebs), at the University of Washington, published a paper on a cAMP-dependent protein kinase.

A protein kinase is an enzyme that facilitates the transfer of phosphate groups from ATP to a protein. After being phosphorylated, the protein assumes a different three-dimensional configuration and its function is altered, too.

Sutherland had worked on glucagon. Krebs focused on epinephrine, which was secreted as a hormone by the adrenal gland and also acted on remote cells to convert glycogen to glucose. Since both hormones had the same effect on glycogen, it seemed likely that the mechanisms were similar. Sutherland had shown that glucagon increased the amount of cAMP in a cell and that cAMP alone could replace the hormone in a test system. Krebs provided the next step when he found that cAMP phosphorylates an enzyme, phosphorylase kinase, which then phosphorylates a second enzyme, the one that breaks down glycogen to glucose.

Greengard moved to Yale in 1968. Inspired by Sutherland and Krebs, he was primed to determine whether cAMP played a role in the activity of neurotransmitters. A decade had passed since Arvid Carlsson had first identified dopamine as a transmitter in the brain in 1957 and 1958. One question investigators needed to answer was how dopamine acted on neurons. It did not take long for Greengard to make the essential observations, which he recorded in two papers in 1969.

He and his associates started with the superior cervical ganglion of the rat,[2] the same ganglion that Julius Axelrod had used to analyze the actions of catecholamines in the brain and pineal gland. The cervical ganglion was desirable because it provided a readily accessible tissue with a configuration suitable for both stimulating the nerves and analyzing the chemistry.

A ganglion is a collection of nerve cells and the nerve fibers (axons) that enter and leave it. In this ganglion, the axons arise in cells of the spinal cord in the neck; the fibers leave those cells and pass through the soft tissues of the neck to enter the ganglion. Some fibers synapse there and some pass through without synapsing. Ultimately, they become the autonomic fibers to the pupils of the eye, the salivary glands in the mouth, or blood vessels of the head. All these are involuntary or "autonomic" functions and part of the sympathetic nervous system.

Greengard and his associates found that preganglionic stimulation of the fibers increased the content of cAMP five-fold. The increase occurred only when there was synaptic activity in the postganglionic neurons. Adding dopamine without prior stimulation also increased the content of cAMP, duplicating the chemical effects of nerve action. As predicted, that effect was achieved by enhancing the activity of the enzyme, adenyl cyclase. In systems elsewhere in the body, dopamine is not always the agent of increasing cAMP; sometimes, catecholamines are. But in the cervical ganglion, they found that both dopamine and other catecholamines could be effective.

Moreover, they found two kinds of response: fast and slow. In the slow responses there was increased activity of a dopamine-sensitive adenylate cyclase. Activity in the dopaminergic slow responses could either potentiate or antagonize the fast responses, which had a different transmitter, acetylcholine. They also found that the increased amount of cAMP activated a cAMP-dependent

PROTEIN PHOSPHORYLATION

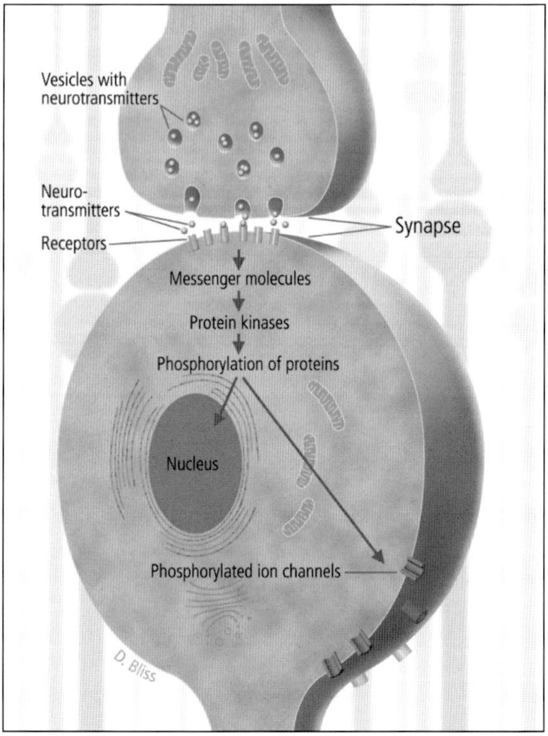

protein kinase (or protein kinase A) in the postganglionic neuron. The resulting phosphorylation altered some proteins and somehow altered membrane permeability to ions and so modified the electrical activity or the action potential of the nerve. The action terminated when other enzymes, called phosphatases, removed the phosphate groups.

What Greengard demonstrated with these experiments was that the state of phosphorylation of a protein depends on the balance of activity between the protein kinases and the phosphatases. All of this takes place in synaptic membranes. These general principles also rule neurons throughout the central nervous system and in other organs.

Greengard remained at Yale from 1969 until 1983, when he left to join the Rockefeller University as Vincent Astor Professor and Head of the Laboratory of Molecular and Cellular Neuroscience; he has remained there ever since. In both positions he continued to pursue phosphorylation and dopamine functions.

Through the years Greengard's group found several different kinases in the brain – cAMP-dependent protein kinase, cyclic guanosine monophosphate (GMP)-dependent protein kinase, calcium-calmodulin-dependent protein kinase, and at least one that functions alone, that is, it is not dependent on some other molecule. The calcium-dependent and GMP-dependent kinases had not been known to exist previously in any organ. Protein kinase A is the most prevalent of all the kinases and the brain content is much higher than that in the liver, which is ordinarily a major source of enzymes. A new world was opening.

But which brain proteins are targets for the kinases? The Greengard team used two approaches to determine which proteins were being phosphorylated. First, they tested known proteins, to find out whether they could be phosphorylated by the action of a kinase and which kinase was most effective.

Then they studied unknown proteins, those that had not yet been characterized. The procedure started by exposing an organ's cells to the action of a kinase in the presence of cAMP tagged with a radioactive label on the phosphate group. Then they carried out a mass extraction of all the proteins in the organ and separated the proteins. Many (but not all) carried the radioactive label, which meant the proteins had been phosphorylated.

Combining both methods, Greengard and his team found more than 100 brain proteins that could be phosphorylated by these kinases. All were present in large amounts in the brain. In contrast, the liver contains only six such proteins and in much lower concentrations. And these phosphorylated proteins could function. Injecting either the kinase or the phosphorylated protein sometimes eliminated the need for nerve stimulation; the phosphorylated proteins could mimic the effects of neurotransmitters, proving that they were essential parts of the system. Greengard knew they were on the track of something important for brain function.

"In a way, I was working alone in this field for 15 years," Greengard has said,[1] because of the division between the electrophysiologists and the general biochemists. Part of the problem had to do with time. Electrical transmission is almost instantaneous; chemical reactions take time. That was one reason why physiologists had difficulty believing transmission could be chemical and preferred to think the process was entirely electrical.

Then it was recognized that there are "fast" and "slow" synapses. Chemical reactions can account for slow transmission and, in turn, slow transmission can enhance or curtail the faster synapses. In more formal terms, chemicals can directly "mediate" slow transmission but they only "modulate" fast transmission indirectly.

By the time Greengard had started in 1968, chemical transmission had prevailed but it was still not known how the chemical neurotransmitter acted on the postsynaptic cell. As we have described, his studies began to illuminate that process and more was to come.

Among the 100 previously unidentified proteins that were amenable to phosphorylation by the cAMP-dependent kinases and the calcium-dependent kinases was a group called synapsins. These proteins are specifically associated with the vesicle membranes in which chemical transmitters are stored in nerve terminals. The dephosphorylated synapsin inhibits release of transmitter. The phosphorylated form enhances release. The synapsins play a role in linking the vesicles to surface membranes and the cell's cytoskeleton, which helps maintain the three-dimensional structure of the cell. Synapsins also function in the embryonic development of nerve terminals.[3] Therefore, the synapsins are essential in maintaining the reserve pool of vesicles and in modifying release of transmitter.[4] Synapsins are the most abundant proteins in the brain but they are not the only players; other proteins have also been considered important in determining the functionality of synaptic vesicles.[5]

Another protein Greengard's team discovered goes by the initials DARPP-32, which stands for *d*opamine and *a*denosine 3'5'-monophosphate *r*egulated *p*hospho*p*rotein (32 kilodaltons, a measure the size of the molecule). The brain content of DARPP-32 is much less than that of the synapsins, which are present in all nerve cells. DARPP-32, in contrast, is found in high concentration only in nerve cells that are activated by dopamine. It is therefore less abundant but also more specific in its functions and it is found in all cells with a dopaminergic input. Synapsins were found in a search for brain-specific phosphorylated proteins, those present only in the brain or in much higher concentration than in other organs.

DARPP-32, on the other hand, was found in a search for region-specific proteins within the brain. DARPP-32 was one of 12 found in an area called the striatum rather than in other parts of the brain; it was the first to be purified.

Greengard considers DARPP-32 "a master molecule"[1,2] that seems to "control everything in the cells." There are multiple receptors for dopamine and the effects depend upon which receptor binds the transmitter. If one is involved, protein kinase A is activated and DARPP-32 is phosphorylated. When DARPP-32 is phosphorylated it inhibits phosphatases, maintaining other proteins in a phosphorylated state. In contrast, if a different dopamine receptor is involved, the effects are just the opposite: protein kinase A is inhibited and a phosphatase is activated, removing phosphate groups from DARPP-32.

In these studies they found that dopamine and glutamate, a different transmitter, had opposing actions, one inhibitory, the other excitatory. The two amino acids also had opposite actions on the state of phosphorylation of DARPP-32.

Other transmitters involve other kinases with different effects on DARPP-32. Which of these actions is taken determines which modifications ensue in the function of other neuronal phosphoproteins in key cellular elements, including transmitter receptors, ion channels, enzymes, and other essential cellular functions.[6]

To analyze the complex functions of DARPP-32, Greengard used genetically engineered mice – DARPP-32-knockouts[7] – that lacked the gene and were therefore totally devoid of the protein in their brains. Anatomically, the brains seemed normal and the animals' behavior seemed normal. However, they differed from normal animals in physiological and pharmacological responses. All the effects of dopamine were abolished – on physiology, biochemistry, and drug responses. Also, all the effects of the antipsychotic drugs were abolished. Greengard therefore had shown that DARPP-32 is essential in all responses to dopamine and to all drugs that act through the dopamine pathway; that included drugs of abuse, such as cocaine and amphetamine.

Greengard has also investigated the role of phosphorylated proteins in Alzheimer disease, but his focus now is largely on dopamine, a key player in four major public health problems: parkinsonism, schizophrenia, drug abuse, and attention deficit disorder. Parkinson disease is on the list because dopamine deficiency seems to be the root cause of symptoms. Schizophrenia is there because drugs that effectively treat the symptoms are those that block dopamine receptors and curtail dopamine overactivity. Drug abuse is intimately related to dopamine, since drugs of abuse allow dopamine to remain in the synapse longer than normal. And attention deficit disorder is there because the most effective drug for treatment is methylphenidate (Ritalin), a dopamine antagonist.

All of this evolved from Carlsson's discoveries that dopamine is a neurotransmitter, a discovery that originated in his visit to Brodie's NIH laboratory. It has been elaborated by Greengard's research, which is the fourth in the line of Nobel Prizes for second messengers – Earl Sutherland (1971), Edward Krebs and Edmond Fisher (1992), and Alfred Goodman Gilman and Martin Rodbell (1994).

Clarifying the complex interactions of transmitters, enzymes, messengers, channels, and drugs is a challenge for the future. Greengard's progress may provide clues to the places where chemical intervention could be therapeutic and offer clues to drug design and development.[8]

Greengard's unique views emerged again when, in honor of the mother he never knew, he donated his portion of the Nobel Prize money to Rockefeller University for an award to outstanding women doing biomedical research.

1 Greengard P. Interview with author, January 8, 2001.

2 Greengard P, Kebabian JW. Role of cyclic AMP in synaptic transmission in the mammalian peripheral nervous system. *Fed Proc* 1974;33:1059-1067.

3 Greengard P, Valtorta F, Czernik AJ, Benfenati F. Synaptic vesicle phosphoproteins and regulation of synaptic function. *Science* 1993;259:780-785.

4 Hilfiker S, Pieribone VA, Czernik AJ, Kao HT, Augustine GJ, Greengard P. Synapsins as regulators of neurotransmitter release. *Phil Transact Roy Soc: Biol Sci* 1999;354:269-279.

5 Südhof TC, Scheller RH. Mechanism and regulation of neurotransmitter release. In Cowan WM, Südhof TC, Stevens CF, eds. *Synapses.* Baltimore: Johns Hopkins University Press, 2001:177-215.

6 Greengard P, Allen PB, Nairn AC. Beyond the dopamine receptor: the DARPP-32/ protein phosphatase-1 cascade. *Neuron* 1999;23:435-447.

7 Fienberg AA, Greengard P. The DARPP-32 knockout mouse. *Brain Res Rev* 2000;31:313-319.

8 Greengard P. Nobel Lecture, 2000.

CHAPTER TWENTY THREE

ERIC R. KANDEL, M.D.

The Nobel Prize in Physiology or Medicine, 2000

Awarded jointly to Arvid Carlsson, Paul Greengard, and Eric Kandel for their discoveries concerning signal transduction in the nervous system.

Eric Kandel is rewarded for his discoveries of how the efficiency of synapses can be modified, and which molecular mechanisms take part. With the nervous system of a sea slug as experimental model he has demonstrated how changes of synaptic function are central for learning and memory. Protein phosphorylation in synapses plays an important role for the generation of a form of short term memory. For the development of a long term memory a change in protein synthesis is also required, which can lead to alterations in shape and function of the synapse.

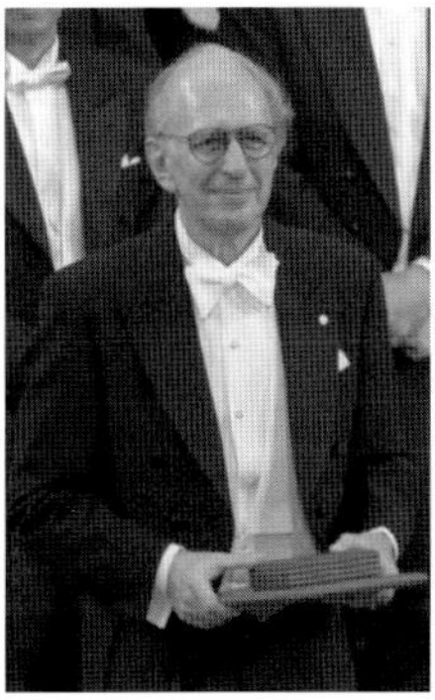

ERIC R. KANDEL, M.D., RECEIVING NOBEL AWARD

Eric Kandel's path to glory was not straightforward. Born in Vienna, he left "through the courtesy of Adolph Hitler."[1,2] At age 9, he and his 14-year-old brother traveled by train from Vienna to Holland and then, by ship, to the United States. For the year before his parents arrived, the brothers lived with relatives in Brooklyn. Eric spoke no English on arrival but, within a few months of school, he caught up to his classmates. After a short time in public school, he transferred to a bilingual school, with classes in Hebrew in the morning and English in the afternoon.

Kandel returned to the public school system at Erasmus Hall High School, which the Dutch had founded in 1787. His interests were broad and he thought about becoming a sports writer. In a New York sports newspaper, *Gotham Sports*, he wrote a column called "Breaking the Tape." He was captain of the school track team. When he graduated, he and the co-captain were the only two from a class of 1,400 who went to Harvard, which then favored students from private schools more than public schools.

At Harvard, Kandel majored in history and literature; he was immersed in the humanities, not science. His thesis was a critical review of prominent German writers in Nazi times. Through personal contact with psychoanalysts Ernst and Marianne Kris, he was introduced to other psychoanalysts. He found them erudite and intellectually stimulating, so much so that he wanted to be an analyst himself. To that end, he thought it appropriate to go to medical school. Because he had taken no science courses in the first years of college, he completed all the premedical requirements in one summer session and his senior year.

In 1952, he enrolled at the New York University (NYU) School of Medicine, where he gradually began to enjoy the clinical courses.

He thought he should know at least something about the brain, but there were then no neuroscientists at NYU. A friend referred him to Harry Grundfest at Columbia, who was said to be "interested in the brain." In fact, Grundfest, a leading neurophysiologist, was more interested in simpler systems, especially the giant axon of the crayfish. Grundfest advised Kandel to team up with a young neurosurgeon-neurophysiologist, Dominick Purpura (later a renowned neuroscientist and now Dean of the Albert Einstein College of Medicine), who had just set up his own laboratory.

Among other experiments, Kandel and Purpura tested a popular theory that schizophrenia might be related to abnormalities in the neurotransmitter serotonin because the popular hallucinogen, lysergic acid diethylamide (LSD), affected that transmitter. They gave cats serotonin intravenously but found that nothing happened to electrical activity in the brain. They learned only later that serotonin does not cross the blood-brain barrier.

Kandel was much taken by Purpura's sense of humor in the laboratory ("like an early version of Woody Allen") and he thought it might be a nice way of life – "doing experiments, not having to wear a necktie, and laughing a lot."

In fact, his devotion to science was almost total by then. But he knew he would have trouble financially if he opted for a career in research. So he consulted his future wife, Denise, who was in graduate school at Columbia, aiming for a Ph.D. in sociology. She said her parents had always wanted her to marry a poor intellectual. Kandel did not know if he qualified as an intellectual but he surely was poor.

When he graduated from NYU in 1956, he interned at the Montefiore Hospital (now Montefiore Medical Center) and returned to the Grundfest laboratory for an elective period. This time around he met Stanley Crain, one of the pioneers in the then-new practice of culturing neurons in dishes and using microelectrodes for experiments with the isolated cells. Kandel was much impressed by both the cultures and the intracellular recordings.

When Kandel completed his internship in 1957, Grundfest recommended him to join the laboratory of NIMH researcher Wade Marshall in the combined NIMH-NINDB program. Earlier, Marshall had been one of the first to study sensory functions in the parietal lobes. At NIH, however, he was interested in *spreading depression*, an enigmatic phenomenon that did not call for microelectrode analysis. However, Kandel assisted Jack Brinley in studying the role of potassium in propagating the wave of spreading depression, a peculiar suppression of brain electrical activity. Kandel says the paper is a classic "among the five people in the world who care."

To start using microelectrodes, Kandel sought the advice of Karl Frank, an innovative spinal cord physiologist who was officially in NINDB, formally a different institute, but had an adjacent laboratory and taught the needed techniques. When W. Alden Spencer arrived in the laboratory, Kandel worried that this new investigator might compete for laboratory space and apparatus. Fortunately, they were both interested in learning and memory.

Working at the University of Oregon before coming to NIH, Spencer had worked on brain connections, especially between the thalamus (a deep structure within the brain) and the cortex on the outer surface. He was also interested in habituation, a form of learning, in the spinal cord of cats. He and Kandel combined to study functions in the hippocampus in cats with intracellular electrodes – which their advisors unanimously pronounced an impossible task. But succeed they did, analyzing both normal and epileptic activity.[3] When they had their first recordings and heard the musical sounds of the electrical activity, Kandel felt it was "a life-changing experience;" he was fully committed to a research career.

Kandel and Spencer became close friends and long-term colleagues but they considered the hippocampus too complicated for the study of memory. There were too many neurons and too many interconnections. Also, it was difficult to keep an electrode within the small cells for the prolonged periods each experiment needed.

After 3 years, Kandel left NIH in 1960 to start psychiatric training in Boston. Dominated by psychoanalysis, the program offered no teaching conferences, journal clubs, required reading, or other accoutrements of a medical residency. The trainees were rarely on call at night. Kandel was disappointed in the lack of biological thinking and the limited educational program, but the leisurely pace gave him time for laboratory work in the evenings. The residency program director, Jack Ewalt, considered this nocturnal research rather unusual, but provided the research facilities.

His reputation grew. In 1961, which was the sole year Seymour Kety headed psychiatry at Johns Hopkins, Kety's eye for talent was again evident when he offered young Kandel a position. Kandel was flattered by this invitation because he had known Kety at NIH. Just a year earlier, he had attended and had been "tremendously impressed" by Kety's famous NIH lecture on the biochemistry of schizophrenia.

Halfway through the residency, Kandel was still interested in memory and sought a system simpler than the hippocampus. He thought about using the neurons of invertebrates such as cockroaches or worms. Ultimately, he chose *Aplysia*, the sea slug, and in 1962, with Ewalt's support, Kandel traveled to Paris on an NINDB fellowship to work in the laboratory of Ladislav Tauc.

Aplysia proved to be the ideal preparation. In contrast to the billions of cells in a mammalian brain, there were only 20,000 in *Aplysia*. And, compared to human neurons, the cells in *Aplysia* were gigantic, the largest in the animal kingdom and ideal for intracellular electrodes. Because the cells were large and relatively

Aplysia

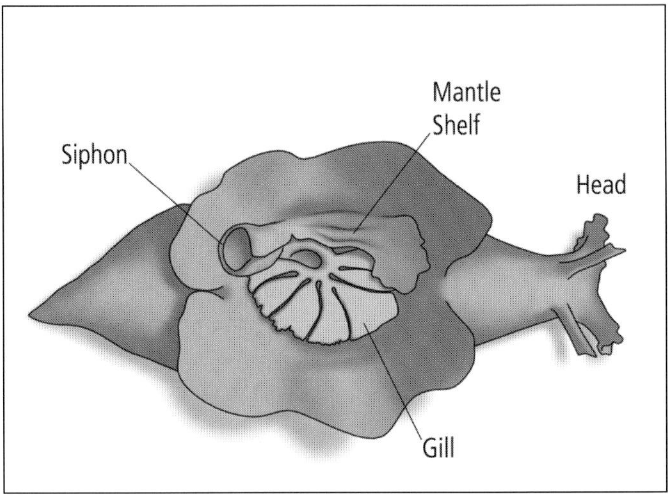

few, the same cells could be identified reliably for repeated tests in the same animal or in different animals. Kandel stayed with *Aplysia* for decades, adapting new methods and new concepts – when they came.

Kandel returned to Harvard in 1963, where he was much impressed by the young investigators assembled by Steve Kuffler in what later became the world's first Department of Neurobiology. The group included two future Nobelists, Torsten Wiesel and David Hubel, as well as Ed Fuhrspan, David Potter, and Ed Kravitz. Kandel interacted extensively with them and began to attract post-doctoral fellows of his own.

In 1965, Kandel accepted a position at NYU. There he was reunited with Alden Spencer, but their reunion was cut short tragically. In 1977, Spencer died at age 46. Ironically, the cause of death was amyotrophic lateral sclerosis (ALS or Lou Gehrig's disease), a disease of the same spinal cord neurons Spencer himself had studied so fruitfully. At NYU, Kandel established his own Division of Neurobiology and Behavior. The choice of words in that title was deliberate because many scientists had considered behavior too complex for reductionist investigation in simple systems. The division's name documented a philosophical belief.

In 1974, Kandel made his last institutional move, this time to Columbia University, where he has been ever since. There, he established a Center for Neurobiology and Behavior. He had appointments in the departments of psychiatry, physiology, biochemistry, and molecular biophysics; combining the methods of all those disciplines, neuroscience had arrived. In recognition of his multiple talents, he was appointed university professor in 1983 and, the next year, he was recruited as a senior investigator of the Howard Hughes Medical Institute. Always committed to teaching, he organized a course on neuroscience and the syllabus became his noted textbook *Principles of Neural Science*, edited with James Schwartz and Thomas Jessell. That book has lured many medical and graduate students worldwide into becoming neurobiologists.

Kandel's detailed studies of Aplysia were the basis for his recognition by numerous awards before the Nobel. Kandel[1,4-7] has summarized that work, which can be divided into three epochs spanning four decades and recorded in hundreds of peer-reviewed papers. His reasoning was direct. In human and animal studies, psychologists had recognized habituation; if a single benign stimulus is given repeatedly, the subject ultimately ignores it. If the same stimulus is innocuous and is given in combination with a strong noxious or rewarding stimulus, the stronger one takes over the original response, as in classic conditioning. If you give the strong stimulus alone repeatedly, the response is enhanced; this is sensitization. Kandel reasoned that by stimulating nerves in a simple system, such as *Aplysia*, he could do the equivalent of psychological experiments.

He said: "What psychologists are doing is simply providing stimulus sequences to an individual. One could do that electrically," making it possible to study habituation, sensitization, and classic conditioning. "You could have an analog of learning, with all the elements of the behavior except for the artificial stimulus."

With time, he and his associates learned to identify and record from the specific cells of *Aplysia*. The structures involved were the gill (for extracting oxygen from water), the siphon (which eliminates waste), and the mantle (which connects the two structures.) If the siphon is touched, the gill and mantle are briskly retracted, a defensive reflex that results from the actions of two groups of nerve cells. First, the sensory neurons detect the touch and convey the message directly or indirectly to the second group of cells, the motor neurons, which activate the muscles involved in withdrawing the gill or the siphon. Because the cells in *Aplysia* are so recognizable, Kandel and his group could map out the precise connections between them.

Kandel recognized that he could study a behavior by analyzing the defensive reflex. Simply touching the siphon was an innocuous stimulus. When it was repeated, the vigor of the withdrawal response lessened, as in habituation. Simultaneously, the electrical activity of the sensory and motor cells diminished also as in habituation. The behavior and the electrical activity moved in parallel.

Facilitation is the mirror image of habituation. If, in contrast to the nonthreatening tactile stimulus, a harmful shock induces an escape response, the withdrawal is more vigorous when it is repeated and the duration of the change depends again on the number of times the animal is shocked. The changes in neuronal firing, an increase in sensitization or a decrease in habituation, are accompanied by parallel changes in the number of molecules of the transmitter glutamate, which is released by sensory neurons and acts on the motor cell.

Kandel and his associates also found that both habituation and facilitation could be of short or long duration. One training session led to brief memory – the more the repetition, the longer the changes lasted. The repeated reflex responses were therefore altering the synaptic connections between nerve cells. If it altered the synapses, the changes must involve "transmitters," chemicals released by the presynaptic (sensory) cell to flow across the tiny gap between the cells and react with receptors on the postsynaptic membrane. As a result of these and other chemical changes that Kandel elucidated, they found that transmitter release was decreased in habituation and enhanced in facilitation.

In addition to habituation and sensitization, Kandel and his associates investigated a third form of learning, classic conditioning, which involves the pairing of two stimuli. A conditional stimulus produces either no overt response or a weak response that is usually unrelated to the response to be learned. The unconditioned stimulus – shock to a leg or food – normally does elicit a visible response. For instance, the animal salivates when food is the stimulus or the leg withdraws after a shock. Responses to unconditioned stimuli are innate; responses to conditioned stimuli are learned. As Pavlov had found, if the conditioned stimulus is the sound of a bell and is followed reliably by the unconditioned stimulus of food, the sound of the bell alone evokes salivation. If the bell is not followed by food, the response gradually disappears.

Kandel and his group began to examine the cellular connections of the gill withdrawal response of *Aplysia*, applying the concepts of classic conditioning. Kandel then turned to the molecular basis of the learned changes with James Schwartz. They wondered if the transmitters might have effects other than on electrical signals. When they injected inhibitors of protein synthesis, there was no effect on the short-term responses, so they considered smaller molecules. Earl Sutherland had shown that some hormones effect responses by increasing the cellular content of cyclic adenosine monophosphate or cAMP.

If the Kandel team injected cAMP directly into the presynaptic neuron, it simulated the sensitizing stimulus. This observation confirmed electrical studies that had shown the key role of the presynaptic nerve cell. Then they collaborated with Greengard, who had found that cAMP activates an enzyme that enhances the addition of phosphate groups to a protein, a protein kinase. If they injected the kinase itself, it had the same action as cAMP and it enhanced release of the neurotransmitter serotonin.

In the *Aplysia* studies, a benign stimulus (touching the siphon or mantle shelf) was combined with and followed a shock to the tail. The resulting facilitation was more pronounced than that evoked when the stimuli were not paired. The mechanism was more complex than simple facilitation and involved several cellular events: calcium metabolism, a calcium-binding protein called calmodulin, and adenyl cyclase, which ultimately potentiated the response to serotonin. The molecular basis of conditioning was therefore an elaboration of the mechanism for sensitization.

For sensitization, a single training session or a single application of serotonin induced short-term changes, lasting a few minutes. This was attributed to strengthening neural connections but did not require new synthesis of proteins. With more training, the effects lasted weeks and did require the synthesis of proteins. This was proven by giving inhibitors of protein synthesis during the learning period, which blocked long-term facilitation. It seemed as though short- and long-term memory were independent but involved overlapping systems. Both modified the strength of synapses. Both enhanced the release of transmitter. Both used the same transmitter, serotonin, in either short- or long-term effects. Both used cAMP. However, the necessity of protein synthesis in long-term facilitation implied the growth of new synaptic connections. How did that happen?

These complicated relationships were unraveled with a formidable combination of the traditional methods of electrophysiology, electron microscopy, and biochemistry. In the next phase of Kandel's research, the newer methods of molecular biology became available for the analysis of long-term storage of memory involved in sensitization and conditioning. In 1979, Kandel met molecular biologist Richard Axel. Later, when he became a Howard Hughes scholar, Kandel decided that he had to transform himself; he too would go molecular, studying the effects of genes as well as proteins.

With Arnold Kriegstein first, and then with Samuel Schacher, Kandel developed a tissue culture system that reproduced the circuitry of *Aplysia* with three cells in a glass dish: a single sensory neuron, a single motor neuron, and a serotoninergic cell. They could even remove the serotoninergic cell and puff the serotonin directly onto the motor neuron – one puff, transient facilitation; five puffs, facilitation lasted more than a day. Long-term effects required protein synthesis; short-term effects did not. They thought the long-term effects would involve kinases.

Then Roger Tsien developed a method for visualizing the location of the kinase within the cultured cells. Together, they found that with repeated pulses of serotonin, the active subunit of the kinase moved into the nucleus, the cellular compartment for DNA. This observation suggested that a transcription factor might be involved. (Transcription factors induce the synthesis of forms of ribonucleic acid or RNA, which is the first step in synthesizing proteins.)

At the time, there was considerable interest in proteins that were targets of cAMP-dependent protein kinases. One was called CREB, which stands for *c*AMP-*r*esponse *e*lement-response-*b*inding protein. So they took the segment of DNA that binds CREB and injected the DNA into the nucleus of a sensory neuron. This maneuver tied up the CREB and selectively blocked long-term facilitation but not the short-term effects. When they isolated the gene for CREB they could produce the protein in amounts sufficient for experiments and they injected the phosphorylated form of CREB. As expected, that maneuver produced the long-term effects. The results implied that CREB enhanced long-term facilitation.

The CREB system became more complicated with the discovery of CREB-2, which inhibited the effects of CREB-1, so that the final result depended on the balance of the activity of the two CREBs, one a stimulator, the other a repressor.[8]

They also documented the production of new synapses in long-term effects. Normally, the sensory neuron has 1,200 connections; after long-term sensitization, there were 2,800. Short-term memory involved the strengthening of synaptic connections; long-term memory involved the creation of new synapses.

Because long-term memory involves the synthesis of new proteins and because genes control the synthesis of proteins, it was logical to seek a genetic control. The genetic evidence was provided by studies in the fruit fly, *Drosophila*, by Seymour Benzer and his colleagues at the California Institute of Technology, and by Tim Tully and Jerry Yin at Cold Spring Harbor, as well as by Kandel in the mouse. The Benzer team found four mutant flies that, in tests of odor recognition, failed to show classic conditioning or sensitization. Three of the four had mutations that affected the cAMP cascade. One mutation depended on cAMP and the associated protein kinase; as in *Aplysia*, both features were critical for learning and short-term memory.

Similarly, Tully and Yin found that both the activator CREB-1 and the repressor CREB-2 were required for long-term memory. Depending on the circumstances, a gene can be deleted or overexpressed by mutation. They found one mutant fly that overexpressed the repressor CREB-2 and could not acquire long-term memory. Conversely, a mutant overexpressing the activator immediately produced long-term memory, even without prolonged training. The molecular basis of memory was therefore similar in *Aplysia* and flies. If the system had been conserved in evolution, it ought to be found in other species, too.

To study memory in mammals, the only class of vertebrates suitable for some forms of recall, Kandel took advantage of methods – which appeared in the 80s and 90s – to create transgenic mice.[9,10] For this project, Kandel returned to the hippocampus, the structure he had long ago studied with Spencer. The immediate object of study was long-term potentiation (LTP).

The hippocampus is a section of the temporal lobe recognized as important in human memory because lesions here selectively affect long-term memory but do not bar acquisition of new facts for the short term. Physiologists had identified three different anatomic systems within the hippocampus that were capable of LTP. The potentiation results when a brief burst of stimuli (a tetanus) increases the amplitude of the action potentials evoked in the target system. This facilitation can last 3 hours after a single tetanus or weeks after multiple tetani. Analysis indicated that CREB was involved, a parallel between LTP and long-term memory. Simple application of cAMP to hippocampal cells led to LTP even without a preceding tetanus, reinforcing the parallelism.

Long-term memory can be more directly studied in the mouse, where some specific hippocampal neurons are responsible for spatial memory. The location of an animal is encoded in the firing pattern of these cells and combinations of cells form new "place fields" whenever the animal moves to a different location. The fields are stable for weeks or months. The rapid formation and long duration are similar to the properties of LTP.

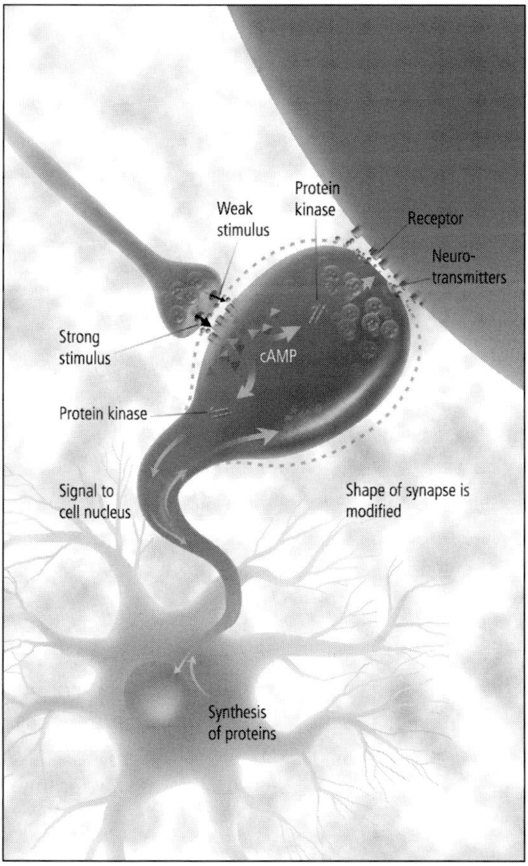

INDUCTION OF SHORT- AND LONG-TERM MEMORY

Kandel's group developed a mouse that lacked a functioning gene for a calcium-activated kinase; LTP could not be induced in these animals. To test spatial memory they used a water maze. A mouse was trained to find a hidden platform beneath the surface of a pool, using markings on the wall of the room for orientation. Injecting an antagonist of a particular neurotransmitter into the hippocampus rendered the animals incapable of finding the submerged platform. Additionally, mice lacking the calcium-activated kinase had no capacity for LTP in hippocampal neurons and could not find their way in the water maze. Other knockout mice lacked a gene for one of three different protein kinases, each needed for LTP; mice devoid of one particular kinase lacked both LTP and long-term memory.

The cAMP pathway is also important in LTP in mice. The early stage of LTP does not require protein synthesis but does require activity of two kinases. The late phase lasts more than 24 hours and requires a third kinase and the synthesis of new proteins. When the gene for CREB was knocked out, short-term memory and early LTP were normal but long-term memory and late LTP were absent.

In all of these experiments the results were consistent in showing the parallels between LTP and long-term memory, as well as the differences between short-term and long-term memory and their molecular basis. In *Aplysia*, *Drosophila*, and mice, the molecular systems are similar. Kandel hopes that the studies may lead to the development of drugs that could improve memory in the failing human brain.

APLYSIA WITH ITS WELL-EARNED PRIZE!

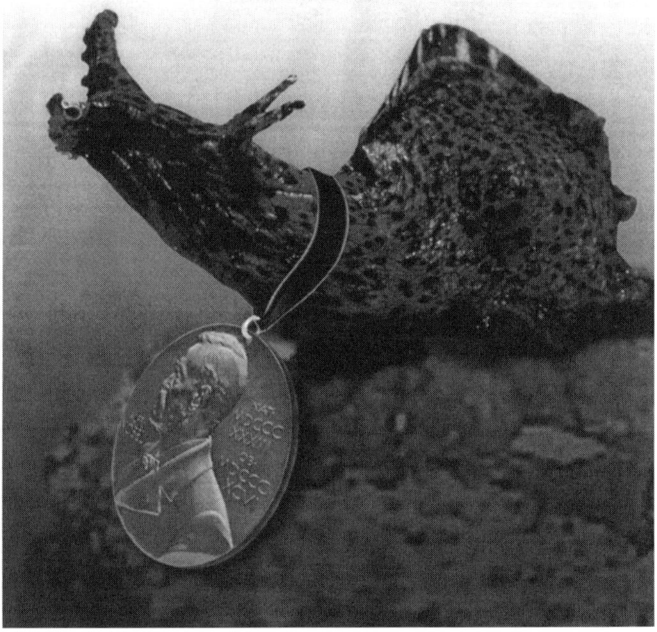

Through all of these new techniques and new concepts, Kandel has been the leader of molecular memory studies. However, he has not forgotten his clinical experiences and he has made a persuasive case for the importance of molecular memory studies for clinical psychiatry,[11] including psychoanalysis.[12,13] And he has championed the re-uniting of psychiatry and neurology.[14,15] His career was studded with honors that anteceded the Nobel Prize and included a Lasker Award and the National Medal of Science.

1 Kandel ER. Interview with author, October 20, 2000.

2 Kandel ER. Nobel Autobiography, 2001.

3 Kandel ER, Spencer WA. Cellular neurophysiological approaches in the study of learning. *Physiology Rev* 1968;48:65-134.

4 Kandel ER. Cellular mechanisms of learning and the biological basis of individuality. In Kandel ER, Schwartz JH, Jessell TM, eds. *Principles of Neural Science,* 4th ed. New York: McGraw-Hill, 2000:1247-1279.

5 Milner B, Squire LR, Kandel ER. Cognitive neuroscience and the study of memory. *Neuron* 1998;20:445-468.

6 Squire LR, Kandel ER. *Memory: From Mind to Molecules.* New York: Scientific American Library, a Division of HPHLP, W. H. Freeman, 1998.

7 Kandel ER. Molecular biology of memory: a dialogue between genes and synapses. Nobel Lecture, 2000. *Science,* in press.

8 Kandel ER. Molecular biology of memory: a dialogue between genes and synapses. Nobel Lecture. *Science,* in press.

9 Mayford M, Kandel ER. Genetic approaches to memory storage. *TIG* 1999; 15:463-470.

10 Kandel ER, Pittenger C. The past, the future, and the biology of memory storage. *Phil Trans R Soc Lond B* 1999;354:2027-2032.

11 Kandel ER. A new intellectual framework for psychiatry. *Am J Psychiat* 1998; 155:457-469.

12 Kandel ER. Psychotherapy and the single synapse: the impact of psychiatric thought on neurobiological research. *N Engl J Med* 1979;301:1028-1037.

13 Kandel ER. Biology and the future of psychoanalysis; a new intellectual framework for psychiatry revisited. *Am J Psychiat* 1999;156:505-524.

14 Cowan WM, Harter DH, Kandel ER. The emergence of modern neuroscience; some implications for neurology and psychiatry. *Annu Rev Neurosci* 2000;23:343-391.

15 Cowan WM, Kandel ER. Prospects for neurology and psychiatry. *JAMA* 2001; 285:594-600.

SECTION 4

CHAPTER TWENTY FOUR

ONE BRAIN SCIENCE, GENOMICS, THE CLINICAL NEUROSCIENCES, AND THE FUTURE OF NINDS

The Balkanization of neuroscience at NIH started long before the word neuroscience was widely used. Now, we have to live with it – at NIH itself and, in the wider world, through the research grants sponsored nationally by NIH.

The first division came through the sequence of birthdays – NIMH preceded NINDB. The distribution of research responsibility was never formally stated. It might have been assumed that neurology research would be more biological while NIMH research would be more psychoanalytic and more sociological. But, from the start, Seymour Kety was making psychiatry research more biological.

He was supported in that effort by NIMH Director Robert Felix who, paradoxically for one with a biological bent, was better known nationally for his strong interest in community psychiatry.[1] Felix had actually appointed neurologists to the staff before Kety came and they started programs in multiple sclerosis research, a field not ordinarily considered psychiatric. Kety continued to hire neuroscientists on the basis of skills, not by institutional affiliation, and their laboratories were mixed together. When Milton Shy came to NINDB in 1953, neuromuscular disease and epilepsy research were initiated.

The next division was loss of the "B" in NINDB. Vision research was logically part of neuroscience and it remained in NINDB from 1950 to 1968. By that time ophthalmology wanted its own institute, and so did vision-related advocacy groups. So the Eye Institute was born. In response, the name NINCDS was contrived as the institute retained responsibility for research on hearing and speech. The "S" laid claim to stroke. Even that did not last long. In 1988, hearing had its own institute for deafness and communicative disorders (NIDCD). By that time there were four neuroscience institutes and three had emerged directly from NINDB (NEI, NIDCD, and NINDS itself). NIMH was the fourth.

But there were to be more: the Aging Institute came in 1974, staking out dementia research. The National Institute of Child Health and Human Development (NICHD) became home for mental retardation and many inherited diseases of the nervous system. The National Institute on Drug Abuse (NIDA) developed its own programs for neurotransmission, transmitter receptors, and brain imaging. The Cancer Institute has dealt with brain tumors, and the Infectious Diseases Institute has had neuro-AIDS and other neurological infections. The Institute for Arthritis and Musculoskeletal and Skin Diseases began to have programs in muscle disease, which had long been the province of neurologists. The Dental Institute, in

NIH parlance, is the "lead center" for pain research. The National Institute of Environmental Health Sciences is involved with neurotoxins and neurodegenerative diseases. In 2001, the National Institute of Biomedical Imaging and Bioengineering emerged and cuts across all of them.

NINDS continues to sponsor research in all neurological diseases. For instance, NINDS supported the research of Dennis Selkoe, Stanley Prusiner, and others. Among the 28 NIH institutes, however, 11 now have both intramural and extramural programs in neuroscience. Is this fragmentation good or bad? The mishmash may seem administratively haphazard and therefore detrimental to creativity, but there has been a long record of research success across the broad span of institutes.

Leaders of NIH have expressed their views about this matter. Some touch the lighter side, as when Steven Hyman (Director of NIMH) explained,[2] that "in basic neuroscience, if a grant application has acetylcholine in the title, it goes to NINDS. If it has serotonin in the title it goes to NIMH. And if it has dopamine in the title, we fight (and NIDA does too). That is not good."

Yet all involved take the matter seriously. Ruth Kirschstein, Acting Director of NIH, put it this way when she was asked about competition between NIMH, NINDS, and NIA for dementia research:[3]

> Q. If we just take Alzheimer disease as an example, is it good, bad, or does it not matter that three institutes have a major interest in it?
>
> R.K. It depends on whether they fight for turf or whether they work together. The three of them work extremely well together.
>
> Q. Now – but there was a time when Mental Health and Neurology . . .
>
> R.K. There was a time when they did not and it matters when they do not work together. It does not matter that they are in competition – if it is a healthy competition. It doesn't matter if one of them wants a particular grant, but it does matter if that one wants to hold onto a grant application and cannot fund it because it does not have enough money or whatever – and prevents (if it is a very good application) the other institute from doing it. We used to have individual "fiefdoms." The Director of NIH really had one job – to keep them from cutting off each other's heads – and to do a little bit of coordination.

Gerald Fischbach, Director of NINDS from 1998 to 2001, has been particularly concerned with the duplication resulting from the diffusion of neuroscience to different institutes. He said:[4] "There are probably over 200 principal investigators at the NIH who are in the field of neuroscience. By one count, almost $300,000,000 a year is spent in the intramural programs that have relevance to neuroscience."

His "vision about the intramural program is that it ought to transcend all the institutes. There ought to be one strong intramural National Neuroscience Research Program that crosses disciplines and brings behavior into contact with molecular biology." He continued: "It is insane for each institute to recruit like Noah's Ark, with two of each kind of person, and then keep them apart so they are not interacting."

Harold Varmus, overall Director of NIH from 1993 to 1999 has recorded the administrative complexity of having so many institutes reporting to the Director.[5] Historically five new institutes have emerged every 10 years. At that rate, there would be 50 institutes in 2040, which he considers an administrative nightmare. His solution: reduce the number by incorporating multiple units into six mega-institutes. Whether that will be possible is a question of modifying the self-interest or perceived self-interest of those in charge of the individual institutes – and their advocacy supporters.

Richard Hodes, Director of the National Institute on Aging, commented about this interpretation:[6]

> I think I understand the sense of what Harold is saying, that so many institutes with different – albeit, overlapping – missions certainly create a greater problem of assignment of individual areas of science to a given institute. It creates greater challenges in terms of the governance and coordination across them. But I think that there are also some very important counteracting arguments that one could argue to favor the existence of multiple institutes and, in effect, underlie the reason why there are so many. That is because there are so many different advocacy issues that the public and to some degree even the scientific community appreciate.

And he continued, noting that:

> This shouldn't be enough to drive a solution that is counterproductive. I'm sure that with either of the alternatives there are advantages and disadvantages. The disadvantage we have now… neuroscience, is in so many institutes that have divided what is all neuroscience – the richness we have, one could argue – means that there are such different perspectives on it. They assure emphasis on these different perspectives. The risk of having so many? That we won't have adequate coordination, that it will be hard to adequately govern and coordinate neuroscience research. I think that what is important and appropriate is to judge – I think it might be interesting to have opinions

expressed – to judge the degree to which having multiple institutes supporting neuroscience is either interfering with neuroscience research or has been part of the stimulus to its growing so well. I don't think that it is obvious whether the net result has been one of interference or benefit – but having these several communities cooperating and interacting has led to a richness that wouldn't exist under a single administrative entity.

In the meantime, the growth of neuroscience has revolutionized theory and practice in psychiatry. The reasons are many: the efficacy of drug therapy for behavioral and mood disorders; the identification of neurotransmitter abnormalities in different diseases; the increasing evidence that complex genetic factors are important in the major psychoses; and the identification of abnormalities in functional brain imaging in several disorders. Progressively, the gap between neurobiology and cognitive science has narrowed.

On the other hand, there is increasing recognition of behavioral and cognitive abnormality in diseases long considered "neurological." For instance, the movement disorder and dementia of Huntington disease may be preceded by alcoholism, depression, and a high risk of suicide. Depression and dementia are recognized as integral parts of Parkinson disease. Abnormal behavior and epileptic seizures run together in some patients. The focal lesions of a stroke may result in behavioral change. And frontotemporal dementia syndromes are recognized by disinhibition and other behavioral abnormalities.

More, several institutes converge in their interests for some diseases. Examples include autism, attention deficit disorder, and Tourette syndrome.

Turk Skirmishes

The story of how Alzheimer disease research came to rest primarily with the Aging Institute instead of NINDS is an example of what happens when an Institute decides not to establish "turf." Outsiders have long believed it was a tactical error for NINDS to "give up" Alzheimer research in 1974 and allow the newly established Aging institute to take it over. But, according to some on the inside, NINDS authorities decided that there was not much dementia research then and there was not much promise of new research, so they conceded it.

Donald Tower was the director of NINDS at the time. In an interview 26 years later, he said:[7]

> We had a big problem with Alzheimer's disease. Bob Terry and Bob Katzman came to me and said: 'You are not doing anything for Alzheimer's and that is important.' I had to agree with them. We had a meeting to which we invited the Aging Institute and other institutes that might relate, plus the lay people. There

> were, I think, four lay groups at that time, none of which were doing very well. They had not gotten a big enough mass of patients' families to make a go of it. The Aging Institute grabbed the ball and ran with it.
>
> I was a little put off, if you will, by this because I thought NINDS ought to be running it from the research standpoint. But under the circumstances, it seemed better that something was being done, rather than to worry about who was doing it. The major outcome of the original meeting was that all the Alzheimer patients' family groups got together and amalgamated into one. They established their group in Chicago and that really got the ball rolling there.

Some historical considerations put the question in perspective. German neuropsychiatrist Alois Alzheimer had described the disease in 1906 as a form of presenile dementia. The human lifespan was not so long in those days and dementia after age 65 was presumed to be vascular in origin – due to hardening of the arteries and lack of nourishment to the brain. As late as 1960, when the AMA published the first edition of the *Index Medicus* (a reference guide to medical literature), the terminology seemed strange and the number of papers was tiny.

If you had looked for "Alzheimer disease" in 1960, you would have been referred to "psychoses, presenile" and you would have found seven papers published that year. You would also have been referred to "psychoses, senile," covered in 62 papers.

However, in 2000, a Medline search for "dementia" or "Alzheimer disease," as words in the title of the paper, produced 888 papers. If the terms were in either the title or the abstract, there were 1,908 papers. The vast difference between these numbers is a measure of the extent of advances in dementia research during the last 40 years.

From the time of Alzheimer himself, research progress was scant. In 1963, two neuropathologists first applied the electron microscope to the study of the brain in Alzheimer disease. Robert Terry at the Albert Einstein School of Medicine and Michael Kidd at the Maida Vale Hospital in London described the characteristic abnormal structures found in the brains, the neurofibrillary tangles, which consist of cytoskeletal elements, the microtubules. That abnormality gave biochemists a target for elucidation and a new field was opened.

Terry's partner at Einstein was Robert Katzman, a neurologist-investigator who arranged to have a prospective study of people living in a chronic care facility. Neuropsychological tests were done on these people and, with some cajoling, 80 percent of the families gave permission for postmortem examination by Terry and his colleagues. In 1974, they had a Center Grant from NINCDS to support that program.

By 1976, Katzman was convinced that Alzheimer disease accounted for most cases of dementia starting after age 65 as well as in younger people. He also noted that life expectancy for patients with the condition was less than their non-demented peers, which meant that Alzheimer disease was the third most common cause of death. He predicted that there would be an epidemic of dementia as people lived longer and longer. He expounded these views in a famous editorial in 1976.[8]

At that time, Katzman and Terry also wrote to NINCDS director Tower, suggesting that the Institute sponsor a workshop. They were unaware that the Aging Institute had already been established. When the conference was held in 1977, there were three institutional sponsors: NINCDS, NIMH, and NIA.

Robert Butler became a central figure in the saga. He was another product of Seymour Kety's Laboratory of Clinical Science. With Kety, Louis Sokoloff, and others he published a 1963 monograph on the cerebral circulation in aging people. His 1976 Pulitzer Prize winning book, *Growing Old in America*,[9] aroused the interest of Congress in research on aging in general, and the aging brain in particular.

Butler had not been involved in the congressional action, but he entered the picture after he was invited to do so by the Director of NIH. When, in 1976, Butler became Director of the National Institute on Aging, he rapidly addressed the question of Alzheimer disease, realizing that it would be important in requesting research funds for his fledgling institute from Congress.[10]

> The way we were going to get resources for the institute was not going to be the way a scientist might wish it, but rather was going to be at least partly driven by politics in terms of health advocacy groups because people don't perceive themselves as dying of molecular biology or basic science. They do perceive themselves as afflicted by whatever. I thought it was justified, since I was already interested in dementia in the broadest sense and Alzheimer's disease in particular, and since Alzheimer's was a common disease. It wasn't as though I was picking telangiectasia, progeria, or something.
>
> Then, at about that time, I was talking to Don Tower and I learned about Robert Katzman and Robert Terry's proposed conference on Alzheimer's disease. I thought that it would be very important for the Aging Institute to join with Neurology and Mental Health to be a part of this. So I can't tell you whether Don Tower kindly turned to me and said, "Would you like to do this?" or whether I, aggressively, turned to him and said, "I would like us to be cosponsor." I really don't remember. But he was very nice to work with. And so we immediately

> became cosponsors of the wonderful contribution that you all made bringing that symposium together.
>
> ... So I really felt that one of the ways to get aging on the map was going to be through Alzheimer's and at the same time I thought it was a massive disease that had to be attended to. So, to me, it was an appropriate conjoining of two events. As you know, now about 45 percent of the NIA budget is for Alzheimer's disease. In fact, I really, frankly think it is out of balance. Not that I think we shouldn't have all those dollars for Alzheimer's, but there are so many other issues.... There has to be more money.[11]

That conference was important for the scientists who were there because it propelled their ideas and collaborations. It also fueled a major increase in research funds because public advocates at the meeting pulled together their separate organizations to form the Alzheimer's Disease and Related Disorders Association, which then had a major impact on Congress. Two of the sponsors of the meeting – Katzman and Katherine Bick – were active in the creation of that organization of advocates. Dr. Bick represented NINDS in planning the conference.

Katherine Bick grew up on a farm in Prince Edward Island, Canada. Her undergraduate work was done at the University of Western Ontario and her doctoral degree was in biology at Brown University in Providence. Her early research was directed to liver failure. In 1959, she moved to the pathology department at UCLA. There she worked with neuropathologist Jann Brown, who had been a contemporary of Bob Terry's when they were fellows with Harry Zimmerman at Montefiore Hospital in New York.

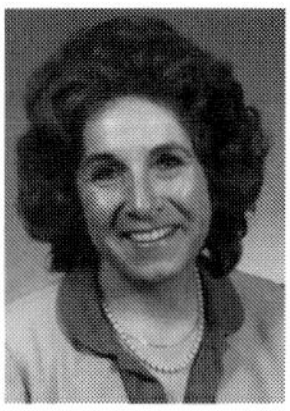

KATHERINE BICK, PH.D.

That was a fruitful time for Bick. She became a skilled electron microscopist and was directed to brain pathology. After years of raising a family and teaching at a state college in California, in 1970 she moved to Georgetown University in Washington, D.C., where she taught undergraduate biology. In April 1976 she was hired to work at NINDS as a Health Scientist Administrator. Her position would now be called a program director in the extramural program. She thought she would be dealing with epilepsy, but within a month after her arrival, Donald Tower assigned her responsibility for organizing the 1977 conference. That experience surely changed her life.

Within a year she became the Deputy Director for the Neurological Disorders Program, which included Alzheimer disease. Her opposite number at the Aging Institute was Zaven Khatchaturian, an energetic proponent of Alzheimer research. Bick rose to become Acting Deputy Director of NINDS in 1980, when Tower retired and Murray Goldstein succeeded him as Director of NINDS. Robert Katzman interviewed Bick in 1999:[11]

RK: Now when you came to NIH in 1976 you became involved in setting up the conference on Alzheimer's disease and apparently Don Tower was very much interested in this area and yet, somehow or another, NIA took this over as their major disease. From your point of view, can you tell me about how that happened and what impact it had on you?

KB: Don Tower is one of the people whom I really admire in this world. He was less concerned about institutional/institute boundaries than others had been at NIH. And Don felt it didn't matter, particularly, what institute's name was on the research grant. He may have miscalculated the territorial ambitions of Bob Butler who, after all, came with a mission to build a new institute and did not come from the old NIH tradition. I think that fragmentation has continued. There are signs that they may be trying to put the neurosciences back together....

...And perhaps naively, Don Tower thought, "it really doesn't matter." And as a matter of fact, it didn't matter, really, in the first years because NIA had the words "Alzheimer's disease" in their legislation (their mission statement, I suppose you could call it). But most of the extramural research at that time was being funded by Neurology. We really had a pretty clear idea in those early days of what the most appropriate division was. I would like to put it on the record that despite what many people have thought must have been great competition between Zaven Khatchaturian and myself, there really never was; at least not on my part and I think Zaven would say the same thing.

Categorical (Disease-Oriented) and General Biomedical Research

The multiplicity of neuroscience institutes is neutral in regards to scientific discovery. Categorical or disease-oriented research may lead scientists into fields far from their original goal, but it creates a shift which has nevertheless been important for advances. Examples suffice to make the point.

Advances in one field may greatly benefit another. We saw that in the story of Arvid Carlsson, who worked in the laboratory of Bernard Brodie in the Heart Institute. Cardiac scientists were interested in serotonin because it was involved in the regulation of blood pressure, but Brodie found that it played a role in the brain. Then Carlsson found that dopamine was involved in some apparent responses to serotonin drugs. That led him to discoveries that were important for a major neurological disorder, Parkinson disease.

Another example concerns Duchenne muscular dystrophy. For more than three decades, starting in 1950, the Muscular Dystrophy Association directed research aimed to cure that group of diseases. At the beginning, little was known about the biology of the diseases except that they were inherited; the organization therefore supported research on any project that promised to provide information about muscle. In the ensuing decades a great deal was learned about muscle – but not much about the diseases, except that muscle surface membranes seemed to be involved in Duchenne dystrophy.

Then came molecular genetics in the 1980s and, as we related in the chapter on voluntary health agencies, a new world opened. Acting on the advice of James Watson, Donald Wood, Scientific Director of the MDA, orchestrated a search for the Duchenne gene. Through the contributions of Kay Davies, Ron Whorton, Ute Francke, and, most notably, Lou Kunkel and his stellar postdocs (Tony Monaco, Marcel Koenig, and Eric Hoffman), the gene for the disease was found in 1987. Their discovery was a landmark in the history of medical genetics since it was the first disease in which the affected gene product was identified by molecular markers without prior knowledge of the function of the protein.

Huntington disease was the first disease to be mapped by positional cloning (in 1983) but it took another ten years to clone the gene and identify *huntingtin*, the gene product, in 1993. The Duchenne gene was mapped in 1987 and, within months, the affected gene product was found to be *dystrophin*, a previously unidentified protein of muscle surface membranes. NINDS supported the laboratories working on both diseases.

But the methods leading to the discovery of the Duchenne gene product did not emerge directly from studies of muscle. Rather, they came from studies of the fundamentals of genetics, which were supported by many NIH institutes – particularly the National Cancer Institute. In his withering attack on the War on Cancer, oncologist-writer Jerome Groopman acknowledged that the fruitless attempts to find a viral cause of cancer in the 1970s nevertheless provided science with the methods of DNA biology. Those were the techniques that led to the two productive decades of the molecular genetics of human disease between 1980 and 2000, as well as the introduction of molecular biology to neuroscience in the same years, including transgenic animals. Ultimately that "fruitless" war on cancer contributed to the success of the Human Genome Project in 2000.

There are other examples of the serendipitous nature of scientific discoveries at NIH. Ronald McKay of the NINDS intramural program has focused on developing stem cell therapy for neurological disease, and he has made progress along those lines. In the process, however, his findings have led him to create pancreatic islet cells that may be useful in the treatment of diabetes mellitus.

The renowned Craig Venter provides another example. He was a laboratory chief in NINDS, using antibodies to identify neurotransmitter receptors, when he was led to methods that would accelerate analysis of the human genome.

Julius Comroe, Jr., and Robert Dripps[12] were highly respected cardiopulmonary physiologists who worked on human subjects. They also made a heroic attempt to do "research on research." They selected ten major clinical advances and then determined there had been 137 "essential bodies of knowledge" in the background. From 4,000 published articles they found 2,500 specific reports that contributed to the 137 bodies of knowledge. Their conclusion was clearly stated: 41 percent of the papers essential for clinical advances were written by investigators who, when they did their work, "expressed no interest in a clinical problem – their goal was knowledge for the sake of knowledge."

Sixty percent of the key articles described basic research, defined as attempts to determine the "mechanisms by which living organisms – including humans – function, or mechanisms by which drugs act." They also emphasized that these reports did not spring from the mind of a single investigator but grew from the accumulation of many prior reports.[13]

From another angle, Shannon and Varmus were surely correct in their view that the business of NIH is research. Yet everyone knows, and the advocacy groups make it emphatic, the enterprise is devoted to "health," as the name emphasizes. It is not a National Institutes of "Science." Leaders of NIH must strike a delicate balance between basic science and disease-oriented research. One of the glories of NIH is that it has done just that.

Multiplex Neuroscience Laboratories in Multiple NIH Institutes

Biomedical research progress is now accelerating. Each new discovery begets many more and the completion of the Human Genome Project will push the frontiers even more rapidly. Does it matter whether all of these institutes are separate? Could we move even faster to find cures or preventive measures for diseases that still defy control?

Logically, it seems that more cooperation would expedite the work. Once, in 1968, an attempt was made to provide a single building for the several institutes doing neuroscience research. That was Building 36, which is now obsolete for modern science. Fischbach noted that "because of the construction of that building, it is really antithetical to the kind of collaborative science we need. The modules are 200 square feet with cinder-block walls and little communication between them. There are no common seminar rooms, no lecture rooms, no library, no sunlight getting into the building. It tends to keep people apart rather than bringing them together."

Led by Drs. Fischbach and Hyman, the ten institute directors have therefore proposed the construction of a National Neuroscience Research Center on the NIH campus in Bethesda, and Congress has

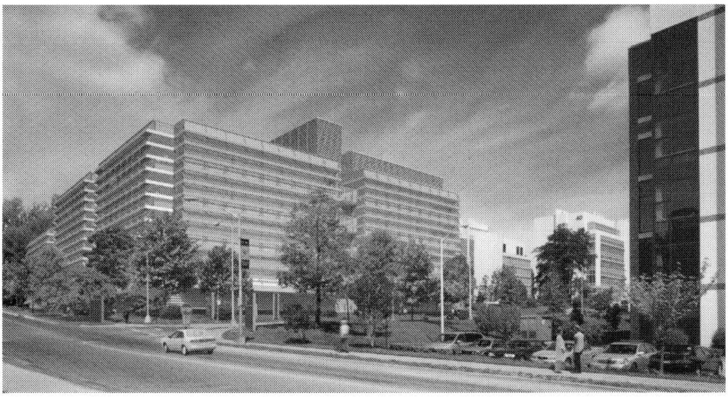

Architect's Sketch of the John Edward Porter Neuroscience Research Center

approved the initial funding. The building is to be named in honor of Senator John Porter of Illinois, who has done so much for NIH in general and neuroscience in particular. The rationale has been stated clearly.[14]

Genomics, the Brain, and Human Disease

The newest revolutionary sets of tools now are genomics and its derivative, proteomics. Genomics techniques and technologies allow researchers to map the location of specific genes and identify and characterize unknown genes. Proteomics offers researchers tools to analyze the proteins that are the products of genetic expression and understand their activities and interactions.

In the past two decades, neuroscience has used the techniques of molecular genetics – based on the predecessors of the Genome Project. The creation of models of human disease in transgenic mice, worms, and fruit flies provided the opportunity to study human disease mechanisms and to understand the basis of memory or fundamental neuronal interactions and pathways. At the same time, human molecular genetics has mapped most of the Mendelian diseases. We have seen the impact of those techniques in the stories of Stanley Prusiner, Eric Kandel, and Paul Greengard.

But the era of molecular genetics has been superseded by the advent of genomics as we opened the new millennium. Whole-genome knowledge now makes it possible to identify and characterize the remaining unknown genes. More than that, it is now possible to do whole-genome searches to determine susceptibility "factors," which may themselves be genetic or environmental.

Francis Collins is the Director of the National Human Genome Research Institute (NHGRI) and leader of the public consortium in the genome projects for humans and other species. He has long asserted that every disease has a genetic component, even diseases that are most often sporadic. The age-related neurodegenerative diseases provide excellent examples. For Parkinson disease, Alzheimer disease, and ALS, the number of familial cases is less than

10 percent; the vast majority of each of these conditions comprises people who have no known family history of the condition. Yet the 10 percent who seem to have inherited the mutation in Mendelian fashion are important because the inherited and sporadic forms seem identical in terms of symptoms and signs, pathology at autopsy, and cellular changes at the molecular level. Twin studies show that there is a genetic component for the apparently sporadic cases. For these non-Mendelian forms of the disorders, more than one gene may play a role ("complex" genetics). To explain why some people get the disease and not others, susceptibility factors are invoked. Susceptibility may be determined by one or more genes, or by environmental agents.

Collins has pointed out that we now have markers throughout the genome and this provides the opportunity to identify these factors. It may even be possible to identify people who are susceptible to a disease and then take measures to prevent the disease from actually developing. This could apply not only to the neurodegenerative diseases but also to schizophrenia and any other disease.

Collins[15] explains how this might work:

> FC: So, most of what we've done until now has been linkage – which means you have to find families. If you can't find families, you find affected sib pairs, you crank through the genome looking for areas that are shared in the affected individuals. Terribly painful, terribly slow, not very powerful – especially if you are limited to affected sib pairs in a polygenic condition, your power is not really very great. But we're going to transition out of that, I think, in the next three or four years to a whole genome association strategy – where, instead of looking for a linkage, we really are going to look in a case-control kind of model for variants that appear in increased frequency in the affected compared to the controls. In the past that has been done as a candidate gene approach. The problem is the candidate genes – usually we don't have the right list. We're not smart enough to know what should be a candidate gene.
>
> Q: But you do not have functions that we haven't conceived of?
>
> FC: Exactly. And things that turn out to be really important in many diseases are genes that you couldn't have guessed because we don't understand the pathway. But now we are at the point where effectively you could look at all the genes as your candidates. We have a million and a half single nucleotide polymorphisms or SNIPS now in public databases. Because the genome is, conveniently for us, not a completely randomized set of those variations but things tend to travel in blocks in what we

> call linkage dysequilibrium. If you scan 500 cases and 500 controls with, say, 100,000 SNIPS, you should find the area that seems to be conferring hereditary susceptibility. The power of that approach is a couple of orders of magnitude better than what you can do with linkage. So we should be able to find more subtle effects than we ever would find using the existing strategies. Yes, it has been frustrating trying to find the genes for common disorders using linkage. It has been very frustrating. But I think it's about to get a lot better with this new approach.

The partner of genomics is proteomics, which means knowing all the proteins encoded in the human genome. Proteomics goes one step beyond genomics. All life depends on the expression of genes and genes determine the nature of proteins, which comprise enzymes, hormones, structural proteins of all cells, and others. It was once thought that "one gene creates one protein."

However, the Human Genome Project uncovered fewer genes than the number of known proteins, so some genes must encode more than one protein. If a gene encodes multiple proteins with different functions, the conformation of the protein or some other physical differences must be responsible for the diverse functions. In other words, the same protein – that is, the same string of amino acids – may have two different functions, depending on different three-dimensional configurations. Variations of the same sequence of amino acids must play a role in many normal functions. A striking example of the consequence of altered conformity is provided by the prion diseases, in which a mutation or some other force changes the three-dimensional structure of the prion protein from a benign influence to a malign poison.

The impact of genomics and proteomics will be felt in all basic cell biology and basic neuroscience, providing information about the control of all cellular functions and how they interact in the brain.

Pharmacogenomics is a third result of the genomic revolution. It is now possible to determine which genes are involved in the metabolism of a drug and to determine which people are likely to benefit from the drug and who is likely to have adverse effects. The impact will be felt on all medicine, not just neurology and psychiatry.

We are entering a new world. After World War II, when NINDB was starting in the 1950s, biochemical genetics developed and so did the multi-faceted neuroscience, which combined the earlier sciences of neuroanatomy, neurochemistry, neurophysiology, neuropathology, and embryology. Then, in 1980, neuroscience was changed by the advent of molecular genetics. Now, we have already seen the beginning of the genomics revolution, one that promises to accelerate neuroscience – both basic and clinical. It is likely to become more difficult to identify or separate "basic" from "clinical."

Neurology and Psychiatry: A Remarriage?

In the first quarter of the twentieth century, clinicians interested in the brain called themselves neuropsychiatrists. Research was confined to neuropathology and treatment was nonexistent – except for the fever therapy of neurosyphilis (which won a 1927 Nobel Prize for Julius Wagner-Jaurreg, but was then totally displaced by penicillin). As late as 1950, neurology trainees were told they would have to invest in a shock box – to give electroconvulsive therapy for depression – if they wanted to earn a living. Neuropsychiatry was still in vogue in mid-century. Throughout the 1920s, however, psychoanalysis had grown dominant in the medical schools of the United States. By 1950, analysts were at their peak of influence, a broad crest that lasted two or three decades. During that interval, psychiatry trainees concentrated on psychotherapy and, in contrast, many neurology trainees disdained psychiatric exposure and so there was little academic interaction between the two disciplines.

During that same period, however, the growth of psychotropic drug therapy and the advance of neuroscience eroded the influence of psychoanalysis, which was much diminished by 1980. Since then, and especially during the 90s – the Decade of the Brain – advances in neuroscience have drawn the clinical disciplines closer. Nobel Prize winner Eric Kandel believes the appreciation and application of neuroscience could actually enhance psychotherapy.

The reunification movement has picked up steam from the forceful lead of prominent neurologists, psychiatrists, and neuroscientists.[16-19] Symposia, celebratory issues of leading science journals, and the appearance of new journals directed to neurologists and psychiatrists are beginning to have an impact. Among the new journals are *Neuropsychiatry*, the *Journal of Neuropsychiatry*, and *Clinical Neuroscience Research*. Some clinicians have advocated a change in terminology from "mental illness" to "brain disease."[20] To expedite the movement, highly respected authorities have recommended more psychiatry training for neurologists and vice versa.[16-19]

However, cross-training in neurology and psychiatry, especially if mandatory, would prolong training and extend even further the already arduous training of clinical investigators. If that happens, educators will have to address the potential consequences. First of all, they will have to ask if prescribed curricula are needed. There is already spontaneous admixture of neurologic and psychiatric research. There are already more and more symposia and journals devoted to overlapping science in the two fields. This is occurring without changes in training curriculum – other than the impact of neuroscience itself.

Great hope is placed on the M.D.-Ph.D. clinical scientists. Their training takes six to eight years for the combined degree, then five years for clinical training in neurology or psychiatry. Fischbach has bemoaned the length of time it takes for Ph.D. neuroscientists to gain the first RO-1 (investigator-initiated) award – now about age 38. It takes even longer for the M.D.-Ph.D.

These are bright young scientists. They may be helped best by giving them freedom to develop their own curricula and shortening clinical training time. They will be doing clinical work for the rest of their lives – however limited that may be – and likely will focus on a disease related to their research.

And times change. When Steven Hyman completed his psychiatric training and sought to learn the methods of molecular biology, he was told by a senior professor at Harvard that he should watch his step, what he was doing in the laboratory was not psychiatry.[21] Now, Hyman is the director of NIMH and the search for the genetic contribution to the major psychoses is a vast enterprise.[22,23]

NINDS in the Twenty-First Century

Landmark discoveries have come with increasing rapidity during the 50 years since NINDS was founded. That process of acceleration will surely continue. Predictions abound[24] about stem cells, gene therapy, bioengineering breakthroughs, robotic surgery, and genomically designed drugs for diseases of all organ systems. It is fitting that a new director of NINDS, soon to be named, will be a major leader in the new era. It will be a wonderworld for NINDS, for all the other neuroscience institutes at NIH, for all of neuroscience, and for all people, everywhere.

1 Grob GN. The forging of mental health policy in America: World War II to New Frontier. *J Hist Med Alliled Sci* 1987;42:410-446.

2 Hyman S. Interview with author, February 27, 2001.

3 Kirschstein R. Interview with author, March 7, 2001.

4 Fischbach G. Interview with author, August 30, 2000.

5 Varmus H. Proliferation of National Institutes of Health. *Science* 2001; 291: 1903-1905.

6 Hodes R. Interview with author, March 23, 2001.

7 Tower DB. Interview with author, July 19, 2000.

8 Katzman R. The prevalence and malignancy of Alzheimer's disease: a major killer. *Arch Neurol* 1976;33:217-218.

9 Butler RN. *Why survive? Being old in America.* New York: Harper and Row, 1975.

10 Butler RN. The National Institutes of Health Respond. In Katzman R, Bick K, eds. *Alzheimer disease: the changing view.* San Diego: Academic Press, 1999:272-293.

11 Bick K. The impact of AD and society's response. The National Institutes of Health respond. In Katzman R, Bick K, eds. *Alzheimer disease; the changing view.* San Diego: Academic Press, 2000: 294-312.

12 Comroe JH Jr, Dripps RD. Scientific basis for the support of biomedical science. *Science* 1976;192:105-111.

13 Comroe JH Jr, Dripps RD. Ben Franklin and open heart surgery. *Circ Res* 1974; 35:661-9.

14 The John Edward Porter Neuroscience Research Center at the National Institutes of Health: A Vision for the Times. Bethesda, MD: The Foundation for the National Institutes of Health, 2001.

15 Collins FS. Interview with author, March 14, 2001.

16 Price BH, Adams RD, Coyle JT. Neurology and psychiatry: closing the great divide. *Neurology* 2000;54:8-14.

17 Kandel ER. A new intellectual framework for psychiatry. *Am J Psychiatry* 1998; 155:457-469.

18 Kandel ER. Biology and the future of psychoanalysis: a new intellectual framework for psychiatry revisited. *Am J Psychiatry* 1999;156:505-524.

19 Cowan WM, Harter DH, Kandel ER. The emergence of modern neuroscience: some implications for neurology and psychiatry. *Annu Rev Neurosci* 2000;23:343-391.

20 Baker M, Menken M. Time to abandon the term mental illness. *British Medical Journal* 2001;322:937.

21 Hyman S. Interview with author, February 27, 2001.

22 Hyman S. Mental illness: genetically complex disorders of neural circuitry and neural communication. *Neuron* 2000;28:321-323.

23 Brown RH Jr, Ross CA, eds. Genetic aspects of psychiatric and neurological disorders. *Clin Neurosci Res* 2001;1:82-169.

24 Nathan DG, Fontanarosa PG, Wilson JD. Opportunities for medical research in the 21st century. *JAMA* 2001;285:499-654.

CELEBRATING 50 YEARS OF BRAIN RESEARCH

50th ANNIVERSARY

SECTION 5

NEUROSCIENCE TIMELINE

The citations in this timeline were selected as "landmarks," contributions that permanently changed neuroscience or clinical practice. Since that definition leaves room for choice, we have undoubtedly omitted some advances that could well be considered landmarks. On the other hand, some of the inclusions could also be debated.

To minimize personal bias, we have relied on the choices of respected award committees, the Nobel, Horwitz, Lasker, Potamkin, Charles E. Dana, Bristol-Myers Squibb, and others. The committees selecting the winners often choose the same investigator. Erroneous salutes are uncommon. Even so, the prizes often lag long behind meritorious research. For instance, the 2000 Nobel Prizes were awarded for work done decades earlier and all three recipients continued to register additional landmark discoveries in the interim. Recognition may be a long time coming. In the meantime, the investigator is not paid formal tribute.

In addition to the prizes, we sought the advice of colleagues about possible landmarks and we relied on comprehensive historical reviews of basic neuroscience,[1-4] including two collections of essays that address specific developments in diverse aspects of the field.[5,6]

In contrast, however, there is a paucity of similar historical reviews of clinical neuroscience. At the celebration of the twenty-fifth anniversary of NINDS, advances in clinical neurosciences were documented in a multi-authored book.[7] However, there has been no such comprehensive review since then. There have been many general and disease-specific texts, but only two[8,9] that specifically compare the present with earlier times.

Another historian of the era is Donald B. Tower, director of NINCDS from 1973 to 1981. He has contributed several reviews[10-13] and, for the twenty-fifth anniversary, he recorded the changes in neuroscience since 1950, including the following moving remarks:[14]

> At the time the NINDB was founded our knowledge of the Krebs cycle of intermediary metabolism was newly established. The importance of vitamin B6 to CNS function was still to be demonstrated. Gamma-amino-butyric acid (GABA), serotonin, and dopamine were still to be discovered. And we knew nothing of reserpine and the subsequent host of psychomimetic drugs. The concept of the mechanism of neuromuscular transmission had just changed from an electrical to a chemical one, and the mechanisms of action of cholinesterase and the anticholinesterase agents were just in the process of elucidation . . . .

> Isotopic tracers were few and not widely used. The liquid scintillation counter and isotopic scintiscanning were still to be developed. The mainstays of modern biochemical analysis, thin-layer chromatography and gas-liquid chromatography, were unknown. The preparative ultracentrifuge was just coming off the drawing boards, so that subcellular fractionation, lysosomes, synaptosomes, and membrane and receptor isolations were far in the future. There were no fluorescence techniques for tracing anatomical pathways, identifying antigen-antibody reactions, or conducting microanalytical quantifications. Computer technology as we know it today was hardly imagined. And that novelty, the electron microscope, had not yet proved applicable to the examination of neural tissues.

Now, it is time to record another 25 years of progress. The staccato format of a timeline can be only superficial. It does not record the impact of computers and the internet, or bioengineering feats that have led to astounding imaging of the brain, fantastic kinds of stereotactic and minimally invasive surgery, pacemakers for deep brain stimulation, tissues for implantation, and endovascular interventions. Molecular genetics has informed clinical practice and transformed neuroscience and cell biology. Now we have the new era of genomic neuroscience and anticipated wonders from stem cells. The annual number of landmarks has increased progressively with the years and the content has become progressively more molecular – more fundamental and more profound in its implications.

The acceleration of research in the past twenty-five years is undoubtedly only a prelude to more rapid change in years to come.

1 Kandel ER, Squire LR. Neuroscience: breaking down scientific barriers to the study of brain and mind. *Science* 2000;290:1113-1120.

2 Cowan WM, Harter DH, Kandel ER. The emergence of modern neuroscience: some implications for neurology and psychiatry. *Annu Rev Neurosci* 2000;23:343-391.

3 Albright TD, Jessell TM, Kandel ER, Posner MI. Neural science: a century of progress and the mysteries that remain. *Neuron* 2000 Feb;25 Suppl:S1-55.

4 Cowan WM, Kandel ER. A brief history of synapses and synaptic transmission. In Cowan WM, Südhof TC, Stevens CF, Davies K. *Synapses.* Baltimore: Johns Hopkins University Press, 2001:1-87.

5 Jessell T, Kandel E. Introduction: one decade of Neuron, six decades of neuroscience. *Neuron* 1998;20:367-369.

6 Hyman S. Mental illness: genetically complex disorders of neural circuitry and neural communication. *Neuron* 2000;28:321-333.

7 Chase TN, ed. *The Clinical Neurosciences.* vol. 2 of Tower DB, ed. *The Nervous System: A Three-Volume Work Commemorating the 25th Anniversary of the National Institute of Neurological and Communicative Disorders and Stroke.* New York: Raven Press, 1975.

8 Waksman BH. Historical perspective and overview. In Antel J, ed. *Clinical Neuroimmunology*, London: Blackwell Science,1988:391-404.

9 Leeds NE, Kiefer SA. Evolution of diagnostic neuroradiology from 1904 to 1999. *Radiology* 2000;217:309-318.

10 Tower DB. A century of neuronal and neuroglial interactions, and their pathological implications: an overview. *Prog Brain Res* 1992;94:3-17.

11 Tower DB. The impact of the NINCDS on the neurosciences: an essay written for the centennial of the NIH. *J Neurosci* 1987;7:1601-1606.

12 Tower DB. The American Society for Neurochemistry (ASN): antecedents, founding, and early years. *J Neurochem* 1987;48:313-326.

13 Tower DB. Neurochemistry – one hundred years, 1875-1975. *Ann Neurol* 1977;1:2-36.

14 Tower DB. Introduction. In Brady RO, *The Basic Neurosciences*, vol. 1 of Tower DB, ed. *The Nervous System. A Three-Volume Work Commemorating the 25th Anniversary of the National Institute of Neurological and Communicative Disorders and Stroke.* New York: Raven Press, 1975: xvii-xx.

FIFTY YEARS OF ADVANCES IN NEUROSCIENCE

The Fifties

1950

- Wilder Penfield and Herbert Jasper report first surgical treatment for temporal lobe epilepsy.
- Eugene Roberts and J. Awapara discover gamma-amino butyric acid.

1951

- Paul Fatt and Bernard Katz discover mini end-plate potentials (Nobel Prize to Katz, 1970).
- Russell Brain describes paraneoplastic cerebellar degeneration.
- Brian McArdle describes abnormal glycogen metabolism in syndrome of recurrent myoglobinuria.
- C. Miller Fisher describes transient ischemic attacks in carotid artery disease.

1952

- Alan Hodgkin and Andrew Huxley discover the ionic mechanism of the nerve impulse (Nobel Prize, 1963, shared with Sir John Carew Eccles).
- Sir John Carew Eccles and colleagues establish that synaptic transmission in the CNS is chemical (Nobel Prize, 1962).
- Intracranial pressure monitoring introduced for critical care of brain trauma and infection.

1953

- Last epidemics of paralytic poliomyelitis in the United States and Europe.
- First widespread use of positive pressure respirators to treat paralytic respiratory failure, forerunner to neurological and respiratory intensive care units.
- James Watson and Francis Crick discover structure of DNA.
- Rapid eye-movement (REM) sleep discovered by Eugene Aserinsky and Nathaniel Kleitner.
- Betty Twarog and Irvine Page find serotonin in brain.
- Enzyme abnormality in phenylketonuria discovered by George Jervis; landmark in biochemical genetics and inherited brain diseases.
- Stephen W. Kuffler determines receptive fields of retinal ganglion cells.

- Leonard Kurland establishes epidemiology unit at NINDS and takes first trip to Guam to investigate high incidence of ALS.

1954

- Robert Bowman invents the spectrophotofluorometer at NHLBI; used by Julius Axelrod in NIMH and by Arvid Carlsson in Sweden to study catecholamines.
- Measles vaccine introduced; leads to elimination of subacute sclerosing panencephalitis by 1955.
- W.J.H. Nauta and P.A. Gygax introduce technique for tracing connections based on the selective staining of degenerative axons.
- E.J. DelCastillo and Bernard Katz discover the quantal release of neurotransmitters and relate this to the discovery of synaptic vesicles by Sanford Palay and George Palade, and Eddy M. DeRobertis and Stanley Bennet (Nobel Prize to Palade, 1974).
- Rita Levi-Montalcini, Stanley Cohen Viktor Hamburger discover the nerve growth promoting factor NGF (Horwitz Prize to all three, 1983; Nobel Prize to Levi-Montalcini and Cohen, 1986).
- Paul Fatt predicts existence of electric transmission in synaptic vesicles.

1955

- Bernard Brodie begins studies of serotonin at the National Heart Institute (Lasker Award, 1967).
- Experimental autoimmune neuritis induced by Byron Waksman and Raymond Adams.
- Seymour Kety, Louis Sokoloff, William Landau and others describe method for measurement of local cerebral blood flow in cats (Lasker Award to Kety, 1999, for related research).

1956

- Kuru recognized in New Guinea.
- Dorothy Andersen describes type IV glycogen storage disease (later identified as glycogen brancher enzyme deficiency).
- Marian Kies (NIMH) and Elizabeth Roboz-Einstein identify myelin basic protein as the antigen in experimental allergic encephalomyelitis.
- William Windle (NINDS) establishes Prenatal Research Laboratory at the University of Puerto Rico to investigate perinatal neurological development in primates (Lasker Award, 1968).
- Edward Lambert and Lee Eaton describe a paraneoplastic myasthenic syndrome that is designated by their eponym, the Lambert-Eaton syndrome.

- Irving S. Cooper accidentally finds that occlusion of anterior choroidal artery improves contralateral parkinsonian signs, then deliberately carries out pallidotomy and thalamotomy.

1957

- D. Carleton Gajdusek (NINDB) begins investigation of kuru in New Guinea, leading to identification of transmissible spongiform encephalopathies such as Creutzfeldt-Jakob disease in humans and bovine spongiform encephalopathy (mad cow disease) in cows (Nobel Prize, 1976).
- Arvid Carlsson finds that dihydroxyphenylalanine (DOPA) reverses the brain symptoms caused by reserpine, shifting attention from serotonin to DOPA as the affected transmitter (Nobel Prize, 2000).
- Vernon Ingram describes first human point mutation (sickle cell disease).
- Vernon Mountcastle discovers the columnar organization of cells in the cerebral cortex (Lasker Award, 1983).
- Neurosurgeon W.B. Scoville and neuropsychologist Brenda Milner describe profound loss of declarative memory in patient HM following bilateral hippocampal removal to treat intractable epilepsy, a landmark of cognitive neuroscience.
- Michael Fuortes and Karl Frank (NINDB) report findings later identified by Eccles as presynaptic inhibition.
- Edward Fuhrspan and David Potter discover electrically transmitting synapses in invertebrates.

1958

- William Hadlow studies scrapie in English sheep and notes resemblance to kuru.
- Stephen Kuffler and associates show that GABA is inhibitory transmitter in crayfish.
- Ulf von Euler establishes that noradrenaline (norepinephrine) is the transmitter in the sympathetic system (Nobel Prize, 1970).
- David Hubel and Torsten Wiesel characterize the receptor field properties of neurons in the visual cortex (Nobel Prize to both, 1981, shared with Roger Sperry).
- Julius Axelrod discovers a key enzyme in the biosynthetic pathway for norepinephrine (Nobel Prize, 1970).
- James Austin describes chronic inflammatory polyneuropathy and response to prednisone.

The Sixties

1960

- Oleh Hornykiewicz's finding that dopamine is depleted in the striatum of patients with Parkinson disease leads to the introduction of levodopa for treatment of the disorder.
- Levodopa approved by U.S. Food and Drug Administration for treatment of Parkinson disease.
- Georg von Békésy summarizes his contributions to the physiology of hearing (Nobel Prize, 1961).

1962

- Seymour Kety and colleagues, using Danish records of twins and their relatives, establish that schizophrenia has a strong genetic component (Lasker Award, 1999).
- Eric Kandel begins studies with sea snail (*Aplysia*) to explore synaptic function in learning and memory (Lasker Award, 1983; Nobel Prize, 2000).
- E. George Gray and Vernon Whitaker isolate synaptosomes which comprise both presynaptic and postsynaptic structures; Gray identifies axo-axonal synapses as basis for presynaptic inhibition.
- Bengt Falck and Nils Hillarp apply fluorescence histochemistry for tracing neuronal projections.
- American Society of Neuroradiology founded.

1963

- Robert Terry and Michael Kidd independently use electron microscope to identify structure of plaques and tangles in Alzheimer disease (Potamkin Prize to Terry, 1988).
- Robert Martin and Guillermo Pilar identify synapses that are both electrical and chemical.

1964

- Clay Armstrong begins publishing work on nerve cell membrane excitability and the elucidation of ion channel gating kinetics (Lasker Award, 1999).
- T. Gerritsen and H. A. Waisman in one report; and another by S.H. Mudd, F. Irrevere, and L. Laster describe enzymatic defect in homocystinuria; leads to recognition of important risk factor for stroke.
- Bertil Hille begins decade-spanning work exploring the gating mechanisms of ion channels (Lasker Award, 1999).

1965

- Ronald Melzack and Patrick Wall publish gate control theory of pain.
- Clarence J. Gibbs transmits kuru to chimpanzee in NINDS lab.
- Roscoe Brady describes enzymatic defects in Gaucher disease.
- Donald Tschudy describes enzymatic abnormality in acute intermittent porphyria.
- M.H. Aprison and Robert Werman provide evidence that glycine is an inhibitory transmitter in spinal cord and brainstem.
- Neurological intensive care units appear.
- A. Cecil Taylor and Paul Weiss demonstrate axonal flow by radiolabeling, later use for tracing CNS connections.
- Sleep laboratories uncover upper airway obstruction as a cause of sleep apnea syndrome.
- Norman Geschwind formulates "disconnection" theory about language disorders.

1966

- Edward Evarts (NIMH) develops methods for studying movement, and Robert Wurtz (NINDB) creates methods for studying perception, in the brain using single-cell recordings in awake primates.
- First publication of *Mendelian Inheritance in Man* by Victor A. McKusick.
- Sydney Brenner introduces *Caenorhabiditis elegans* (round worm) as a model system for studying development of nervous system (Lasker Award, 1971; Lasker Special Achievement in Medical Science, 2000).
- Seymour Benzer describes behavioral mutants in *Drosophila* (Lasker Award, 1971).

1967

- Roger Sperry summarizes findings for both experimental work and human subjects with "split-brains" on the independent functions of the two cerebral hemispheres (Nobel Prize, 1981, shared with Hubel and Wiesel).
- Michael Bennett, George Pappas, and Y. Nakajima show structure of electrical synapses in vertebrates.
- J. Wada and Theodore Rasmussen describe intracarotid injection of barbiturate to determine which hemisphere is dominate for speech.

- Catheter angiography introduced, replacing direct puncture of carotid artery for diagnosis of brain diseases.

1968

- George Cotzias reports benefit of large doses of levodopa for Parkinson disease (Lasker Award, 1969).
- Peter Dyck and associates define diagnostic criteria for chronic inflammatory demyelinating polyneuropathy.

1969

- Society for Neuroscience founded.
- Roger Guillemin and Andrew Schally report discovery of the first hypothalamic releasing hormones (Nobel Prize, 1977; Lasker Award, 1975).
- Louis Sokoloff, Martin Reivich, and David Kuhl develop labeled radioactive ligands; Sokoloff perform first animal blood flow experiments with ^{14}C-deoxyglucose.
- First successful randomized controlled therapeutic trial for multiple sclerosis (adrenocorticotrophin).
- Melvin D. Yahr, Roger C. Duvoisin, et al., report first controlled therapeutic trial of levodopa in Parkinson disease.
- S. Tarui describes muscle phosphofructokinase deficiency as a cause of recurrent myoglobinuria, extending list of diseases of glycogen metabolism.

The Seventies

1970

- Noise analysis by Bernard Katz and Ricardo Miledi used to analyze opening and closing of acetylcholine receptor channels.
- Eric Kandel finds that habituation and sensitization alter strength of synaptic connections in *Aplysia*, providing a cellular basis for memory.

1972

- Rodolfo Llinas confirms role of calcium influx in transmitter release.
- H.R. Muller describes use of Doppler ultrasound to diagnosis occlusion of internal carotid artery.
- Jerome B. Posner initiates reports that found the field of neuro-oncology, comprising metastases to CNS, primary CNS tumors, complications of therapy, and delineation of paraneoplastic syndromes from molecular to clinical.

- Fred Plum and Jerome B. Posner publish *The Diagnosis of Stupor and Coma*, which altered the practice of neurology and initiates development of criteria for brain death and persistent vegetative state; contributes to transplantation surgery and end-of-life ethics.
- New methods for tracing connections in the brain based on the anterograde and retrograde transport of isotopically labeled proteins and other markers introduced by Cowan and colleagues and by LaVail and LaVail.

1973

- T.V. Bliss and T. Lømo discover long-term potentiation (LTP) thought to be the cellular basis of learning and memory.
- James Patrick and Jon Lindstrom show that antibodies against the acetylcholine receptor can cause myasthenia gravis.
- First CT scanners available commercially (Nobel Prize, 1979 to Allan Cormack and Godfrey Houndsfield, 1979).
- John Heuser and Thomas Reese (NINDS) show recycling of synaptic vesicles.
- Candace Pert and Solomon Snyder locate opioid receptors in the brain (Lasker Award to Snyder, 1978; Bristol-Myers Squibb Award to Snyder, 1996).
- Michael Merzenich describes use of cochlear prosthesis and begins long-term studies of hearing and related behavior.

1974

- Michael Phelps, Edward Hoffman, and Michael Ter Pogossian develop PET scanning to study brain function in conscious human subjects.
- MRI scanners become available for clinical use.
- Seymour Benzer, with W.G. Quinn and W.A. Harris, opens the field of neurogenetics of memory.

1975

- Paul Greengard discovers the significance of protein phosphorylation in synaptic transmission mediating the effects of neurotransmitters (Nobel Prize, 2000).
- Louis Sokoloff develops deoxyglucose method for studying oxygen utilization in the brain (Lasker Award, 1981).
- Pasko Rakic documents "neuronal migration" outward from the ventricular or subventricular layers of the brain in embryonic development.
- PET shows seizure focus in patients with epilepsy.

- Hugo Moser identifies accumulation of very long chain fatty acids as cause of adrenoleukodystrophy.
- Neurology-Neurosurgery Intensive Care Units founded at Massachusetts General Hospital, Johns Hopkins University, University of Virginia, Washington University, and New York Neurological Institute; establishes new specialty of critical care neurology.
- Hughes identifies first morphine-like peptide in brains; later referred to as opiods.

1976

- Erwin Neher and Bert Sakmann invent patch-clamping as a method for recording activity in single ion channels or receptors (Nobel Prize, 1991).
- Robert Katzman identifies Alzheimer disease as cause of late-onset as well as "presenile" dementia and a leading cause of death; predicts increasing incidence as an epidemic (Potamkin Prize, 1992).

1977

- Dale McFarlin and Marian Kies show role of activated T-cells in transfer of experimental allergic encephalomyelitis (EAE).
- J. Storm-Mathisen finds that glutamate is an excitatory transmitter.
- Horwitz Prize to Elvin A. Kabat for lifetime work in quantitative immunology, including 1948 discovery that CSF levels of (γ-globulin are increased in multiple sclerosis, a lasting contribution to diagnosis of MS and autoimmune causation.

1978

- Roscoe Brady determines the basis of lipid storage diseases and shows that affected cells can be treated by appropriate enzyme transfer (Lasker Award, 1982).
- Bert Sakmann and H.R. Brenner apply patch-clamp to analyze currents in neuromuscular transmission by channels in acetylcholine receptor.
- Pak Chan and Robert A. Fishman describe role of polyunsaturated fatty acids and free radicals in causing brain edema.

1979

- Nancy Wexler makes first trip to Lake Maracaibo, Venezuela to identify families with Huntington disease (Lasker Award, 1993).

The Eighties

1980

- Huntington Disease Commission (NINDS) sets need for gene mapping.
- Combined radiotherapy and chemotherapy improves survival for malignant gliomas (brain tumors).
- Jean-Pierre Changeux and Arthur Karlin analyze structure of acetylcholine receptor; transmitter binding site and ionic channel are recognized as different components of receptor.
- Norman Latov and associates find antibodies to myelin-associated glycoprotein in patients with monoclonal gammopathy.

1981

- James Gusella and Joseph Martin start mapping Huntington disease gene.
- Lambert-Eaton syndrome, a paraneoplastic myasthenic syndrome, is transmitted to mice with serum from patients by John Newsom-Davis, Angela Vincent, and colleagues.
- Soluble contrast agents replace iodinated lipids for myelography with CT, reducing adverse effects of contrast agents.
- First cases of AIDS appear.
- Kathleen M. Foley evaluates treatment of cancer pain, leading to national movement revising palliative care of chronic diseases.

1982

- AIDS and neuro-AIDS recognized.
- Stanley Prusiner formulates prion hypothesis as the basis of spongiform encephalopathies like Creutzfeldt-Jakob disease and kuru.
- Irwin Kopin and James Langston identify MPTP as an environmental toxin that can cause a Parkinson-like syndrome.
- Creutzfeldt-Jakob disease transmitted to non-human primates by C.J. Gibbs and D.C. Gajdusek, injecting brain tissue from patients.
- Dennis Selkoe initiates biochemical approach to analysis of amyloid plaques in Alzheimer disease (Potamkin Prize, 1989, with George Glenner).
- Audrey S. Penn, Chris Bever, Hai Won Chang, and others provide evidence that penicillamine may alter the structure of the acetylcholine receptor to induce clinical myasthenia gravis rather than the dominant theory, which holds that the drug primarily interacts with T-cell antigens to cause myasthenia.

1983

- James Gusella and colleagues identify a locus on chromosome 4 that is altered in Huntington disease (Metropolitan Life Foundation Award, 1987; Dana Award, 1998).
- MRI shows lesions in patients with multiple sclerosis with no relation to clinical symptoms; provide marker of progression or recovery.
- Fernando Nottebohm discovers formation of new neurons in brains of song-birds.

1984

- George Glenner identifies Alzheimer brain deposits as amyloid, opens molecular research (Potamkin Prize, 1989, with Dennis Selkoe).
- MRI available; myelography gradually eliminated; angiography less commonly used.
- Corey Goodman and associates determine signals for axonal development and guidance.
- Timothy A. Pedley, Ronald Emerson, and colleagues describe diagnostic usefulness of somatosensory-evoked potentials.

1985

- Dennis W. Choi begins studies of glutamate toxicity to neurons after ischemia or other injury.

1986

- S. Numa and colleagues succeed in cloning the genes for sodium and other ion channels.

1987

- Genes associated with familial Alzheimer disease identified by Rudolph Tanzi, James Gusella, G.A.P. Bruns, and Peter St. George-Hyslop (Potamkin Prize, 1990, to Masters and Keyreuther; Potamkin Prize, 1996, to Tanzi and St. George-Hyslop).
- Gene for Duchenne muscular dystrophy identified by Louis Kunkel, Anthony Monaco, Eric Hoffman, and Marcel Koenig (Dana Award to Kunkel, 1998).
- Stanley Prusiner proves that prions cause Creutzfeldt-Jakob disease and bovine spongiform encephalopathy – mad cow disease (Lasker Award, 1994; Nobel Prize, 1997).
- Steven E. Hyman initiates molecular studies of addiction and psychiatric disorders.
- Patricia Goldman-Rakic and co-workers demonstrate role of prefrontal neurons in remembering places within visual field; eye movements can be used to monitor working memory.

- Mitchell Brin, Stanley Fahn, and associates find benefit from injections of botulinum toxin in torticollis, spastic dysphonia, and other focal dystonias.

1988

- Mutations in mitochondrial genes identified as the basis for Leber Hereditary Optic Atrophy and other disorders by Douglas Wallace, and by Anita Harding and colleagues.
- Thomas Masaryk introduces magnetic resonance angiography, a noninvasive method that makes intra-arterial injection unnecessary.
- PET scanning used to study human cognitive and motor functions by Michael Posner, Marcus Raichle, the Damasios, and Richard Frakowiac.
- Guy McKhann, John W. Griffin, David Cornblath, and associates report that plasmapheresis accelerates recovery from Guillain-Barré syndrome.

1989

- Cloning of the first glutamate receptor subunits by Stephen Heinemann and colleagues.
- Demonstration of mutation of prion protein gene in human disease (Gerstmann-Sträussler-Scheinker syndrome) by Karen Hsaio and Stanley Prusiner, major confirmation of prion theory.

The Nineties

1990

- President George Bush signs proclamation declaring the 1990s the Decade of the Brain.
- Clinical trial by Michael Bracken and colleagues shows that methylprednisolone significantly improves recovery after spinal cord injury.
- First of the disorders known as channelopathies identifed by Bertrand Fontaine.
- Andrew G. Engel describes first of many congenital syndromes of myasthenia gravis with mutations in the genes for acetylcholine receptor subunits.
- Segi Ogawa and Bruce Rosen develop functional MRI for the non-invasive study of human brain function.
- Cornelia Bargmann initiates molecular studies of smell and chemosensory functions in *C. elegans*.

1991

- E.J. Kremer, Steve Warren, Tom Caskey, and A.J. Verkerk find trinucleotide repeat in fragile X syndrome, a cause of mental retardation.
- James Lupski and associates, and Philip Chance and associates, describe duplication of gene for peripheral myelin protein gene PMP-22 in hereditary sensorimotor neuropathy (Charcot-Marie-Tooth disease).
- Stereotactic radiosurgery recommended for treatment of arteriovenous malformations.
- Larry Squire, Morton Mishkin, and their associates create animal model of human amnesia for declarative memory by making lesions of the hippocampus and adjacent brain.

1992

- U.S. Food and Drug Administration approves interferon beta-1b for treatment of relapsing-remitting multiple sclerosis.
- Kenneth Fischbeck, Steve Warren, Tom Caskey, and others identify "trineucleotide repeats" as the basis of a number of neurological disorders
- Charles G. Gross identifies "face-cells" in the temporal lobe that selectively respond to images of heads and faces.

1993

- Gene for Huntington identified by HD Collaborative Research group (Dana Award, 1998 to Gusella).
- Allen Roses and W.J. Strittmatter identify apolipoprotein E ε4 as a risk factor for late-onset Alzheimer disease.
- U.S. Food and Drug Administration approves interferon therapy for multiple sclerosis.
- New anti-epileptic drugs approved by U.S. Food and Drug Administration after 20-year hiatus.
- U.S. Food and Drug Administration approves tacrine (a cholinergic drug) the first drug for treatment of Alzheimer disease.
- E. Tournier-Lasserve and colleagues describe hereditary syndrome of stroke and dementia – CADASIL (for Cerebral Autosomal Dominant Arteriopathy, with Subcortical Infarcts and Leucoencephalopathy); map to chromosome 19q12 and notch gene.
- Linda Buck and Richard Axel identify large family of genes that encode olfactory sensory receptors.

- Thomas Jessell and colleagues identify "hedgehog" genes; elucidate proteins and molecular mechanisms involved in CNS development in the mammalian embryo (Bristol-Myers Squibb Award to Jessell, 2000).
- Magnetic resonance spectroscopy; echo-planar, diffusion weighted, and perfusion imaging extend range of diagnostic MRI.
- Justin C. McArthur, Jr., and associates, and Bradley A. Navia, Barry D. Jordan, and Richard W. Price describe HIV-dementia.

1994

- Kirk Wilhelmsen and Timothy Lynch and colleagues describe syndrome of frontotemporal dementia, disinhibition, parkinsonism, and amyotrophy linked to chromosome 17.
- M. Tessier-Lavigne identifies first protein involved in directed outgrowth of axons in CNS.
- J.R. Jack and colleagues introduce pre-surgical mapping of speech area with fMRI.
- Genetic basis of programmed cell death in nematodes identified by H. Robert Horvitz and colleagues. Later shown also in human B cell lymphomas by Korsmeyer (Horwitz Prize in 2000, with Stanley J. Korsmeyer).
- John Newsom-Davis, Angela Vincent, and associates discover calcium channel autoantibodies in Lambert-Eaton paraneoplastic myasthenic syndrome.
- Huda Zoghbi and Harry Orr identify trinucleotide repeats in different types of spinocerebellar ataxia.

1995

- FDA advisory panel recommends approval of interferon β-1a for treating remitting-relapsing multiple sclerosis.
- NINDS clinical trial recommends use of t-PA for the treatment of acute ischemic strokes.
- Antonio Damasio uses fMRI to demonstrate importance of the amygdala in emotional learning.
- Riluzole is first approved drug by the U.S. Food and Drug Administration for treating amyotrophic lateral sclerosis (Lou Gehrig's disease).
- R. Sherrington and colleagues, the Alzheimer Disease Collaborative Group, and others map gene for presenilin-1 in Alzheimer disease. E. Levy-Lahad and colleagues, and others, map gene for presenilin 2 in different families with Alzheimer disease.

- Gerard D. Schellenberg discovers mutations in genes for presenilins 1 and 2 (Potamkin Prize, 1994).
- High field magnets available for magnetic resonance imaging.
- Kevin Campbell and colleagues identify mutations in genes for a number of dystrophin-associated proteins as the basis of other forms of muscular dystrophy.
- Eric P. Hoffman introduces term "channelopathies" to group hereditary diseases of nerve or muscle with mutations in genes for sodium, potassium, chloride, or calcium channels.
- Eric Kandel and colleagues discover role of CREB (Cyclic AMP-response element binding protein) in long-term potentiation and memory.
- Kay Redfield Jamison publishes *An Unquiet Mind*, describing her personal experience with bipolar disease; book influences public policy and medical research.

1996

- Alim-Louis Benabid finds benefit in treating parkinsonism with deep brain stimulation of the subthalamic nucleus.
- New variant Creutzfeldt-Jakob disease found in United Kingdom associated with eating beef from cattle suffering from "mad cow disease."
- Microarrays for whole genome scanning introduced.
- Transgenic mice carrying presenilin mutations for Alzheimer disease created by Karen Hsaio and Karen Duff.
- J. DeRisi and colleagues introduce microarray-based expression monitoring.
- Thomas Jessell and associates define developmental determinants of cell types in spinal cord.
- Lisa M. DeAngelis and associates find response of primary CNS lymphoma to initial treatment with chemotherapy.

1997

- Mutation in α-synuclein identified by Mihael Polymeropoulos and Robert Nussbaum as basis for familial Parkinson disease. Followed in 1998 by identification of a second gene *parkin* by Kitada and associates.
- Gerald Fischbach and associates describe *neuroregulins* as influences in development of postsynaptic structures of neuromuscular juncture.
- Donald L. Price, Sangram S. Sisodia, and David R. Borchelt summarize information from transgenic animal models of ALS, Alzheimer disease, and trinucleotide repeat diseases (Potamkin Prize, 1992 to Price).

- Edward H. Oldfield and co-workers (NINDS) use retroviral vectors to deliver herpes simplex gene for thymidilate kinase, rendering human brain tumors susceptible to the antiviral drug, gangciclovir; methods for delivery of gene need improvement.

1998

- P.S. Eriksson and colleagues, and Fred Gage and colleagues, establish evidence for neurogenesis in the adult human hippocampus.
- Rod McKinnon and colleagues describe the first 3-D structure of an ion channel (Lasker Award, 1999).
- Research groups led by Michael Hutton, Maria Spillantini, and L.N. Clark independently identify tau mutations in chromosome-17 related frontotemporal dementia syndromes (Potamkin Award, 2000, to Hutton and Spillantini).
- R. Waterston and J. Sulston complete genome sequence of *C. elegans*.
- William A. Catterall describes voltage-sensitive ion channels.
- John Gearhart and associates report the cloning of the first human embryonic stem cells.
- M. Pandolfo and associates add Friedreich ataxia to list of trinucleotide repeat mutations.

1999

- Dale Schenk demonstrates that vaccination against amyloid prevents development of animal model of Alzheimer disease.
- First use of cloned stem cells to treat model neurological disorders in mice by groups led by Ronald McKay, Evan Snyder, and Louis Kunkel.
- J.W. McDonald and associates find that stem cells accelerate recovery from experimental spinal cord injury.
- Ten new anti-epileptic drugs approved by the U.S. Food and Drug Administration during the Decade of the Brain.

The New Millennium

2000

- Near complete sequencing of the human genome by public and private groups announced.
- Human Genome Project results reported, open new era.
- Second gene described in familial ALS (with frontotemporal dementia).
- M. Schwab and colleagues identify a protein, Nogo, released after CNS injury that blocks effective axon regeneration. In animals, antibodies to Nogo found to promote CNS regeneration.

- René Hen, Ai Yamamoto, and associates, study transgenic mice with a conditional model of HD (one in which gene expression can be turned off by the antibiotic doxycicline); mice express mutated huntingtin protein and show neuronal inclusions that disappear when expression is blocked; conclude that continuous supply of mutated protein is necessary for disease; findings offer a new approach to treatment.
- Jeffrey Kordower and associates use viral vector carrying glial-derived neurotrophic growth factor to protect against nigro-striatal degeneration in an animal model of toxin-induced Parkinson disease.
- Fourth gene for familial Alzheimer disease found on chromosome 10 by Rudolph Tanzi and colleagues.
- Robert Friedlander, Serge Przedborski, and colleagues test theory that proteolytic enzymes, the caspases, are important in the neuronal cell death of mice bearing a mutant gene for familial ALS; a powerful caspase-inhibitor prolonged life of the animals.
- Edward Oldfield and colleagues demonstrate benefit from simple decompressive surgery of syringomyelia and suggest that commonly associated anomaly of cerebellum (Chiari malformation) is acquired not congenital.

2001

- Vaccination with amyloid protein found to significantly improve function and eliminate plaques in mouse models of Alzheimer disease by different research groups.
- Stanley Fahn, Curt Fried, and associates demonstrate that transplanted embryonic dopamine neurons survive in the brains of Parkinson disease patients; dopamine production is normal at first and then accelerates and worsens symptoms; debate follows as some still advocate cell implantation therapy.
- Whole-population study in Iceland indicates genetic susceptibility for Parkinson disease regardless of age at onset.
- Ronald McKay (NINDB) and associates find that nestin, a microtubular protein used as a marker of developing neurons, also identifies precursors of insulin-secreting pancreatic cells.
- H. Shimura, Kenneth Kosik, Dennis Selkoe, and colleagues report interactions between parkinsonian gene products previously thought to act independently: synuclein, parkin, and ubiquitin.
- Dennis Selko proposes that presenelin may be the long-sought amyloid precursor protein.

- F.C. Nucifora, Ted and Virginia Dawson, Chris Ross, and colleagues find *huntingtin* in polyglutamine aggregates of neurons; the expanded polyglutamine repeats interfere with CBP-activated gene transcription.
- C. Zuccato and colleagues report that mutant *huntingtin* lacks beneficial effect; cell death may not be solely a toxic gain of function.
- Robert Desimone and associates find that synchronous neuronal firing in visual cortex may be a fundamental mechanism for boosting brain signals, bringing to attention behaviorally relevant stimuli.
- Jay P. Mohr leads multicenter study to find that warfarin and aspirin are equivalent in safety and efficacy in preventing recurrence of ischemic stroke.
- Daniel McGowan and associates describe reversal by antiretroviral treatment of an ALS-like syndrome in HIV infection.

CELEBRATING 50 YEARS OF BRAIN RESEARCH

50th

ANNIVERSARY

APPENDICES

NIH INSTITUTES, OFFICES, AND CENTERS SEPTEMBER 2001

CC	Warren Grant Magnuson Clinical Center
CIT	Center for Information Technology
CSR	Center for Scientific Review
FIC	John E. Fogarty International Center
NCCAM	National Center for Complementary and Alternative Medicine
NCI	National Cancer Institute
NCMHD	National Center on Minority Health and Health Disparities
NCRR	National Center for Research Resources
NEI	National Eye Institute
NHLBI	National Heart, Lung, and Blood Institute
NHGRI	National Human Genome Research Institute
NIA	National Institute on Aging
NIAAA	National Institute on Alcohol Abuse and Alcoholism
NIAID	National Institute of Allergy and Infectious Diseases
NIAMS	National Institute of Arthritis and Musculoskeletal and Skin Diseases
NICHD	National Institute of Child Health and Human Development
NIDCD	National Institute on Deafness and Other Communication Disorders
NIDCR	National Institute of Dental and Craniofacial Research
NIDDK	National Institute of Diabetes and Digestive and Kidney Diseases
NIBIB	National Institute of Biomedical Imaging and Bioengineering
NIDA	National Institute on Drug Abuse
NIEHS	National Institute of Environmental Health Sciences
NIGMS	National Institute of General Medical Sciences
NIMH	National Institute of Mental Health
NINDS	National Institute of Neurological Disorders and Stroke
NINR	National Institute of Nursing Research
NLM	National Library of Medicine
OD	Office of the Director

NDS EXTRAMURAL PROGRAM DIRECTORS
PTEMBER 2001

Extramural Research

Constance W. Atwell, Ph.D.
Director, Division of Extramural Research

W. Gahan Breithaupt
Acting Deputy Director, Division of Extramural Research

Robert W. Baughman, Ph.D.
Associate Director for Technology Development

Alfred W. Gordon, Ph.D.
Associate Director for Minority Health and Research

John R. Marler, M.D.
Associate Director for Clinical Trials

Program and Office Directors

Toby Behar, Ph.D.
Glial cell biology and stroke

Daofen Chen, Ph.D.
Channels, synapses, and circuits

Arlene Y. Chiu, Ph.D.
Stem cells

Kirkland L. Davis
Chief, Contracts Management Branch

Emmeline Edwards, Ph.D.
Neurobehavioral disorders

Robert Finkelstein, Ph.D.
Genetics and development

Peter R. Gilbert, Sc.M.
Clinical trials

Katrina Gwinn-Hardy, M.D.
Neurogenetics and clinical neurology

Joellen M. Harper
Chief, Grants Management Branch

Jill Heemskerk, Ph.D.
Neurodegeneration

William J. Heetderks, M.D., Ph.D.
Repair and plasticity, neural prostheses

Deborah Hirtz, M.D.
Developmental disorders, autism and child neurology

Margaret P. Jacobs
Epilepsy

Thomas P. Jacobs, Ph.D.
Stroke, imaging and CNS tumors

Gayathri Jeyarasasingam, Ph.D.
Office of Minority Health and Research

A.P. Kerza-Kwiatecki, Ph.D.
MS, neuroimmunology, neurovirology (AIDS)

Henry Khachaturian, Ph.D.
Training and career development

Cheryl A. Kitt, Ph.D.
Pain, neurotoxicology, and neuroendocrinology

Naomi Kleitman, Ph.D.
Spinal cord injury and repair

Piotr B. Kozlowski, M.D., Ph.D.
AIDS

Dennis Landis, M.D.
Training and career development

Gabrielle Leblanc, Ph.D.
Genetics and neural development

Yuan Liu, Ph.D.
Channels, synapses and circuits

Laura A. Mamouna, Ph.D.
Repair and plasticity

Mary Ellen Michel, Ph.D.
Repair and plasticity

Claudia Moy, Ph.D.
Clinical Research Project Manager

Diane Murphy, Ph.D.
Neurodegeneration

Paul L. Nichols, Ph.D.
Neuromuscular disorders, sleep and circadian rhythms

Eugene J. Oliver, Ph.D.
Alzheimer, Parkinson, and Huntington diseases

Jennifer Pinto-Martin, Ph.D.
Epidemiology

Lillian M. Pubols, Ph.D.
Chief, Scientific Review Branch

Bernard Ravina, M.D.
Clinical trials

Paul A. Sheehy, Ph.D.
Neurodegeneration

Giovanna M. Spinella, M.D.
Developmental and neurodegenerative disorders

James Stables
Anticonvulsant Screening Program

Randall Stewart, Ph.D.
Channels, synapses, and circuits

Danilo Tagle, Ph.D.
Neurogenetics

Ursula Utz, Ph.D.
Immunology and virology

NINDS INTRAMURAL RESEARCHERS SEPTEMBER 2001

Intramural Research

Story C. Landis, Ph.D.
Director, Division of Intramural Research

Basic Neuroscience Program

Story C. Landis, Ph.D.
Acting Chief, Laboratory of Central Nervous System Studies

Lynn D. Hudson, Ph.D.
Chief, Laboratory of Developmental Neurogenetics

Alan P. Koretsky, Ph.D.
Chief, Laboratory of Functional and Molecular Imaging

Ronald D.G. McKay, Ph.D.
Chief, Laboratory of Molecular Biology

Richard H. Quarles, Ph.D.
Chief, Laboratory of Molecular and Cellular Neurobiology

Eugene O. Major, Ph.D.
Chief, Laboratory of Molecular Medicine and Neuroscience

Robert E. Burke, M.D.
Chief, Laboratory of Neural Control

Thomas S. Reese, M.D.
Chief, Laboratory of Neurobiology

Harold Gainer, Ph.D.
Chief, Laboratory of Neurochemistry

Jeffery L. Barker, M.D.
Chief, Laboratory of Neurophysiology

Judith Davis
Chief, Animal Health and Care Section

Clinical Neurosciences Program

Henry F. McFarland, M.D.
Acting Director, Clinical Neurosciences Program

James M. Dambrosia, Ph.D.
Chief, Biostatistics Branch

Roscoe O. Brady, M.D.
Chief, Developmental and Metabolic Neurology Branch

William H. Theodore, M.D.
Head, Epilepsy Research Section

Thomas N. Chase, M.D.
Chief, Experimental Therapeutics Branch

Mark Hallett, M.D.
Chief, Medical Neurology Branch

Karin B. Nelson, M.D.
Chief, Neuroepidemiology Branch

Kenneth H. Fischbeck, M.D.
Chief, Neurogenetics Branch

Henry F. McFarland, M.D.
Chief, Neuroimmunology Branch

Marinos C. Dalakas, M.D.
Chief, Neuromuscular Diseases Section

John M. Hallenbeck, M.D.
Chief, Stroke Branch

Edward Oldfield, M.D.
Chief, Surgical Neurology Branch

	Director	Assistant Director/Deputy Director	Extramural Director	Intramural Research or Scientific Director	Director of Clinical Research (Clinical Director)
1951	Pearce Bailey, M.D., Ph.D			Seymour Kety, M.D. combined w/ NIMH	
1952	Pearce Bailey, M.D., Ph.D.			Seymour Kety, M.D. combined w/ NIMH	
1953	Pearce Bailey, M.D., Ph.D.			Seymour Kety, M.D. combined w/ NIMH	G. Milton Shy, M.D.
1954	Pearce Bailey, M.D., Ph.D.			Seymour Kety, M.D. combined w/ NIMH	G. Milton Shy, M.D.
1955	Pearce Bailey, M.D., Ph.D.			Seymour Kety, M.D. combined w/ NIMH	G. Milton Shy, M.D.
1956	Pearce Bailey, M.D., Ph.D.			Seymour Kety, M.D. and Robert B. Livingston, M.D.	G. Milton Shy, M.D.
1957	Pearce Bailey, M.D., Ph.D.	Richard L. Masland, M.D.		Robert B. Livingston, M.D. combined w/ NIMH	G. Milton Shy, M.D.
1958	Pearce Bailey, M.D., Ph.D.	Richard L. Masland, M.D.		Robert B. Livingston, M.D. combined w/ NIMH	G. Milton Shy, M.D.
1959	Pearce Bailey, M.D., Ph.D. Richard L. Masland, M.D. (9/59)	Richard L. Masland, M.D.		Robert B. Livingston, M.D. combined w/ NIMH	G. Milton Shy, M.D.
1960	Richard L. Masland, M.D.	William F. Windle, Ph.D.		Robert B. Livingston, M.D. combined w/ NIMH	G. Milton Shy, M.D.
1961	Richard L. Masland, M.D.	William F. Windle, Ph.D.	Murray Goldstein, D.O.	G. Milton Shy, M.D. appointed scientific director, NINDB	Maitland Baldwin, M.D.
1962	Richard L. Masland, M.D.		Murray Goldstein, D.O.	Maitland Baldwin, M.D.	Maitland Baldwin, M.D.

	Director	Assistant Director/Deputy Director	Extramural Director	Intramural Research or Scientific Director	Director of Clinical Research (Clinical Director)
1963	Richard L. Masland, M.D.		Murray Goldstein, D.O.	Maitland Baldwin, M.D.	Maitland Baldwin, M.D.
1964	Richard L. Masland, M.D.	Eldon L. Eagles, M.D., Ph.D.	Murray Goldstein, D.O.	Maitland Baldwin, M.D.	Maitland Baldwin, M.D.
1965	Richard L. Masland, M.D.	Eldon L. Eagles, M.D., Ph.D.	Murray Goldstein, D.O.	Maitland Baldwin, M.D.	Maitland Baldwin, M.D.
1966	Richard L. Masland, M.D.	Eldon L. Eagles, M.D., Ph.D.	Murray Goldstein, D.O.	Henry G. Wagner, M.D.	Maitland Baldwin, M.D.
1967	Richard L. Masland, M.D	Eldon L. Eagles, M.D., Ph.D.	Murray Goldstein, D.O.	Henry G. Wagner, M.D.	Maitland Baldwin, M.D.
1968	Richard L. Masland, M.D. Edward F. MacNichol, Jr., M.D.	Eldon L. Eagles, M.D., Ph.D.	Murray Goldstein, D.O.	Henry G. Wagner, M.D.	Maitland Baldwin, M.D.
1969	Edward F. MacNichol, Jr., M.D.	Eldon L. Eagles, M.D., Ph.D.	Murray Goldstein, D.O.	Henry G. Wagner, M.D.	Maitland Baldwin, M.D.
1970	Edward F. MacNichol, Jr., M.D.	Eldon L. Eagles, M.D., Ph.D.	Murray Goldstein, D.O.	Henry G. Wagner, M.D.	Maitland Baldwin, M.D.
1971	Edward F. MacNichol, Jr., M.D.	Eldon L. Eagles, M.D., Ph.D.	Murray Goldstein, D.O.	Henry G. Wagner, M.D.	John M. Van Buren, M.D., Acting
1972	Edward F. MacNichol, Jr., M.D.	Eldon L. Eagles, M.D., Ph.D.	Murray Goldstein, D.O.	Henry G. Wagner, M.D.	John M. Van Buren, M.D., Acting
1973	Edward F. MacNichol, Jr., M.D	Eldon L. Eagles, M.D., Ph.D.	Murray Goldstein, D.O.	Henry G. Wagner, M.D.	John M. Van Buren, M.D., Acting
1974	Donald B. Tower, M.D., Ph.D.	Eldon L. Eagles, M.D., Ph.D.	Murray Goldstein, D.O.	Henry G. Wagner, M.D.	John M. Van Buren, M.D., Acting Donald B. Calne, D.M.
1975	Donald B. Tower, M.D., Ph.D.	Eldon L. Eagles, M.D., Ph.D.	Murray Goldstein, D.O.	Thomas N. Chase, M.D.	Donald B. Calne, D.M.
1976	Donald B. Tower, M.D., Ph.D.	Eldon L. Eagles, M.D., Ph.D.	Murray Goldstein, D.O.	Thomas N. Chase, M.D.	Donald B. Calne, D.M.
1977	Donald B. Tower, M.D., Ph.D.	Eldon L. Eagles, M.D., Ph.D.	K. Kenneth Hisaoka, Ph.D.	Thomas N. Chase, M.D.	Donald B. Calne, D.M.
1978	Donald B. Tower, M.D., Ph.D.	Murray Goldstein, D.O.	K. Kenneth Hisaoka, Ph.D. (5/78) John C. Dalton, Ph.D. (6/78)	Thomas N. Chase, M.D.	Donald B. Calne, D.M.
1979	Donald B. Tower, M.D., Ph.D.	Murray Goldstein, D.O.	John C. Dalton, Ph.D.	Thomas N. Chase, M.D.	Donald B. Calne, D.M.
1980	Donald B. Tower, M.D., Ph.D.	Murray Goldstein, D.O.	John C. Dalton, Ph.D.	Thomas N. Chase, M.D.	Donald B. Calne, D.M.

	Director	Assistant Director/Deputy Director	Extramural Director	Intramural Research or Scientific Director	Director of Clinical Research (Clinical Director)
1981	Donald B. Tower, M.D., Ph.D. (2/81) Murray Goldstein, D.O., Acting	Murray Goldstein, D.O. Katherine L. Bick, Ph.D., Acting	John C. Dalton, Ph.D.	Thomas N. Chase, M.D.	Donald B. Calne, D.M.
1982	Murray Goldstein, D.O., Acting until appointed Director 12/82	Katherine L. Bick, Ph.D., Acting	John C. Dalton, Ph.D.	Thomas N. Chase, M.D.	Dale E. McFarlin, M.D., Acting
1983	Murray Goldstein, D.O.	Katherine L. Bick, Ph.D.	John C. Dalton, Ph.D.	Irwin J. Kopin, M.D.	Paul L. Kornblith, M.D., Acting
1984	Murray Goldstein, D.O.	Katherine L. Bick, Ph.D.	John C. Dalton, Ph.D.	Irwin J. Kopin, M.D.	Mark Hallett, M.D.
1985	Murray Goldstein, D.O.	Katherine L. Bick, Ph.D.	John C. Dalton, Ph.D.	Irwin J. Kopin, M.D.	Mark Hallett, M.D.
1986	Murray Goldstein, D.O.	Katherine L. Bick, Ph.D.	John C. Dalton, Ph.D.	Irwin J. Kopin, M.D.	Mark Hallett, M.D.
1987	Murray Goldstein, D.O.	Katherine L. Bick, Ph.D. Roger J. Porter, M.D.	John C. Dalton, Ph.D.	Irwin J. Kopin, M.D.	Mark Hallett, M.D.
1988	Murray Goldstein, D.O.	Roger J. Porter, M.D.	John C. Dalton, Ph.D.	Irwin J. Kopin, M.D.	Mark Hallett, M.D.
1989	Murray Goldstein, D.O.	W. Watson Alberts, Ph.D., Acting (7/89-6/90)	John C. Dalton, Ph.D.	Irwin J. Kopin, M.D.	Mark Hallett, M.D.
1990	Murray Goldstein, D.O.	Roger J. Porter, M.D.	John C. Dalton, Ph.D.	Irwin J. Kopin, M.D.	Mark Hallett, M.D.
1991	Murray Goldstein, D.O.	Roger J. Porter, M.D.	John C. Dalton, Ph.D.	Irwin J. Kopin, M.D.	Mark Hallett, M.D.
1992	Murray Goldstein, D.O.	Roger J. Porter, M.D. Patricia Grady, Ph.D., Acting	Edward M. Donohue, Acting	Irwin J. Kopin, M.D.	Mark Hallett, M.D.
1993	Murray Goldstein, D.O. (9/93) Patricia A. Grady, Ph.D., Acting	Patricia Grady, Ph.D. Richard Sherbert, Acting	Edward M. Donohue, Acting	Irwin J. Kopin, M.D.	Mark Hallett, M.D.
1994	Patricia A. Grady, Ph.D., Acting Zach W. Hall, Ph.D. (9/94)	Richard Sherbert, Acting Patricia A. Grady, Ph.D.	Constance W. Atwell, Ph.D., Acting	Harold Gainer, Ph.D., Acting	Mark Hallett, M.D.
1995	Zach W. Hall, Ph.D.	Patricia A. Grady, Ph.D. until 11/95 Audrey S. Penn, M.D. appointed 12/95	Constance W. Atwell, Ph.D.	Harold Gainer, Ph.D., Acting Story C. Landis, Ph.D.	Mark Hallett, M.D.
1996	Zach W. Hall, Ph.D.	Audrey S. Penn, M.D.	Constance W. Atwell, Ph.D.	Story C. Landis, Ph.D.	Mark Hallett, M.D.

	Director	Assistant Director/Deputy Director	Extramural Director	Intramural Research or Scientific Director	Director of Clinical Research (Clinical Director)
1997	Zach W. Hall, Ph.D.	Audrey S. Penn, M.D.	Constance W. Atwell, Ph.D.	Story C. Landis, Ph.D.	Mark Hallett, M.D.
1998	Audrey S. Penn, Acting (1/98-7/98) Gerald D. Fischbach, M.D. (8/98)	Constance W. Atwell,Ph.D., Acting (1/98-7/98) Audrey S. Penn, M.D.	Constance W. Atwell, Ph.D.	Story C. Landis, Ph.D.	Mark Hallett, M.D.
1999	Gerald D. Fischbach, M.D.	Audrey S. Penn, M.D.	Constance W. Atwell, Ph.D.	Story C. Landis, Ph.D.	Mark Hallett, M.D.
2000	Gerald D. Fischbach, M.D.	Audrey S. Penn, M.D.	Constance W. Atwell, Ph.D.	Story C. Landis, Ph.D.	Mark Hallett, M.D. (until 5/00) Guy McKhann, M.D., Acting (6/00)
2001	Gerald D. Fischbach, M.D. (1/01) Audrey S. Penn, M.D., Acting (2/01)	Kevin E. Kirby, M.S., Acting (2/01)	Constance W. Atwell, Ph.D.	Story C. Landis, Ph.D.	Guy McKhann, M.D. (1/01-4/01) Henry McFarland, M.D., Acting (5/01)

ACKNOWLEDGEMENTS

Ellsworth C. Alvord, M.D., and *Robert Lisak, M.D.*, for information on Marian Kies, Ph.D.

Jules Asher, NIMH, for locating forgotten photographs

Jeffrey L. Barker, M.D., Chief, Laboratory of Neurophysiology, for detailed information about antibodies, transmitter receptors, and Craig Venter

Roscoe O. Brady, M.D., for advice and support throughout

Catherine Carlson, National Multiple Sclerosis Society

Richard Cohen, producer of National Public Broadcasting System program on Mary Lasker

Jason Credle and *Matt Bridell*, NINDS computer wizards, for advice and practical help

William Davis, National Archives and Records Administration, for advice about finding congressional hearings

Lois DeBakey, former editor of JAMA, for advice about her brother Michael DeBakey, M.D., and his relationship to Mary Lasker

Barbara B. Dillon, Metroplitan Life Foundation

James Fordyce, for advice about his aunt Mary Lasker

Frank Forster, M.D., one of the four founders of the American Academy of Neurology

Barbara Gill, The Charles A. Dana Foundation

Paul Girolami, NINDS, for advice

James Goldman, M.D., for information about postmortem examination of George Balanchine

Harry Gottlieb, NIH Library, for assistance with microfiche records

William Heetderks, M.D., Ph.D., NINDS program director, neural prostheses, for information about cochlear implants and other advice

Marvene Horwitz, NINDS

Kristi L. Hunter, Mayo Clinic, for help with photographs

Lawrence C. Kolb, M.D., phone conversation about the origin of NINDB

Edith Langner, M.D., physician to George Balanchine

Jan Lazarus, National Library of Medicine

Hildegarde Mahoney, The Charles A. Dana Foundation

Andrea Mayer, The Lasker Foundation

Leila Melson, Archivist of the American Neurological Association; Librarian, Bowman-Gray School of Medicine

Mary Monti, NINDS

John Nemmers, Assistant Archivist, Senator Claude D. Pepper Library

Sheila Paul, The Charles A. Dana Foundation

Gregory Pike, *Sarah Leavitt*, and *Peg Dillon*, History Associates, Incorporated

Steven Reingold, National Multiple Sclerosis Society

Mark Renovitch, Franklin Delano Roosevelt Library

Lisa Russell, Government Documents Division of the University of Maryland McKeldon Library, for assistance finding records on the congressional hearings that led to the formation of NINDB

Louis Sokoloff, M.D., for advice and support throughout

Seymour Solomon, M.D., for information about George Balanchine

Randy Sowell, Harry S. Truman Library

Marcy Sugar, Assistant to Ann Landers for advice about Mary Lasker

Bernard Taber, biographer of George Balanchine

Angelique Tronvere, NIH Library, for assistance with microfiche records

Melvin D. Yahr, phone conversation about the origin of NINDB

The staff of the World Federation of Neurology

PHOTO AND ILLUSTRATION CREDITS

Chapter One

Page 3
President Franklin D. Roosevelt formally dedicates the NIH campus, October 31, 1940
The NIH History Office and DeWitt Stetten, Jr. Museum of Medical Research, National Institutes of Health

Page 6
Mary Lasker and Senator Claude Pepper, 1980
Claude Pepper Library, Florida State University

Page 7
Florence Mahoney
The National Library of Medicine

Page 9
Robert H. Felix, M.D.
The National Library of Medicine

Chapter Two

Page 19
Seymour Kety, M.D.
Lewis P. Rowland, M.D.

Page 22
Building T-6
The NIH History Office and DeWitt Stetten, Jr. Museum of Medical Research, National Institutes of Health

Page 24
Wilder Penfield, M.D., and Maitland Baldwin, M.D.
The National Library of Medicine

Chapter Three

Page 28
NINDS Funding Compared to NIH Funding, 1951-2000
NIH Almanac 2000

Page 29
Representative John Fogarty, Senator Lister Hill, and President John F. Kennedy
The National Library of Medicine

Page 30
James A. Shannon, M.D., Ph.D.
The National Library of Medicine

Page 33
Luther Terry, M.D., Senator Lister Hill, and HEW Secretary Anthony Celebrezze greet President Lyndon B. Johnson
The National Library of Medicine

Chapter Four

Page 41
Richard L. Masland, M.D., receiving Award of Merit from President John F. Kennedy
The National Library of Medicine

Chapter Six

Page 68
Norman Goldstein, M.D.
The Mayo Clinic

Page 69
Ellsworth C. Alvord, Jr., M.D., and Marian Kies, Ph.D.
Ellsworth C. Alvord, Jr., M.D.

Chapter Seven

Page 98
NINDS Extramural Funding, 1951-2000
NIH Almanac 2000

Chapter Nine

Page 124
Leonard Kurland, M.D.
The Mayo Clinic

Page 126
Leonard Kurland, M.D., and Donald Mulder, M.D.
Leonard Kurland, M.D.

Page 130
William F. Windle, Ph.D., Sc.D.
The Albert and Mary Lasker Foundation

Chapter Ten

Page 139
David Mahoney
The Dana Foundation

Page 139
President George Bush signing Proclamation of the Decade of the Brain
The National Library of Medicine

Page 141
Neuroscientists Maxwell Cowan, M.D., Albert Aguayo, M.D., and James Watson, M.D., at the 1992 Cold Spring Harbor meeting
The Dana Foundation

Page 142
Brain Awareness Week logo
The Dana Foundation

Chapter Eleven

Page 146
Sylvia Lawry and her brother Bernard Lawry
The National MS Society

Chapter Thirteen

Page 157
Seymour S. Kety, M.D.
McLean Hospital

Chapter Fourteen

Page 163
Louis Sokoloff, M.D.
The National Library of Medicine

Page 166
Deoxyglucose autoradiograph
Laboratory of Cerebral Metabolism, NIMH

Chapter Sixteen

Page 177
Myelin sheath and nerve fiber
Donald Bliss, NIH Medical Illustration

Chapter Seventeen

Page 189
Carleton Gajdusek, Joe Gibbs, and Vin Zigas
Clarence Gibbs, Ph.D.

Chapter Eighteen

Page 200
Theoretical progression of the transmission of bovine spongiform encephalopathy (BSE or "mad cow" disease) from cattle to humans via BSE prions
Donald Bliss, NIH Medical Illustration

Chapter Nineteen

Page 203
Chemical structure of the major neurotransmitters dopamine, norepinephrine, and epinephrine
Donald Bliss, NIH Medical Illustration

Chapter Twenty

Page 207
Julius Axelrod in the laboratory at NIMH, 1976
The National Library of Medicine

Page 208
Bernard Brodie, M.D. (NHLBI)
The National Library of Medicine

Page 213
Chemical composition of LSD
Donald Bliss, NIH Medical Illustration

Page 214
Prototype of the spectrophotofluorometer
The NIH History Office and DeWitt Stetten, Jr. Museum of Medical Research, National Institutes of Health

Chapter Twenty One

Page 219
Arvid Carlsson, M.D. giving his Nobel acceptance speech
©2000 The Nobel Foundation, photo: Hans Mehlin

Page 224
Dopamine pathways in the brain
Donald Bliss, NIH Medical Illustration

Chapter Twenty Two

Page 229
Paul Greengard, Ph.D., receiving his Nobel Award
©2000 The Nobel Foundation, photo: Hans Mehlin

Page 234
Protein phosphorylation
Donald Bliss, NIH Medical Illustration

Chapter Twenty Three

Page 239
Eric R. Kandel, M.D., receiving his Nobel Award
©2000 The Nobel Foundation, photo: Hans Mehlin

Page 242
Aplysia
Donald Bliss, NIH Medical Illustration

Page 247
Induction of short- and long-term memory
Donald Bliss, NIH Medical Illustration

Page 248
Aplysia with its well-earned prize!
Eric R. Kandel, M.D.

Page 263
Architect's sketch of the John Edward Porter
Neuroscience Research Center
Rafael Viñoly Architects PC

INDEX